T0259254

Complications in Sinus and Skull Base Surgery: Prevention & Management

Guest Editors

SAMUEL S. BECKER, MD
ALEXANDER G. CHIU, MD

OTOLARYNGOLOGIC CLINICS OF NORTH AMERICA

www.oto.theclinics.com

August 2010 • Volume 43 • Number 4

SAUNDERS an imprint of ELSEVIER, Inc.

W.B. SAUNDERS COMPANY

A Division of Elsevier Inc.

1600 John F. Kennedy Boulevard • Suite 1800 • Philadelphia, Pennsylvania 19103-2899

http://www.theclinics.com

OTOLARYNGOLOGIC CLINICS OF NORTH AMERICA Volume 43, Number 4
August 2010 ISSN 0030-6665, ISBN-13: 978-1-4377-2412-7

Editor: Joanne Husovski
Development Editor: Donald Mumford

Otolaryngologic Clinics of North America (ISSN 0030-6665) is published bimonthly by Elsevier, Inc., 360 Park Avenue South, New York, NY 10010-1710. Months of issue are February, April, June, August, October, and December. Business and Editorial Offices: 1600 John F. Kennedy Blvd., Suite 1800, Philadelphia, PA 19103-2899. Customer Service Office: 6277 Sea Harbor Drive, Orlando, FL 32887-4800. Periodicals postage paid at New York, NY and additional mailing offices. Subscription prices is $290.00 per year (US individuals), $527.00 per year (US institutions), $142.00 per year (US student/resident), $382.00 per year (Canadian individuals), $662.00 per year (Canadian institutions), $429.00 per year (international individuals), $662.00 per year (international institutions), $219.00 per year (international & Canadian student/resident). Foreign air speed delivery is included in all *Clinics*' subscription prices. All prices are subject to change without notice. **POSTMASTER:** Send address changes to *Otolaryngologic Clinics of North America*, Elsevier Health Sciences Division, Subscription Customer Service, 3251 Riverport Lane, Maryland Heights, MO 63043. **Telephone: 1-800-654-2452 (U.S. and Canada); 314-447-8871 (outside U.S. and Canada). Fax: 314-447-8029. E-mail: journalscustomerservice-usa@elsevier.com (for print support); journalsonlinesupport-usa@elsevier.com (for online support).**

Reprints. For copies of 100 or more of articles in this publication, please contact the Commercial Reprints Department, Elsevier Inc., 360 Park Avenue South, New York, NY 10010-1710. Tel.: 212-633-3812; Fax: 212-462-1935; E-mail: reprints@elsevier.com.

Otolaryngologic Clinics of North America is also published in Spanish by McGraw-Hill Interamericana Editores S.A., P.O. Box 5-237, 06500 Mexico D.F., Mexico.

Otolaryngologic Clinics of North America is covered in *MEDLINE/PubMed (Index Medicus), Current Contents/Clinical Medicine, Excerpta Medica, BIOSIS, Science Citation Index,* and *ISI/BIOMED.*

Printed and bound in the United Kingdom
Transferred to Digital Print 2011

Contributors

GUEST EDITORS

SAMUEL S. BECKER, MD
Director of Rhinology, Becker Nose and Sinus Center, LLC, Voorhees, New Jersey

ALEXANDER G. CHIU, MD
Associate Professor, Director, Rhinology and Skull Base Surgery Fellowship Program, Division of Rhinology, Department of Otorhinolaryngology–Head and Neck Surgery, University of Pennsylvania, Philadelphia, Pennsylvania

AUTHORS

TALAL ALANDEJANI, MD, FRCSC
St Paul's Sinus Centre, ENT Clinic, St Paul's Hospital, University of British Columbia, British Columbia, Canada

VIJAY K. ANAND, MD, FACS
Department of Otolaryngology, Weill Medical College of Cornell University, New York-Presbyterian Hospital, New York, New York

MARCELO B. ANTUNES, MD
Resident, Department of Otorhinolaryngology–Head and Neck Surgery, University of Pennsylvania School of Medicine, Philadelphia, Pennsylvania

SAMUEL S. BECKER, MD
Director of Rhinology, Becker Nose and Sinus Center, LLC, Voorhees, New Jersey

BENJAMIN S. BLEIER, MD
Clinical Instructor, Division of Rhinology, Department of Otolaryngology–Head and Neck Surgery, Medical University of South Carolina, Charleston, South Carolina

RICARDO L. CARRAU, MD, FACS
John Wayne Cancer Institute; Neuroscience Institute, Saint John's Health Center, Santa Monica, California

RAKESH K. CHANDRA, MD
Associate Professor, Department of Otolaryngology–Head and Neck Surgery, Northwestern University, Feinberg School of Medicine, Chicago, Illinois

ALEXANDER G. CHIU, MD
Associate Professor, Director, Rhinology and Skull Base Surgery Fellowship Program, Division of Rhinology, Department of Otorhinolaryngology–Head and Neck Surgery, University of Pennsylvania, Philadelphia, Pennsylvania

CHRISTOPHER A. CHURCH, MD
Associate Professor, Department of Otolaryngology–Head and Neck Surgery, Loma Linda University School of Medicine, Loma Linda, California

NOAM A. COHEN, MD, PhD
Assistant Professor, Division of Rhinology, Department of Otorhinolaryngology–Head and Neck Surgery, Hospital of the University of Pennsylvania, University of Pennsylvania School of Medicine, Philadelphia, Pennsylvania

JAMES A. DUNCAVAGE, MD
Professor, Division of Rhinology, Department of Otolaryngology, Vanderbilt University Medical Center, Nashville, Tennessee

JUAN FERNANDEZ-MIRANDA, MD
Department of Neurosurgery, University of Pittsburgh Medical Center, Pittsburgh, Pennsylvania

SATISH GOVINDARAJ, MD
Assistant Professor, Department of Otolaryngology–Head and Neck Surgery, Mount Sinai Medical Center, New York, New York

JOSEPH K. HAN, MD
Associate Professor, Director of Rhinology and Endoscopic Sinus and Skull Base Surgery, Medical Director of Allergy Center, Department of Otolaryngology–Head and Neck Surgery, Eastern Virginia Medical School, Norfolk, Virginia

RICHARD J. HARVEY, MD
Clinical Associate Professor, Department of Otolaryngology/Skull Base Surgery, Rhinology and Skull Base, St Vincent's Hospital, Darlinghurst, Sydney, New South Wales, Australia

AMIN R. JAVER, MD, FRCSC, FARS
Director, St Paul's Sinus Centre, St Paul's Hospital; Associate Clinical Professor, University of British Columbia, British Columbia, Canada

AMIN B. KASSAM, MD
John Wayne Cancer Institute; Neuroscience Institute, Saint John's Health Center, Santa Monica, California

AMY S. KETCHAM, MD
Department of Otolaryngology–Head and Neck Surgery, Eastern Virginia Medical School, Norfolk, Virginia

ESTHER KIM, MD
Instructor, Division of Rhinology, Department of Otolaryngology, Vanderbilt University Medical Center, Nashville, Tennessee

CARL W. MOELLER, MD
Department of Otolaryngology–Head and Neck Surgery, Loyola University School of Medicine, Maywood, Illinois

KENNETH E. MORGENSTERN, MD
Morgenstern Center for Orbital and Facial Plastic Surgery, Wayne, Pennsylvania

YEW KWANG ONG, MD
Department of Otolaryngology, University of Pittsburgh Medical Center, Pittsburgh, Pennsylvania

JAMES N. PALMER, MD
Associate Professor, Director, Division of Rhinology, Department of Otorhinolaryngology–Head and Neck Surgery, University of Pennsylvania, Philadelphia, Pennsylvania

RICHARD D. PARKINSON, MD
Department of Neurosurgery and Neuroendovascular Surgery, St Vincent's Hospital, Darlinghurst, Sydney, New South Wales, Australia

ANKIT M. PATEL, MD
ENT Surgical Consultants, Joliet, Illinois

ZARA M. PATEL, MD
Assistant Professor, Department of Otolaryngology–Head and Neck Surgery, Mount Sinai Medical Center, New York, New York

DAVID M. POETKER, MD, MA
Assistant Professor, Division of Rhinology and Sinus Surgery, Department of Otolaryngology and Communication Sciences, Medical College of Wisconsin; Department of Surgery, VA Medical Center, Milwaukee, Wisconsin

DANIEL M. PREVEDELLO, MD
John Wayne Cancer Institute; Neuroscience Institute, Saint John's Health Center, Santa Monica, California

VIJAY R. RAMAKRISHNAN, MD
Assistant Professor, Department of Otolaryngology, University of Colorado Denver, Denver, Colorado

EVAN R. RANSOM, MD
Resident, Department of Otorhinolaryngology–Head and Neck Surgery, University of Pennsylvania, Philadelphia, Pennsylvania

DOUGLAS D. REH, MD
Assistant Professor, Division of Rhinology and Sinus Surgery, Department of Otolaryngology–Head and Neck Surgery, Johns Hopkins Medical Institutions, Baltimore, Maryland

PAUL T. RUSSELL, MD
Assistant Professor, Division of Rhinology, Department of Otolaryngology, Vanderbilt University Medical Center, Nashville, Tennessee

RAYMOND SACKS, MD
Associate Professor, Department of Otolaryngology/Head and Neck Surgery, Concord General Hospital, Macquarie & Sydney Universities, Sydney, Australia

MADELEINE R. SCHABERG, MD, MPH
Department of Otolaryngology, Weill Medical College of Cornell University, New York-Presbyterian Hospital, New York, New York

RODNEY J. SCHLOSSER, MD
Professor, Division of Rhinology, Department of Otolaryngology–Head and Neck Surgery, Medical University of South Carolina, Charleston, South Carolina

THEODORE H. SCHWARTZ, MD, FACS
Department of Otolaryngology Neurosurgery and Neurology and Neuroscience, Weill Medical College of Cornell University, New York-Presbyterian Hospital, New York, New York

EUGENE P. SNISSARENKO, MD
Department of Otolaryngology–Head and Neck Surgery, Loma Linda University School of Medicine, Loma Linda, California

CARL H. SNYDERMAN, MD
Department of Otolaryngology, University of Pittsburgh Medical Center, Pittsburgh, Pennsylvania

C. ARTURO SOLARES, MD
Department of Otolaryngology, Medical College of Georgia, Augusta, Georgia

THOMAS E. STILL ESQ, JD
Partner, Hinshaw Law Firm, Hinshaw, Draa, Marsh, Still & Hinshaw, Saratoga, California

BRUCE K. TAN, MD
Assistant Professor, Department of Otolaryngology–Head and Neck Surgery, Northwestern University, Feinberg School of Medicine, Chicago, Illinois

MARC A. TEWFIK, MD, MSc, FRCSC
Rhinology Fellow, Department of Otolaryngology–Head and Neck Surgery, The Queen Elizabeth Hospital, Woodville South, South Australia, Australia

DANIEL TIMPERLEY, MD
Fellow, Department of Otolaryngology/Skull Base Surgery, Rhinology and Skull Base, St Vincent's Hospital, Darlinghurst, Sydney, New South Wales, Australia

WINSTON VAUGHAN, MD
Director, California Sinus Centers, Atherton, California; Department of Otolaryngology–Head and Neck Surgery, Stanford University Medical Center, Stanford, California

KEVIN C. WELCH, MD
Assistant Professor, Department of Otolaryngology–Head and Neck Surgery, Loyola University School of Medicine, Maywood, Illinois

PETER-JOHN WORMALD, MD, FRCS, FRACS
Professor and Chair, Department of Otolaryngology–Head and Neck Surgery, The Queen Elizabeth Hospital, Woodville South; Department of Otolaryngology–Head and Neck Surgery, Adelaide and Flinders Universities, Adelaide, South Australia, Australia

ADVISORS TO OTOLARYNGOLOGIC CLINICS 2010:

BRIAN KAPLAN, MD
Ear, Nose, and Throat Associates; Baltimore, Maryland

JOHN KROUSE, MD, PhD
Temple University Medicine; Philadelphia, Pennsylvania

ANIL KUMAR LALWANI, MD
New York University Langone Medical Center; New York, New York

ARLEN MEYERS, MD, MBA
University of Colorado; Denver, Colorado

MATTHEW RYAN, MD
University of Texas Southwestern Medical Center, Dallas, Texas

RALPH TUFANO, MD
Johns Hopkins Medicine; Baltimore, Maryland

Contents

Prevention and Management of Complications in Sinus and Skull Base Surgery **xvii**

Samuel S. Becker and Alexander G. Chiu

Perioperative and Intraoperative Maneuvers to Optimize Surgical Outcomes in Skull Base Surgery **699**

Daniel Timperley, Raymond Sacks, Richard D. Parkinson, and Richard J. Harvey

There are many approaches to obtaining a workable endoscopic surgical field in sinus surgery. With extended sinus and transdural endoscopic surgery, a more rigid approach must be taken. There are 3 main factors that invariably lead to poor surgical outcomes in endoscopic sinus and skull base surgery: bleeding, inadequate access, and unidentified anatomic anomalies. Bleeding is arguably the most common reason for incomplete resection. An understanding of microvascular and macrovascular bleeding allows a more structured approach to improve the surgical field in extended endoscopic surgery. The endoscopic surgeon should always be comfortable in performing the same procedure as an open operation. However, converting or abandoning an endoscopic procedure should rarely occur because much of this decision making should take place preoperatively. Along with poor hemostasis, inadequate access is an important cause of poor outcome. Evaluation of the anatomy involved by pathology but also the anatomy that must be removed to allow adequate exposure is important. This article reviews the current techniques used to ensure optimal surgical conditions and outcomes.

Preoperative Computed Tomography Evaluation in Sinus Surgery: A Template-Driven Approach **731**

Samuel S. Becker

Anatomic abnormalities in the paranasal sinuses and skull base are not uncommon. Awareness of these abnormalities may be of assistance in preoperative planning. This content presents a template-driven approach to the analysis of computed tomography scans in preparation for endoscopic sinus surgery.

A Comprehensive Review of the Adverse Effects of Systemic Corticosteroids **753**

David M. Poetker and Douglas D. Reh

Corticosteroids are widely used in otolaryngology to treat many disorders; however, the nature and extent of possible complications may not be completely understood. A comprehensive review of the physiology of systemic corticosteroids and literature discussing the known side effects associated with their use is presented. The pathophysiology and the clinical impact of these side effects are reviewed. There are various potential side effects from the use of corticosteroids. Practitioners using corticosteroids should be familiar with these and obtain the patient's informed consent when appropriate.

Medial rectus injury is an uncommon but often devastating complication of functional endoscopic sinus surgery. Prevention of these types of injuries is predicated on a thorough preoperative assessment of the position and integrity of the medial orbital wall coupled with excellent surgical technique. The use of powered instrumentation has led to more severe injuries and thus should be used with caution near critical structures such as the lamina papyracea. Early recognition and management of medial rectus and associated orbital injuries is critical to improve outcomes and prevent associated complications. Despite optimal surgical and medical interventions, the prognosis is relatively poor and patients should be counseled that the primary goal of these interventions is to reestablish a binocular single visual field.

Skull base defects and injuries are rare, but may occur during endoscopic sinus surgery, as a result of facial trauma, or as a result of tumors in the anterior cranial fossa. Injury to the skull base can lead to catastrophic outcomes such as meningitis, brain abscess, neurological deficits, brain hemorrhage, and death. The content presents ways in which a surgeon may work to prevent or minimize injury to the skull base and describes management of skull base injuries when they do occur, reviews the current literature, and describes various reconstruction techniques used in free tissue grafts and pedicled grafts.

In the past 2 decades, endoscopic sinus surgery has been widely used as a safe and effective treatment for disorders of the paranasal sinuses that are refractory to medical therapy. Advances in surgical technique, including powered instrumentation and stereotactic image-guided surgery, have improved the efficiency and safety of this procedure. These techniques have been further expanded to manage skull base pathologies. This expansion has been facilitated by a better understanding of the endonasal skull base anatomy. Despite these advances, complications are still encountered. Vascular injuries are particularly troublesome. Interior ethmoid artery injuries during sinus surgery that led to orbital hematoma were discussed extensively in a recent issue of this journal. Therefore, this article focuses mainly on inadvertent carotid artery injuries during routine sinus surgery and vascular injuries during endoscopic skull base surgery.

surgeon to take great care in ensuring sound surgical principles. Understanding the potential areas in which surgery can fail will help tremendously in preventing complications.

Prevention and Management of Complications in Intracranial Endoscopic Skull Base Surgery **875**

Evan R. Ransom and Alexander G. Chiu

Development of minimally invasive approaches has become a significant driver across surgical specialties in recent years. Purely endoscopic resections with proper attention to oncologic margins are now possible, with the potential benefit of decreased perioperative morbidity and improved cosmesis compared with traditional open transfacial or craniofacial approaches. Efforts to reduce perioperative morbidity and mortality have been applied with increasing sophistication in the most complex anatomic regions of the human body, including the head and neck. These efforts have resulted in an expanded role of purely endoscopic approaches to the paranasal sinuses, the anterior skull base, and the anterior cranial fossa. This article reviews the current understanding and available literature regarding the diagnosis and management of complications associated with endoscopic anterior skull base surgery.

Complications and Management of Septoplasty **897**

Amy S. Ketcham and Joseph K. Han

Septoplasty is a common procedure in otolaryngology used to address nasal obstruction caused by a deviated nasal septum. It is often accompanied by inferior turbinate reduction. Complications that may arise from this procedure include excessive bleeding; cerebrospinal fluid rhinorrhea; extraocular muscle damage; wound infection; septal abscess; toxic shock syndrome; septal perforation; saddle nose deformity; nasal tip depression; and sensory changes, such as anosmia or dental anesthesia. Local and general anesthetics have been used to successfully perform septoplasty and the operation may be done either endoscopically or open. Overall, good intraoperative visualization is a key factor in preventing complications and achieving a functional nasal airway.

Medicolegal Issues in Endoscopic Sinus Surgery **905**

Ankit M. Patel, Thomas E. Still Esq, and Winston Vaughan

Endoscopic sinus surgery is one of the most litigated areas in otolaryngology. Physicians typically receive little education regarding medicolegal issues during training and may find themselves in an unfamiliar territory during litigation. This article reviews the scope of the problem and provides strategies to improve patient care and mitigate medicolegal risk in endoscopic sinus surgery.

FORTHCOMING ISSUES

Meniere's Disease: Current Diagnostic and Treatment Methods
Jeffrey Harris, MD, and
Quyen Nguyen, MD,
Guest Editors

Oral Medicine
Arlen Meyers, MD, MBA, and
Vincent Eusterman, MD, DDS,
Guest Editors

Head and Neck Ultrasound
Joseph Sniezek, MD, and
Robert Sofferman, MD,
Guest Editors

RECENT ISSUES

Rhinology: Evolution of Science and Surgery
Rodney J. Schlosser, MD, and
Richard J. Harvey, MD, *Guest Editors*
June 2010

Thyroid and Parathyroid Surgery
Sara I. Pai, MD, PhD, and
Ralph P. Tufano, MD, *Guest Editors*
April 2010

Cough: An Interdisciplinary Problem
Kenneth W. Altman, MD, PhD, FACS,
and Richard S. Irwin, MD, *Guest Editors*
February 2010

RELATED INTEREST

In Neuroimaging Clinics, August 2009
Skull Base and Temporal Bone Imaging
Vincent Fook-Hin Chong, MBBS, MBA, *Guest Editor*

Prevention and Management of Complications in Sinus and Skull Base Surgery

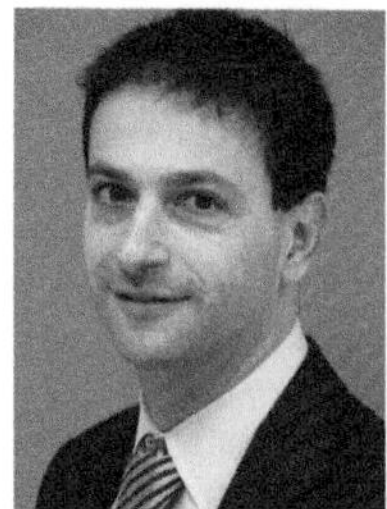
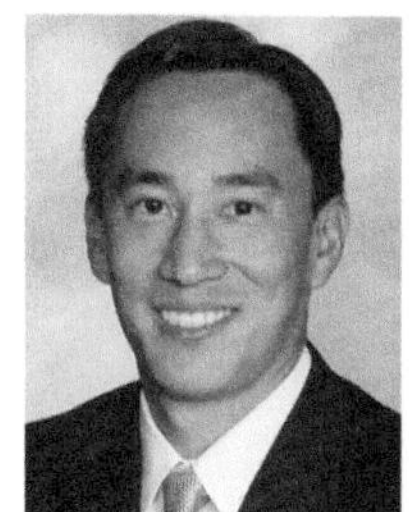

Samuel S. Becker, MD Alexander G. Chiu, MD
Guest Editors

Every surgical procedure involving the paranasal sinuses and skull base carries the risk of complication. Complications can occur despite surgery that has been technically well performed; however, at every step of the surgical pathway there are opportunities to minimize complications.

Medical management, including oral steroids, is often used in the diagnostic and preoperative setting. Steroids and other commonly used medications have the potential for significant side effects, and prescribing physicians should be well versed in their mechanisms of action and potential complications.

Once a decision to operate has been made, the informed consent process is critical to ensure that patients have a reasonable understanding of the potential risks, benefits, and complications involved. Before surgery, the CT scan should be evaluated by the surgeon to help plot a surgical plan and to identify anatomic "danger zones." Intraoperatively, attention to patient positioning and anesthetic techniques has been shown to help improve outcomes and limit complications. During surgery on the nose, sinuses, and skull base, complications may involve any of the 4 sinuses—maxillary, ethmoid, sphenoid, and frontal. Surrounding structures, such as the lacrimal duct, orbit, skull base, and surrounding vasculature, may also be damaged during intranasal surgery. After surgery, proper postoperative care is important to the healing process to avoid scarring and an eventual unfavorable outcome.

When complications occur, physicians should be prepared to appropriately manage the situation. Once the situation is stabilized, a surgeon must be prepared to discuss what has occurred with appropriate members of the patient's family.

In this issue of *Otolaryngologic Clinics of North America*, expert rhinologists and endoscopic skull base surgeons address the prevention and management of

Otolaryngol Clin N Am 43 (2010) xvii–xviii
doi:10.1016/j.otc.2010.04.024
0030-6665/10/$ – see front matter
oto.theclinics.com

complications in sinus and skull base surgery. We would like to thank the authors for their contributions, the editor for her guidance, the publisher for their support, and the readers for their attention.

Samuel S. Becker, MD
Becker Nose and Sinus Center
2301 Evesham Road
Suite 404 Voorhees, NJ 08043, USA

Alexander G. Chiu, MD
Division of Rhinology
Department of Otorhinolaryngology–Head and Neck Surgery
University of Pennsylvania
Philadelphia, PA, USA

E-mail addresses:
Sam.s.becker@gmail.com (S.S. Becker)
Alexander.Chiu@uphs.upenn.edu (A.G. Chiu)

Perioperative and Intraoperative Maneuvers to Optimize Surgical Outcomes in Skull Base Surgery

Daniel Timperley, MD[a], Raymond Sacks, MD[b], Richard J. Parkinson, MD[c], Richard J. Harvey, MD[a,*]

KEYWORDS

• Endoscopic • Skull base • Tumor • Sinonasal
• Angiofibroma • JNA • Inverted papilloma • Osteoma

There are 3 main factors that invariably lead to poor surgical outcomes in endoscopic sinus and skull base surgery: bleeding, inadequate access, and unidentified anatomic anomalies.

Bleeding is arguably the most common reason for incomplete resection, and not just for endoscopic cases. Poor hemostasis can lead to increased difficulty in recognizing the most important anatomic landmarks and identifying the sinus outflow pathways. It enhances the risks of intraoperative complications and postoperative scarring. Most importantly, it can lead to an incomplete operation. Inadequate access is often a product of incomplete exposure and failure to identify the limitations of the endoscopic approach in preoperative assessment and planning. The paranasal sinus anatomy represents one of the most highly variable anatomic areas within the body.[1] Since the beginning of sinus surgery, surgeons have stressed the importance of preoperative radiographic assessment of potential anatomic anomalies. Failure to identify simple abnormalities, such as dehiscent medial orbital walls and orbital contents in the ethmoid, can lead to lifelong debilitating diplopia.[2]

[a] Rhinology and Skull Base, Department of Otolaryngology/Skull Base Surgery, St Vincent's Hospital, 354 Victoria Street, Sydney, NSW 2010, Australia
[b] Department of Otolaryngology, Concord General Hospital and Sydney University, Hospital Road, Sydney, NSW 2139, Australia
[c] Department of Neurosurgery and Neuroendovascular Surgery, St Vincent's Hospital, 438 Victoria Street, Sydney, NSW 2010, Australia
* Corresponding author.
E-mail address: richard@sydneyentclinic.com

Otolaryngol Clin N Am 43 (2010) 699–730
doi:10.1016/j.otc.2010.04.002 oto.theclinics.com
0030-6665/10/$ – see front matter.

This article discusses bleeding control and access as it relates to endoscopic sinus and skull base surgery. Much has been written about careful radiologic evaluation for anatomic anomalies, and this will be addressed in a separate article.

HEMOSTASIS

There are many approaches to obtaining a workable endoscopic surgical field for sinus surgery. However, with extended sinus and transdural endoscopic surgery, a more rigid approach must be taken.

Diffferent techniques are required for control of arterial, venous, or microvascular bleeding. These include topical and local vasoconstriction, patient positioning, anesthetic technique, dissection techniques to reduce bleeding, surgical control of large vessels, embolization, and agents to control venous and microvascular bleeding.

The Vascular System of the Nose

The vascular system of the nose is supplied by large arteries, the most clinically important of which are the sphenopalatine and anterior ethmoid. These progressively divide into smaller arteries, then arterioles. The arterioles are the resistance vessels, and regulate blood flow into capillary beds and arterovenous anastomoses.[3] The main adrenergic receptor subtype is α_1, which has implications for the use of vasoconstrictive agents.[4] There is a copious system of fenestrated capillaries under the nasal mucosa. In addition, there are venous sinuses or capacitance vessels that have a thick layer of smooth muscle. The blood volume within the capacitance vessels to a large extent determines swelling of the nasal lining, such as in the nasal cycle.[3] The predominant adrenergic receptor subtype in these vessels is believed to be α_2.[4,5] In addition to these capacitance vessels, there are many arterovenous anastomoses, which are believed to bypass the capillary beds and capacitance vessels and have a role in temperature and humidity control.[3] Postcapillary venules, also predominantly α_2, drain the capillary beds, capacitance vessels, and arterovenous anastomoses. In addition to the adrenergic receptors, there are other receptor types and neural control of the nasal mucosa.[5] An understanding of this adrenergic organization is important in determining vasoconstrictor use.

Exposure of bone, intentionally through drilling and unintentionally through mucosal stripping, has a significant effect on hemostasis. The bone haversian canal system comprises 15 to 20 μm–wide endothelial-lined structures. These blood-filled channels have no smooth muscle (and thus are not responsive to adrenergic stimulation) or elastic fibers.[6] Hemostasis only occurs with clotting pathway activation.

Microvascular Control (Capillary, Postcapillary Venules, and Small Arterioles)

Preoperative

Reducing obstructive inflammation and infective processes The use of preoperative antibiotics and steroids is common, although there is only a small evidence base for their use. Anecdotally, the authors have found that large tumors predispose to obstructive inflammatory sinus changes. This predisposition results in a moderate degree of edema in the mucosal lining of areas not directly involved with tumor. Preoperative steroids are potent antiinflammatory agents, potentially reducing intraoperative bleeding. In addition to their antiinflammatory actions they potentiate the effect of adrenalin on smooth muscle, possibly prolonging topical vasoconstriction.[7] Sieskiewicz and colleagues[7] found an improvement in surgical field in 18 patients with severe nasal polyposis undergoing endoscopic sinus surgery (ESS) with preoperative steroid treatment compared with placebo.

Preoperative antibiotic use is intended to reduce bacterial load (or treat overt infection) and resultant inflammation to reduce intraoperative bleeding and optimize postoperative healing.

This practice affords better operative conditions and earlier recovery of regenerating mucosa. Comorbidities allowing, the authors start oral prednisone and antibiotics for 7 days before surgery. This decision is based on endoscopic and radiological assessment and not on clinical symptoms.

Bleeding diathesis The hemostatic system is a complex cascade of enzyme activation and inhibition that results in a balance between pro- and anticoagulation. It consists of 3 main components: platelets and other blood cells, plasma proteins, and the vessel wall.[8] The response to vascular injury consists of platelet adherence and plug formation (primary hemostasis), protein activation and the coagulation cascade (secondary hemostasis), feedback mechanisms to control coagulation, and lysis and recannulation.[9]

Inherited coagulopathies The most common inherited abnormalities of the coagulation system are von Willebrand disease and hemophilia (**Table 1**). Von Willebrand disease is a heterogeneous, autosomally inherited condition affecting 1% to 2% of the population in which there is a defect in production of von Willebrand factor (vWF). VWF has 2 functions: to act as glue between platelets and subendothelial collagen, thereby promoting formation of the platelet plug, and to transport factor VIII (FVIII). Defects in vWF can result in impaired platelet adhesion and reduced levels of FVIII.[10] Most cases are mild, with severe disease occurring in 1:10,000 to 2:10,000 people.[10] Patients are often asymptomatic and present only after surgery, or may present with mucosal bleeding, petechiae, and purpura. There are several subtypes of vWD depending on the type (quantitative vs qualitative) and severity of the defect in vWF (see **Table 1**). Most cases will respond to desmopressin (DDAVP) (intravenous infusion of 0.3 μg/kg over 20 to 30 minutes; nasal use is variable and not recommended preoperatively[9]), which causes release of vWF, FVIII, and plasminogen activator from storage sites. Type III is not responsive to DDAVP and use in type IIB is debated because of platelet aggregation resulting in a reversible reduction in platelet count. A test dose can be given with measurement of FVIII and vWF: ristocetin cofactor at 30 minutes after infusion to determine responsiveness.[10]

Hemophilia A and B are X-linked recessive deficiencies of FVIII and factor IX (FIX) respectively. There is a spectrum of disease from mild to severe. Presentation is typically with muscle hematomas and hemarthrosis, in contrast to platelet disorders and vWD. Treatment of hemophilia A may be with DDAVP in mild cases, or with FVIII concentrates in moderate to severe cases. FIX concentrate is used for hemophilia B.[10] Other, rare conditions of primary and secondary hemostasis are summarized in **Table 2**.

Acquired coagulopathies Clotting abnormalities can be due to a wide variety of conditions and a thorough medical and drug history should be taken (**Tables 3** and **4**). Anticoagulant and antiplatelet medications are a common cause of clotting abnormalities (**Table 5**). Antiplatelet and anticoagulant agents should be stopped for surgery. Most patients will have strong indications for anticoagulation and require the use of bridging medications (heparin, low molecular weight heparin, or nonsteroidal antiinflammatory drugs [NSAIDs]).[11,12] The authors generally cease bridging therapy within 7 days for extradural and between 7 and 14 days for intradural procedures.

Many alternative therapies and dietary supplements have reported or potential effects on coagulation (see **Table 1**). Their use is ubiquitous, with up to 27% of presurgical patients taking supplements or alternative therapies that are believed to affect

Table 1
Dietary supplements and alternative therapies affecting coagulation or anesthesia

Name	Effect
Alfalfa	Contains coumarins Also high levels vitamin K
Arnica	Platelet aggregation inhibitor Contains coumarins
Bilberry	Platelet aggregation inhibitor
Black currant	Platelet aggregation inhibitor
Bladderwrack	Platelet aggregation inhibitor Fibrin formation inhibitor
Black cohosh	Bradycardia, peripheral vasodilation
Capsicum	Platelet aggregation inhibitor Contains coumarins Hypertension
Cayenne fruit	Platelet aggregation inhibitor Fibrin formation inhibitor
Celery	Platelet aggregation inhibitor Contains coumarins
Chamomile	Contains coumarins
Da huang	Platelet aggregation inhibitor
Dandelion root	Inhibits clotting
Danshen	Platelet aggregation inhibitor
Devil's claw	Platelet aggregation inhibitor
Dong quai	Platelet aggregation inhibitor
Ephedra	Arrhythmias, myocardial infarction, stroke
Evening primrose seed oil	Platelet aggregation inhibitor
Fenugreek	Contains coumarins
Feverfew	Platelet aggregation inhibitor
Fish oil	Platelet aggregation inhibitor
Flax seed oil	Platelet aggregation inhibitor
Garlic	Platelet aggregation inhibitor Fibrin formation inhibitor
Ginger	Platelet aggregation inhibitor Bradycardia
Gingko	Platelet aggregation inhibitor (inhibits platelet activation factor)
Ginseng	Platelet aggregation inhibitor Fibrin formation inhibitor Hypertension
Grape seed extract	Platelet aggregation inhibitor
Horse chestnut	Contains coumarins
Horseradish	Contains coumarins
Kava kava	Platelet aggregation inhibitor May cause liver failure Sedative

(*continued on next page*)

Table 1
Dietary supplements and alternative therapies affecting coagulation or anesthesia (*continued*)

Name	Effect
Licorice	Platelet aggregation inhibitor Contains coumarins Hypertension Hypokalemia
Meadowsweet	Platelet aggregation inhibitor
Motherwort	Contains coumarins
Papaya	Platelet aggregation inhibitor
Passionflower	Contains coumarins
Poplar	Platelet aggregation inhibitor
Red clover	Contains coumarins
St John's wort	Cytochrome P450 inducer; increases metabolism of many drugs including warfarin
Sweet clover	Contains coumarins
Tamarind	Increases bioavailability of aspirin and ibuprofen
Tumeric	Platelet aggregation inhibitor
Valerian	Potentiate sedative effects of anesthesia
Vitamin E	Platelet aggregation inhibitor
Willow bark	Platelet aggregation inhibitor

Data from Refs.[8,13,14,16,131]

bleeding, whereas 70% of patients do not report their use to their doctor.[13,14] The American Society of Anesthesiologists recommends cessation of all herbal medications 2 to 3 weeks before surgery, although more specific recommendations are available for certain products.[15,16]

Preoperative assessment of bleeding risk A careful history should be taken to assess the risk of bleeding. Medical conditions and the use of medications and alternative therapies should be assessed as well as a specific bleeding history (see **Table 3**). The routine use of coagulation studies in asymptomatic patients has not been shown to be of any benefit in predicting the risk of bleeding, changing management, or altering outcomes.[17–19] In patients with a history suggestive of bleeding tendency, laboratory testing may be indicated.

Testing of platelet function has traditionally been with platelet count and an assessment of bleeding time; however, the reliability of bleeding time testing is low and it has not been found to predict operative bleeding.[20] Tests of clot viscoelastic strength, such as the thromboelastogram (TEG) and the Sonoclot, test all the components of the coagulation system and are better at predicting perioperative bleeding than routine tests.[20] Results from the platelet-activated clotting factor test (PACT, Coulter Electronics, Hialeah, FL) and the PFA100 (Dade International, Miami, FL) are mixed and they are believed to be less sensitive than the TEG.[17,20]

Suggested tests in patients with a history suggestive of a bleeding abnormality include activated partial thromboplastin time (APTT), prothrombin ratio (PR), platelet count, fibrinogen, and vWD panel (see **Table 1**)[17] or TEG.[20] If abnormalities are detected, specific factor assays can be performed to further evaluate the bleeding abnormality.

Table 2
Hereditary disorders of hemostasis

Disorder	Types	Mechanism	Typical Presentation	Inheritance	Incidence/Prevalence	Treatment
von Willebrand disease	All	Defects in vWF with secondary FVIII deficiency	Mucosal bleeding, petechiae, purpura may be asymptomatic, basic laboratory tests variable, may be normal or have abnormal PFT		Prevalence mild: 1%–2% severe: 1:5000–10,000	Antifibrinolytics (tranexamic acid, ε-aminocaproic acid) may be useful for mucosal bleeding
	I	Quantitative vWF deficiency			70%–80% of cases	DDAVP
	IIA	Qualitative vWF deficiency	Specific tests: vWF:Ag vWF:RCo vWF:CB vWF:FVIIIB	Autosomal dominant with variable penetrance	15%–20% of cases, IIa most common	DDAVP
	IIB					Cryoprecipitate or concentrates containing vWF DDAVP debated; causes drop in platelet count
	IIM					DDAVP
	IIN			Autosomal recessive		DDAVP
	III	Severe quantitative vWF and secondary FVIII deficiency	May present as hemophilia	Autosomal recessive	5% of cases	Cryoprecipitate or concentrates containing vWF Not responsive to DDAVP
Hemophilia	A	FVIII deficiency	Hemarthrosis, muscle hematomas	X-linked recessive	1:5000 male births	DDAVP for mild cases FVIII concentrate
	B	Factor IX deficiency	APTT prolonged PR normal	X-linked recessive	1:25,000 male births	FIX concentrate or cryoprecipitate
	C	Factor XI deficiency	As mild hemophilia A	Autosomal recessive	Rare	FXI concentrate

(*continued on next page*)

Table 2
Hereditary disorders of hemostasis (*continued*)

Disorder	Types	Mechanism	Typical Presentation	Inheritance	Incidence/Prevalence	Treatment
Rare clotting factor defects		Factor I (fibrinogen) deficiency	Severe cases: difficulty with implantation of embryo into uterine wall, miscarriage, bleeding	Autosomal recessive	All rare. FVII deficiency most common, FII deficiency least common	Fibrinogen
		Factor II (prothrombin) deficiency	As hemophilia			Plasma or prothrombin complex concentrate
		Factor V deficiency		All autosomal recessive, heterozygotes may be mildly symptomatic		Plasma
		Combined FV and FVIII deficiency	Prolonged PR and APTT			Plasma or FVIII concentrate
		Factor VII deficiency	PR prolonged, APTT normal			FVII concentrate
		Factor X deficiency	PR and APTT prolonged			Plasma or prothrombin complex concentrate
		Factor XIII deficiency	PR and APTT prolonged			Plasma or FXIII concentrate
Rare platelet defects	Adhesion defects (eg, Bernard-Soulier syndrome	Gp Ib-X deficiency (platelet membrane receptor for vWF)	Mucosal bleeding, petechiae, purpura	Autosomal recessive	Rare	Platelet transfusions if required
	Aggregation defects (eg, Glanzman thrombasthenia)	Gp IIb–IIIa deficiency (platelet membrane receptor for fibrinogen)				
	Secretion defects (storage pool disorders)	Defective release of mediators		Variable		

Abbreviations: APTT, activated partial thromboplastin time; BT, bleeding time; CB, collagen binding; DDAVP, desmopressin; F, factor, prostaglandin; FVIIIB, factor VIII binding; PFT, platelet function tests; PR, prothrombin ratio; RCo, ristocetin cofactor; vWF, von Willebrand factor; vWF:Ag, vWF level.

Data from Refs.[8,10,132,133]

Table 3
Bleeding history

Bleeding Type	Suggestive of:
Epistaxis	Very common; does not necessarily indicate bleeding disorder but is most common presentation of vWD Hereditary hemorrhagic telangectasia
Oral mucosal bleeding	Platelet disorders/vWD Bleeding with tooth eruption suggestive of moderate to severe hemophilia
Excessive bruising	Platelet abnormality/vWD Blood vessel abnormalities (Ehlers-Danlos syndrome, chronic steroid use, aging)
Muscle hematomas or hemarthroses	Hemophilia/factor deficiencies
Excessive bleeding after surgery or trauma	Nonspecific
Menorrhagia	Nonspecific
Postpartum hemorrhage	Nonspecific

Data from Konkle BA. Bleeding and thrombosis. In: Fauci AS, Braunwald E, Kasper DL, et al, editors. Harrison's principles of internal medicine. 17th ed: McGraw-Hill; 2008.

Table 4
Classification of acquired causes of clotting defects

Component	Problem	Causes	Examples
Platelet plug	Decreased production	Drugs Nutritional deficiencies Infections Bone marrow disorders	Alcohol, thiazides, cytotoxics Vitamin B_{12}, folate HIV Aplastic anemia, myelodysplastic syndromes, leukemia, lymphoma
	Decreased survival	Autoimmune Drug induced Infections Sequestration Consumption	Primary: idiopathic thrombocytopenic purpura Secondary: SLE Heparin, quinine, vancomycin HIV, infectious mononucleosis Hypersplenism Thrombotic microangiopathies, giant hemangiomas, DIC
	Impaired function	Autoimmune Drug induced Uremia; complex effects on adhesion, aggregation, and secretion	Acquired vWD (autoantibodies vs vWF; see **Table 5**)
Clotting factors	Decreased production	Drugs Nutritional deficiency Liver failure	Warfarin Vitamin K deficiency
	Decreased survival	Consumption Autoimmune	DIC Inhibitory autoantibodies
	Impaired function	Drugs	Heparin

Abbreviations: DIC, disseminated intravascular coagulation; HIV, human immunodeficiency virus; SLE, systemic lupus erythematosus.

Data from Refs.[8,133,134]

Table 5
Anticoagulant and antiplatelet medications

Medication	Actions	Stop Before Surgery	Antidote
Warfarin	Inhibits vitamin K–dependent clotting factor synthesis (factors VII, IX, X, II) Also inhibits protein C synthesis (procoagulant effect); can result in hypercoagulable state in first 24 h of therapy	2–4 d	Vitamin K Fresh frozen plasma or factor IX complex (purified factor IX preparations do not contain II, VII, and X)
Heparin	In combination with antithrombin III, inactivates factors Xa and IIa Risk of heparin-induced thrombocytopenia (HIT, up to 30%) Type I most common, mild, direct effect of heparin on platelets. Onset 1–4 d after commencement of therapy Type II: antibody-mediated activation of platelets resulting in severe intravascular coagulation. Onset 7–11 d after commencement of therapy	6 h	Protamine
Low molecular weight heparin	As heparin, major action on factor Xa Low risk of HIT but contraindicated in patients who have had HIT	12–24 h	Protamine (partial reversal)
Aspirin and NSAIDs	Blocks production of thromboxane A2 in platelets by inhibiting cyclooxygenase. Aspirin, irreversible inhibition; NSAIDs, reversible	Aspirin: 7–10 d	None
Thienopyridines (clopidogrel, ticlopidine)	Inhibit ADP-induced platelet aggregation by altering a platelet receptor for ADP	Clopidigrel: 5–10 d Ticlodipine: 10 d	None
Gp IIb/IIIa receptor antagonists	Bind to Gp IIb/IIIa receptor inhibiting platelet binding to fibrinogen and vWF	24–72 h	None (Tirofiban; hemodialysis)

Abbreviation: NSAIDs, nonsteroidal anti-inflammatory drugs.

Data from Samama CM, Bastien O, Forestier F, et al Antiplatelet agents in the perioperative period: expert recommendations of the French Society of Anesthesiology and Intensive Care (SFAR) 2001 – summary statement. Can J Anaesth 2002;49(6):S26–35 [Guideline Practice Guideline]; Slaughter TF. Coagulation. In: Miller RD, editor. Miller's anesthesia. Maryland Heights (MO): Churchill Livingstone; 2009. p. 1767–81.

Intraoperatively

Anesthetic technique Anesthetic techniques can potentially affect bleeding and the surgical field. These include the type of airway, the degree of hypercapnia, and the anesthetic agents used.

The airway used in ESS is typically a reinforced laryngeal mask airway (LMA) or endotracheal tube (ETT). Early concerns regarding airway protection with the LMA have not been borne out, with one study showing significantly fewer instances of blood in the upper airway with LMA compared with ETT (20% vs 85%). There was a trend toward increased blood in the distal airway with LMA but no complications related to this.[21] The pressor effect of LMA insertion is significantly lower than for ETT.[22,23] Atef and Fawaz[24] compared LMA with ETT in ESS. The ETT group had higher heart rate (HR) and blood pressure (BP) and worse surgical field at 15 minutes, which resolved by 30 minutes after insertion.[23]

The use of spontaneous ventilation may result in normal to high CO_2 levels, whereas the use of muscle relaxants and mechanical ventilation allows normal or low levels to be achieved. Increasing CO_2 levels cause smooth muscle relaxation and vasodilation, potentially increasing bleeding. However, Nekhendzy and colleagues[25] examined the effect of different end tidal CO_2 levels on the surgical field and blood loss in patients undergoing ESS. There was no difference in blood loss or surgical field between hyper-, hypo-, or normocapnia groups. However, the hypocapnia group had significantly greater requirements for remifentanyl and antihypertensive medications, suggesting limited benefit for the use of hypocapnic techniques.

A summary of studies of the effects of various anesthetic techniques on bleeding in ESS is given in **Table 6**. Nine studies compared an intravenous propofol/opioid-based anesthetic with an inhalational agent supplemented with opioid. Seven favored the propofol arm, with lower blood loss or improved surgical field. Of the remaining 2 studies, 1 compared 3 arms and showed improved surgical field with propfol/remifentanyl and sevoflurane/sufentanil compared with isoflurane/fentanyl. There was no difference in BP and the HR was not reported in this study.[38] The final study in this group compared propofol/fentanyl with sevoflurane/fentanyl. There was no difference in surgical field or, importantly, HR between the 2 groups.[27]

The importance of relative bradycardia is shown in several other studies. A correlation between decreased HR and improved surgical field has been shown.[39,44] Hypotension achieved with infusion of esmolol (a short acting β-blocker) or magnesium sulfate,[35] or premedication with clonidine[40] or dexmedetomidine[32] (centrally acting α_2 agonists that, acting on the presynaptic α_2 receptor, result in decreased sympathetic tone) result in lower HR and improved surgical field. In contrast, hypotension achieved with the use of vasodilators (nitroprusside or prostaglandin E_1) results in reflex tachycardia and no improvement in the surgical field or blood loss (respectively) compared with normotensive anesthesia.[36,40]

Many anesthetic agents also have effects on platelet function. Of the inhalational anesthetics, isoflurane and desflurane do not seem to affect platelet function, whereas sevoflurane and nitrous oxide seem to inhibit platelet aggregation.[46] Of the intravenous agents, propofol is believed to inhibit platelet aggregation, whereas the opioids do not.[46] A direct comparison of the effects of propofol, isoflurane, and sevoflurane in sinus surgery found propofol to have a larger inhibitory effect than sevoflurane or isoflurane.[31] However, the clinical significance seems to be minimal in the operative setting.

In summary, the optimal anesthetic technique seems to be relative bradycardia with associated hypotension. All groups in which these conditions were met showed benefit, whereas no group with an increased HR had improved field or blood loss.

Patient positioning The reverse Trendelenberg position is used to reduce venous pressure and thus improve bleeding (**Fig. 1**). Between 5° and 15° of reverse Trendelenberg tilt is sufficient to reduce central venous pressure from an average of 9.2 mm Hg to 1.7 mm Hg.[47] At 25° of reverse Trendelenberg tilt, the mean pressure in the confluums sinuum is zero.[48] Cerebral perfusion pressure is the difference between mean arterial pressure (MAP) and intracranial pressure (ICP). Positional decreases in MAP are offset by decreased ICP, probably due to increased venous outflow and hydrostatic displacement of cerebrospinal fluid (CSF), therefore cerebral perfusion and blood flow are preserved up to 20 to 30° of tilt.[49–51]

Position also affects mucosal blood flow. Gurr and colleagues[52] showed a 38% decrease in blood flow to the head of the inferior turbinate with 20° of reverse Trendelenberg tilt with a corresponding increase in blood flow in the head-down position. Ko and colleagues[53] found an improvement in blood loss and surgical field in ESS with 10° of reverse Trendelenberg tilt compared with patients laid supine.

Topical vasoconstriction A variety of topical agents have been used alone or in combinations. Adrenalin causes a dose-dependent response at α_1 and α_2 receptors, resulting in vasoconstriction of arterial and capacitance vessels.[4] Topical use in up to 1:1000 concentration has been widely used without evidence of systemic hemodynamic response.[54,55] Cocaine blocks the reuptake of noradrenalin at the nerve ending, resulting in a vasoconstrictive effect in addition to its local anesthetic properties. However, it has not been shown to be superior to other agents and has been associated with dose-related and idiosyncratic reactions including cardiac arrhythmias and death.[56–59] Oxymetazoline and phenylephrine are partial α agonists, with predominantly α_1 effects.[4] They therefore have limited effect on the capacitance vessels and are likely to be less effective in hemostasis. Theoretically, the use of one of these partial agonists may result in competitive inhibition with adrenalin, reducing its effect. For these reasons, the authors' preference is to use adrenalin alone as a topical nasal preparation.

Local infiltration Infiltration of the nasal mucosa, commonly with adrenalin containing local anesthetics, has complex hemodynamic effects. There is a hypotensive response to injection of low doses of adrenalin, probably due to activation of high-sensitivity β_2 receptors in skeletal muscle, causing vasodilation. At higher doses, increasing vasoconstriction in skin, mucosa, and kidney, as well as activation of cardiac β_1 receptors, results in increased BP. Lignocaine also has a hypotensive effect, and the relative influences of adrenalin and lignocaine infiltration are difficult to separate in the current literature[54,55,60,61] Cohen-Kerem and colleagues[54] compared saline with lignocaine/adrenalin injection. There was an improved surgical field and lower requirement for topical adrenalin in the lignocaine/adrenalin group. There was a hypotensive response to the lignocaine/adrenalin injection, and a tachycardic response to the saline injection. Increased MAP was correlated with plasma noradrenalin levels, which were lower in the lignocaine/adrenalin group. These findings were believed to be to the result of decreased sympathetic stimulation (less pain) in the lignocaine/adrenalin group.[54]

Infiltration of the pterygopalatine fossa (PPF) via the greater palatine canal has been proposed to reduce blood flow to the nasal cavity by inducing vasoconstriction or compression of the terminal branches of the maxillary artery. PPF injection with lignocaine/adrenalin has been shown to improve the surgical field in sinus surgery.[45] Other clinical studies have shown PPF injection to be effective in posterior epistaxis with plain xylocaine, water, or glycerine, presumably on the basis of physical compression of the artery.[52,62–64] PPF injection may have limited effect

Table 6
Published studies of anesthetic techniques in ESS

Study	Comparison	Outcome Measures	n	Findings
Ahn et al, 2007[26]	Total intravenous anesthetic (TIVA) (P/R) vs S/R	Blood loss Surgical conditions (numeric rating scale 1–10)	40	BP: no significant difference (NSD) HR: lower in propfol/remifentanyl group Lund-Mackay ≤ 12: NSD Lund-Mackay>12: Blood loss: P/R significantly improved Surgical field: P/R significantly improved
Atef and Fawaz, 2008[24]	Laryngeal mask vs endotracheal intubation (all TIVA with P/R)	HR, BP Surgical field: Boezaat rating scale	60	Laryngeal mask: shorter time to achieve target BP Lower doses of remifentanyl required
Beule et al, 2007[27]	S/F vs P/F Lund-Mackay>12	HR Blood loss Blood loss/min Platelet function Surgical field (VAS)	52	HR: NSD Blood loss: NSD Blood loss/min: NSD Surgical field: NSD Platelet function: impaired in both groups, worse in P/F group
Blackwell et al, 1993[28]	P vs I. Retrospective review, groups different age, sex, weight	Blood loss	25	Blood loss: improved in P group
Boezaart et al, 1995[29]	Sodium nitroprusside vs esmolol. Hypotension induced and assessments made at 5 mm BP increments	Surgical field: rating scale 0–5 at different BPs	20	Esmolol group: HR lower Surgical conditions improved
Cincikas and Ivaskevicius, 2003[30]	Normotension vs hypotension (induced with captopril premedication and GTN infusion) Unblinded	HR Surgical field: Boezaart rating scale Blood loss	52	Hypotension group: HR lower Surgical field significantly improved Blood loss lower
Dogan et al, 1999[31]	I, S, P	In vitro effects on platelet aggregation	30	P, S: inhibit platelet aggregation. No difference between groups I: no effect

(*continued on next page*)

Table 6
Published studies of anesthetic techniques in ESS (*continued*)

Study	Comparison	Outcome Measures	n	Findings
Durmus et al, 2007[32]	Dexmedetomidine (α2-receptor agonist) vs placebo in tympanoplasty and septorhinoplasty	HR, BP Bleeding score (nonvalidated 1–4)	40	Dexmedetomidine group: Reduced requirements for anesthetic agents HR, BP lower Surgical field improved
Eberhart et al, 2003[33]	TIVA (P/R) vs I/A	BP, HR Surgical conditions: VAS+Boezaart scale Dryness of field: VAS Blood loss	90	BP: NSD TIVA: HR lower Surgical conditions improved Blood loss: NSD
Eberhart et al, 2007[34]	D/R vs R/D: comparison between D-accentuated and R-accentuated anesthesia	Surgical conditions: VAS+Boezaart scale HR, BP, postoperative recovery	100	Surgical conditions, HR, BP: NSD Dryness: improved in D-accentuated group Recovery: slightly faster in R-accentuated group, no difference at 1 h after operation Summary: NSD between techniques
Elsharnouby and Elsharnouby, 2006[35]	$MgSO_4$ vs saline (both groups S/F)	HR, BP Surgical field (Boezaart rating scale)	60	MgSO4 group: HR, BP lower Surgical field improved Decreased requirements for F,S Emergence time increased
Jacobi et al, 2000[36]	Normotension vs nitroprusside+ captopril induced hypotension	BP Dryness of field ACTH, AVP, cortisol	32	Hypotensive group: HR higher BP lower Surgical field: NSD ACTH, AVP, cortisol: NSD
Kaygusuz et al, 2008[37]	D/R vs I/R in tympanoplasty and sinus surgery	HR, BP, blood loss Surgical field: VAS Postoperative recovery	64	Blood loss, HR, BP: NSD Recovery: quicker with D
Manola et al, 2005[38]	Sufentanil/S vs TIVA(P/R) vs I/F	BP Surgical field (Boezaart scale) Blood loss	71	BP: NSD HR not reported Surgical field significantly better in sufentanil/S and TIVA groups

(*continued on next page*)

Table 6
Published studies of anesthetic techniques in ESS (*continued*)

Study	Comparison	Outcome Measures	n	Findings
Nair et al, 2004[39]	Metoprolol vs placebo premedication	HR, BP Surgical field (Boezaart scale)	80	HR: lower in metoprolol group Surgical field: NSD between groups correlated with HR Significantly better with HR <60 Not correlated with BP
Nekhendzy et al, 2007[25]	Hypercapnia vs hypocapnia vs normocapnia	Blood loss Surgical field	180	Blood loss: NSD Surgical field: NSD Hypocapnia group: higher requirements for antihypertensives Increased blood loss with increased CT score, duration of surgery
Okuyama et al, 2005[40]	Hypotension with prostaglandin E1 (PGE1) and diazepam premedication vs normotension with clonidine premedication vs normotension with diazepam premedication (control group)	BP, HR Blood loss	24	PGE1 group: lower BP, higher HR, blood loss NSD from control Clonidine group: BP NSD, HR lower, blood loss lower than control
Pavlin et al, 1999[41]	TIVA (P/A) vs I/A	Blood loss Surgical field Postoperative recovery HR, BP not reported	56	Surgical field: better in P group Blood loss: NSD Postoperative recovery: shorter time to discharge in P group
Sivaci et al, 2004[42]	P/F vs S/F	BP, HR Blood loss	32	BP, HR: NSD Blood loss: lower in P/F group
Tirelli et al, 2004[43]	TIVA (P/R) vs I/F	BP, HR Surgical field (Boezaart)	64	Surgical field: better with TIVA HR, BP: NSD (trend to be lower in TIVA group)
Wormald et al, 2005[44]	TIVA (P/R) vs S/F	BP, HR Surgical field (Boezaart)	56	TIVA: Surgical field improved Improved field correlated independently with lower BP and lower HR
Wormald et al, 2005[45]	Pterygopalatine fossa injection vs no injection (compared sides in same patients)	BP, HR, Surgical field (Boezaart)	55	Injection: improved surgical field BP, HR: NSD Field correlated independently with HR

Abbreviations: GTN, glyceryl trinitrate; P/R, propofol/remifentanyl; S/R, sevoflurane/remifentanyl; VAS, visual analogue scale.

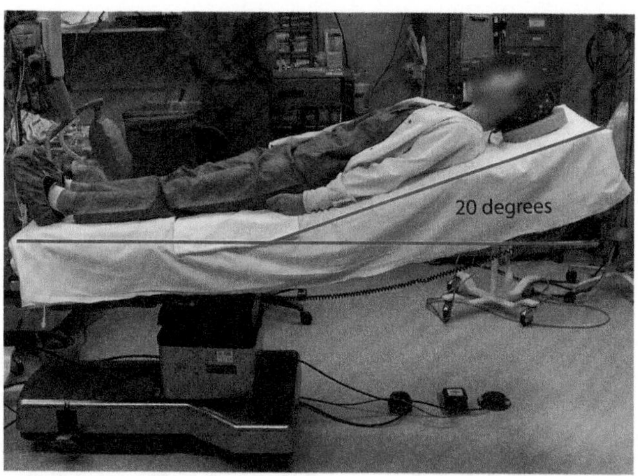

Fig. 1. The reverse Trendelenberg position.

in the anterior nose. Laser Doppler studies have shown only a 4% reduction in blood flow to the head of the inferior turbinate following PPF injection with bupivicaine.[52]

Irrigation Warm-water irrigation has been advocated for hemostasis in nasal mucosa, and warm saline is used in some skull base centers to control diffuse bleeding.[65,66] We use copious irrigation at room temperature, which not only removes excess blood but also seems to have a hemostatic effect.

Hemostatic materials A wide variety of hemostatic materials are available to provide intraoperative and postoperative hemostasis (**Table 7**). In general, it seems that microfibrillar collagen, FloSeal, poly-*N*-acetylglucosamines, and fibrin glues are more effective than Surgicel or gelfoam in hemostasis.[76] The main drawbacks of these agents are the potential for postoperative granulation and adhesion formation (see **Table 7**); however, not all have been studied in the nose and, of the studies available, many are small or uncontrolled. The use of human blood products such as thrombin and fibrinogen raises the possibility of transmission of viral diseases, whereas the use of bovine thrombin is associated with a high rate of antibody development, with reports of anaphylaxis and coagulopathy.[72,76]

The intraoperative use of topical agents (as opposed to at the end of the procedure) is not well studied. Avitene (microfibrillar collagen) with pressure via a cottonoid has been advocated for control of venous and low-flow arterial bleeding in skull base cases.[65]

Macro Vascular Control (Larger Arterioles, Muscular Arteries, and Venous Plexuses)

Preoperative

Embolization Tumor embolization, particularly of juvenile nasopharyngeal angiofibroma (JNA), is important in surgical resection.[96,97] Blood supply is determined by the size and extension of most sinonasal tumors. In the initial stages, there is usually vascular supply from the distal branches of external carotid artery via the internal maxillary artery. In anterior or large tumors, the tumor may receive important vessels from the internal carotid artery (ICA), especially from collateral (especially the posterior ethmoidal artery) branches of the ophthalmic artery.[98,99] Skull base tumors may also recruit pial collaterals from the adjacent brain. Preoperative selective internal and

Table 7
Topical hemostatic agents

Type	Agent/Manufacturer	Mechanism	Hemostatic Effectiveness	Adhesion/Scar Formation
Porcine gelatin (with thrombin)	Surgiflo (Ethicon Inc, Somerville, NJ) combined with thrombin	Gelatin: poorly understood; tamponade effect due to swelling of particles and surface interactions with platelets and clotting factors Addition of thrombin activates final common pathway	Hemostasis median 1 min in 29/30 patients undergoing ESS (prospective, uncontrolled trial)[67]	No synechiae in 30 patients[67]
	FloSeal (Baxter International, Deerfield, IL)		Hemostasis average 2 min in 17/18 patients undergoing ESS (prospective, uncontrolled trial[58] Hemostasis within 3 min, equal to merocel pack in ESS[69]	Increased granulation tissue, adhesions, scarring and incorporation of particles into healing mucosa[70,71] Antisdel, 2008[78]
	Gelfoam (Pharmacia & Upjohn) with thrombin		Effective[70]	Low compared with FloSeal[70]
Antifibrinolytics	ε-Aminocaproic acid (Amicar, Lederle Parenterals, Carolina, Puerto Rico)	Inhibit plasmin formation from plasminogen; reduce breakdown of fibrin clots	Ineffective compared with saline in ESS (RCT)[73]	Not reported Probably low
	Tranexamic acid (Cyclokapron, Pfizer, New York)		Better than saline or amicar in ESS (RCT)[73] Also effective systemically in ESS and tooth extraction[74,75]	
Microporous polysaccharide hemospheres	(MPH, Medafor, Minneapolis, MN)	Dehydrate blood, concentrating platelets, RBC, and clotting factors	Poor in animal studies[76] Hemostasis in 30–45 s in ESS (uncontrolled study)[77]	Low[78] Synechiae: 12% (requiring treatment: 3%)[77]
Carboxymethylcellulose	Surgicel (Arthrocare, Glenfield, United Kingdom)	Surface interactions with proteins and platelets Activation of clotting pathways	No effect on postoperative bleeding in ESS (mesh or gel)[79] Low in vitro[80] Some effect in venous/capillary bleeding (non-nasal surgery)[76]	Low[81] Surgicel granulomas reported[76]

Platelet gel	(PPAI Medical, Fort Myers, FL)	Autologous concentrated platelets, release of procoagulant factors	No postoperative bleeding in 16 patients (retrospective study, historical controls)[82]	No synechiae in 16 patients[82]
Microfibrillar collagen	Avitene (Davol, Warwick, RI), Colgel, others	Activate clotting pathway Platelet aggregation and activation	High in vitro[80] More effective than Surgicel in cardiac surgery[83] More effective than fibrin glue (animal studies)[76]	Granuloma formation reported (no sinonasal studies)[76] Possibly high[84]
Chitosan gel	(University of Otago, Dunedin, New Zealand)	Poorly understood Vasoconstriction Mobilization of RBC, clotting factors, and platelets due to positive charge	Average 4 min to hemostasis, effective compared with no treatment (animal study of ESS)[85] No effect in vitro[76]	Low[86]
Hyaluronic acid	MeroGel (Medtronic Xomed, Jacksonville, FL)	Possible tamponade effect	Unknown	Conflicting reports High (animal studies)[87,88] Low (clinical trial)[89]
	Sepragel sinus (Genzyme Biosurgery, Cambridge, MA)		Minimal[90]	Low[90]
Fibrin glues (thrombin/fibrinogen)	Quixil (Ethicon), others	Forms crosslinked fibrin clot independent of host clotting factors	Effective in ESS compared with merocel[91] Effective in nasal surgery and epistaxis[92–94] Highly effective in animal studies and nonsinus surgery[76]	Low[95]
Poly-*N*-acetylglucosamine	Syvek (Marine Polymer Technologies, MA)	Release of vasoactive substances Platelet activation Concentration of RBC	Highly effective in vitro, in animal studies and in cardiac catheterization[76]	Unknown (no nasal studies)

Abbreviations: A, alfentanyl; BP, blood pressure; D, desflurane; F, fentanyl; HR, heart rate; I, isoflurane; NSD: no significant difference; P, propofol; R, remifentanyl; RBC, red blood cells; RCT, randomized controlled trial; S, sevoflurane; TIVA, total intravenous anesthetic.

external carotid and occasionally superselective angiography greatly assists in determining the vascular contributions to the tumor and to identify significant arteriovenous shunts.[97–99] Careful bilateral internal and external carotid, and occasionally vertebral arteriography is recommended to identify blood supply, collateral circulation and shunting. Even with high-resolution angiography, only blood vessels with diameters exceeding 200 μm can be visualized.[97] Arteriovenous shunts of smaller caliber may not be identified with angiography and present a potential risk during embolization.[97,98] JNA can have a high incidence of arteriovenous shunts and larger particles (≥140 μm in caliber) of polyvinyl acetate (PVA) are recommend for preoperative embolization.[100] Some investigators argue for the need to perform direct intratumoral embolization in addition to preoperative embolization in cases of JNA with significant vascular contribution from the ICA.[98] However, concerns about shunting with potential cerebrovascular consequences versus early revascularization will influence the use of coils versus particle embolization. Particles may be used and a proximal coil as well for this reason. Careful evaluation of the retinal blood supply is also essential as it can occasionally arise from the external carotid circulation, making embolization hazardous. At our institution, if there is good access laterally to feeding tumor vessels then embolization is not essential, but for large tumors for which a structured approached to the vascular control is not available, then embolization is used. Preoperative sacrifice of an internal or external carotid artery can be performed after an occlusion test.[135] Evaluation by an experienced neuro-interventionalist is essential.

Intraoperative

The principles of hemostasis in endoscopic skull base surgery differ little from those of the microsurgical era. Prevention of bleeding is the best solution. Tumor debulking, extracapsular sharp dissection, and countertraction using gentle suction form the foundation of cerebrovascular control.[65] Standard neurosurgical bayonets are often not appropriate via the long surgical corridor of endoscopic skull base surgery, and specialized instrumentation is essential. Monopolar cautery should not be used in the sphenoid sinus, on the skull base, or intracranially because of the risk of neurovascular injury.[65] If bleeding is anticipated, for example in resection of a vascular tumor, preemptive proximal control should be obtained if possible.

Arterial

Sphenopalatine and maxillary arteries The sphenopalatine artery (SPA) can be ligated at its foramen, posterior to the crista ethmoidalis. There are 2 or more branches entering the nose in up to 97% of patients,[101] so care should be taken to control all branches. If more proximal control is required, the maxillary artery can be ligated in the pterygopalatine or infratemporal fossa by removal of the posterior wall of the maxillary sinus (**Fig. 2**).

Anterior and posterior ethmoid arteries The anterior ethmoid artery is more difficult to access surgically, with only 20% of arteries able to be clipped successfully transnasally in a cadaver series.[102] Endoscopic removal of the lamina papyracea allows identification of the anterior and posterior ethmoid arteries between periorbita and skull base (**Fig. 3**).[65,103,104] Alternatively, an external approach via Lynch incision can be used.

Carotid artery An assessment of the cerebral collateral circulation should be done preoperatively by examination of a CT or MR angiography of the head and neck. If there is a high risk of internal carotid injury, preoperative occlusion testing can be

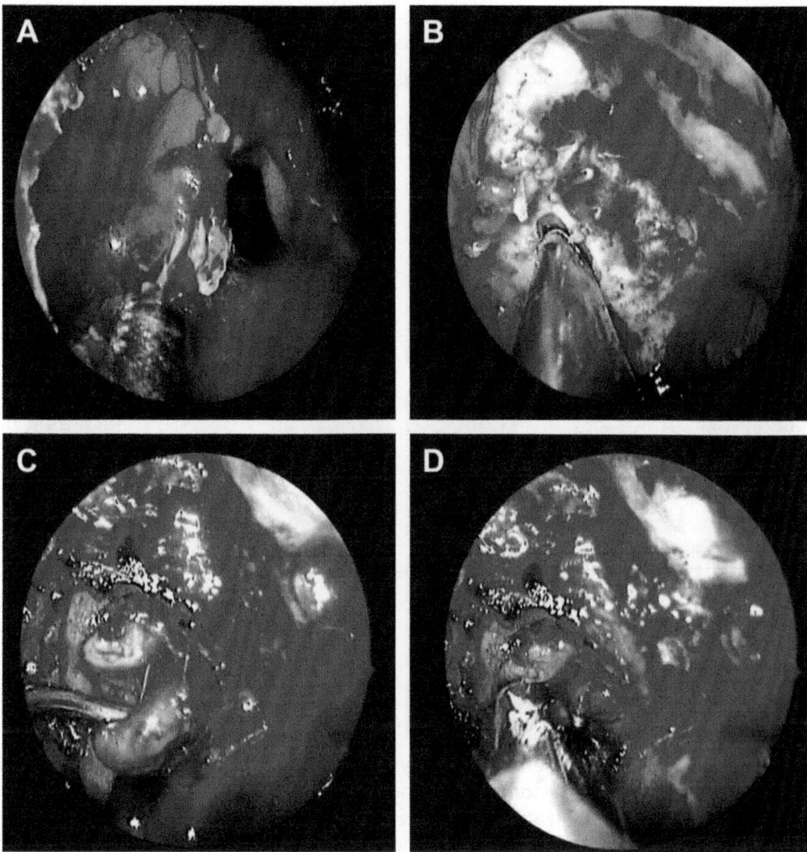

Fig. 2. Ligation of the maxillary artery in the infratemporal fossa. (*A*) Modified medial maxillectomy provides access to the posterior wall of the maxillary sinus. (*B*) Removal of the posterior wall of the maxillary sinus using a 2-mm Kerrison rongeur. (*C*) The maxillary artery is identified. (*D*) Artery is clipped with at least 2 clips then cauterized.

performed.[135] This technique is useful where the artery is involved with tumor, where the operative approach involves a high risk to the artery or if a planned sacrifice is to be undertaken. Proximal control may be achieved via an external lateral approach or extended endoscopic approach with mobilization of the petrous carotid. However, in the event of an ICA injury, conversion to an open approach, whether lateral or anterior, is time consuming and may not provide significantly improved ability to control the bleeding. Management of ICA injury therefore revolves around endovascular techniques once immediate control is gained by focused bipolar cautery or packing. At present, coiling of the ICA is performed, although newer malleable stents may provide an alternative.[65,105] If adequate collateral circulation is not present, a vascular bypass procedure may be attempted.[65] Endovascular temporary intraoperative balloon occlusion techniques are well described[136] and can be performed rapidly in the operating room with little preparation. Arterial reconstruction using flow diverting stent technology such as the older Jo-Med and newer Pipeline stents is feasible if arterial sacrifice is not possible, but full heparinization and antiplatelet cover is essential as soon as possible to avoid in stent thrombosis. Stenting needs to be done in an angiography suite. It is usually recommended to have the neck exposed if an open skull

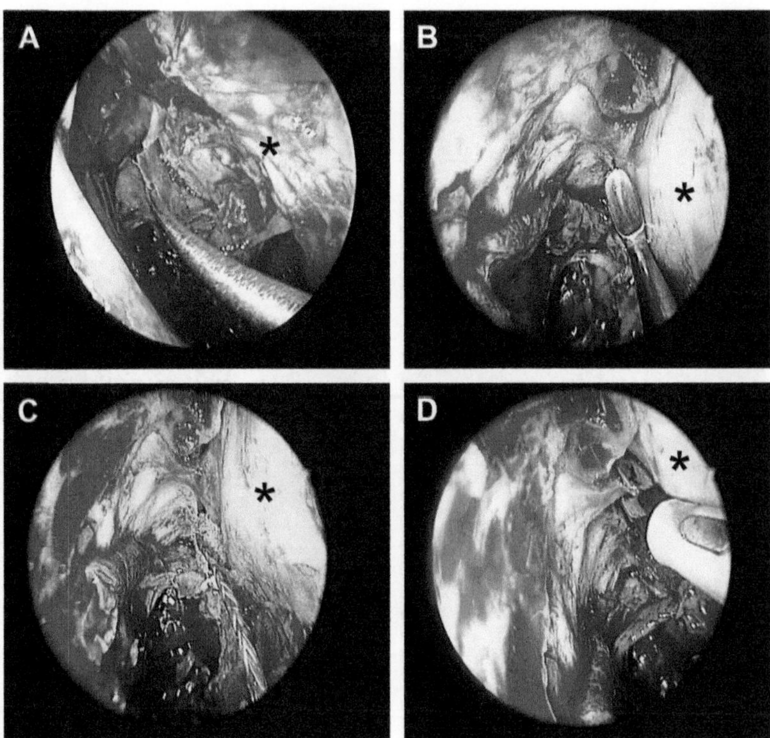

Fig. 3. Ligation of the anterior ethmoid artery. (*A*) Removal of the lamina papyracea up to the skull base (after ethmoidectomy). (*B*) Exposure of the anterior ethmoid artery in the skull base. (*C*) Further mobilization to allow access for cautery or ligation. (*D*) Bipolar cautery of the anterior ethmoid artery. * Medial orbital wall/periorbita. *From* Harvey RJ, Gallagher RM, Sacks R. Extended endoscopic techniques for sinonasal resections. Otolaryngol Clin North Am. 2010;43:613–38; with permission.

base carotid exposure is done, and a neurovascular opinion sought if significant large arterial bleeding occurs. If acute carotid sacrifice is required, this can be done with coils or devices such as the Amplatzer plug which can be rapidly deployed.[137]

Arterial bleeding Once bleeding occurs, control requires precise identification of the site of bleeding and control with cautery. This may require a suction bipolar device or a 2-surgeon approach to keep the bleeding site free of blood.[65] Focal packing may be used, but, in skull base cases, this may result in the bleeding continuing intracranially or intracerebrally, and is generally avoided.[65]

Venous The most important hemostatic technique, especially in venous bleeding, may be patience. Bleeding from the dural sinuses can be troublesome. Surgicel packing and patience will control most venous bleeding. Persistent manipulation often hinders hemostasis. Venous hemostasis should be achieved before intradural dissection.

ACCESS ASSESSMENT

Imaging

The preoperative computed tomography (CT) scan is used as a diagnostic tool to establish the individual patient's anatomy, and possibly for image guidance. Its strengths are the ability to delineate bony anatomy and abnormalities in 3 dimensions, and it is adequate for diagnosis in most sinusitis cases and fibro-osseous lesions.[106,107] Examination of the CT scan preoperatively is essential to identify areas of potential risk during the surgery. It also allows delineation of patient anatomy, particularly in the frontal recess.

Magnetic resonance imaging (MRI) is useful in the delineation of soft tissues. In sinusitis, it is useful in evaluation of intraorbital or intracranial complications. In cases of sinonasal masses or skull base defects, MRI can characterize the soft tissues and differentiate soft tissue from retained secretions. In neoplastic disease, it is also useful in evaluating orbital and cranial involvement as well as perineural spread of disease.[106,107] The use and evaluation of preoperative imaging is discussed in the article in this publication by Sam Becker, "Pre-operative CT Evaluation to Optimize Surgical Outcomes."

Surgical Planning

Anterolateral access

We predefine the regions or zones that will require endoscopic access and resection (**Fig. 4**; **Table 8**). Easy disorientation can occur during open or endoscopic surgery within the complex anatomy of the skull base. The limits of tissue removal may too easily align with surgeon comfort rather than anatomic boundaries defined by the presurgical clinical and radiological examination. Common areas of residual disease are summarized in **Box 1**. Open craniofacial surgery and the principles of en bloc resection from its oncologic foundations in managing malignant disease are often followed, by some surgeons, to ensure that the appropriate margins have been reached. With

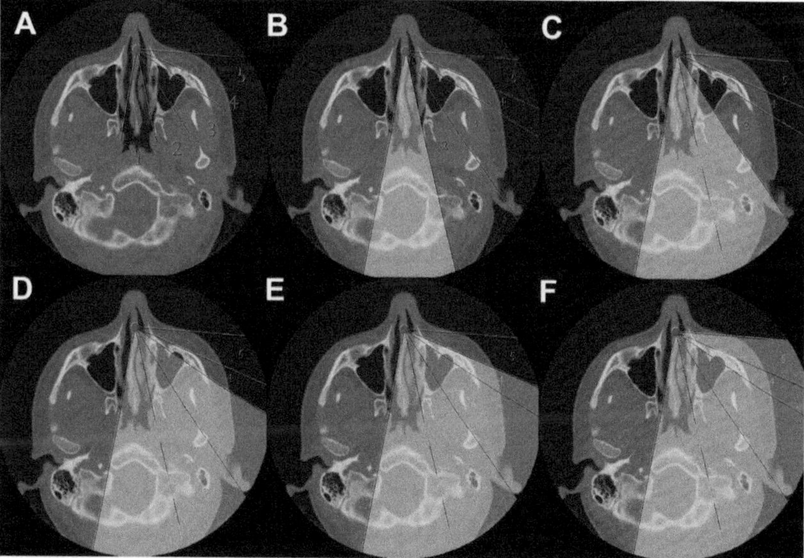

Fig. 4. (*A*) MUSC surgical resection zones. (*B*) Zone 1. Tumor is limited to septum, turbinates, middle meatus, ethmoid, frontal, sphenoid sinuses, and medial orbital wall. (*C*) Zone 2. Tumor extends to involve maxillary sinus medial to the inferior orbital nerve (ION), limited posterior wall, or maxillary floor. (*D*) Zone 3. Tumor involves maxilla lateral to ION and up to the zygomatic recess. (*E*) Zone 4. Tumor involves anterior maxillary wall without extension into premaxillary soft tissue. (*F*) Zone 5. Tumor involves premaxillary tissue or skin. *From* Harvey RJ, Sheahan PO, Schlosser RJ. Surgical management of benign sinonasal masses. Otolaryngol Clin North Am 2009;42:353–75; with permission.

Table 8
Surgical resection zones

Muscle Zone	Anatomic Region	Surgery Techniques	Instrumentation
Zone 1	Tumor limited to septum, turbinates, middle meatus, ethmoid, frontal, sphenoid sinuses, medial orbital wall (IP, hemangioma, chondroma)	Surgery includes turbinectomies, and septectomy	Basic ESS instrumentation
Zone 2	Tumor extends to involve maxillary sinus medial to the inferior orbital nerve (ION), limited posterior wall, or maxillary floor (IP, JNA)	MMA, frontal recess surgery (Draf 1–3, trephine or osteoplastic), sphenoid, ethmoid surgery. Some sinus surgery to include SPA management or modified EMM needed for tumor surveillance	Angled instrumentation and bipolar diathermy/endoscopic clip applicators. Maxillary trephination may be used. Rongeurs or chisel required for bone removal
Zone 3	Tumor involves NLD, medial buttress, or maxilla lateral to ION and up to the zygomatic recess (IP, JNA)	Requires DCR, possible transseptal approach, possible endoscopic Denker maxillotomy or open approach (sublabial Caldwell-Luc type approach)	Angled instrumentation has limitations in access. Standard ESS instruments via transseptal approach or maxillary trephine may be required
Zone 4	Tumor involves anterior maxillary wall with minimal extension into premaxillary soft tissue	Surgery requires transseptal approach, endoscopic Denker maxillotomy or premaxillary ESS approach. Sublabial open type approach. Open lateral rhinotomy/midface degloving	ESS instruments via transseptal approach or maxillary trephine may be required. Angled ipsilateral endoscopic instruments of little usefulness
Zone 5	Tumor involves premaxillary tissue or skin	Surgery requires open approach	Open surgical instrumentation

Abbreviations: DCR, dacrocystorhinostomy; EMM, endoscopic medial maxillectomy; IP, inverted papilloma; JNA, juvenile nasopharyngeal angiofibroma; MMA, Middle meatal antrostomy; NLD, nasolacrimal duct.

From Harvey RJ, Sheahan PO, Schlosser RJ. Surgical management of benign sinonasal masses. Otolaryngol Clin North Am 2009;42(2):353–75; with permission.

Box 1
Common sites of residual disease

Common sites for residual disease

Dental roots

Frontal sinus and recess

Lateral sphenoid

Anterior maxillary wall

Nasolacrimal duct

Infratemporal fossa extension (including PPF and infraorbital foramen [IOF])

careful planning and preoperative evaluation of radiology, it is possible to define the zone of resection likely to be required. **Table 8** outlines our current surgical approach to endoscopic resection. This was defined from practical surgical experience and based on current limitations of the transnasal route. These zones were developed and are used at the Medical University of South Carolina (MUSC) Rhinology and Skull Base and St Vincent's Rhinology and Skull Base Divisions when planning surgical access in endoscopic tumor removal (see **Fig. 4**A). They are defined as: zone 1, in which the tumor is limited to septum, turbinates, middle meatus, ethmoid, frontal, sphenoid sinuses, medial orbital wall. Surgery may include turbinectomies; septectomy; middle meatal antrostomy (MMA); and frontal, sphenoid, and ethmoid surgery. Basic ESS instrumentation is required (see **Fig. 4**B). In zone 2, the tumor extends to involve maxillary sinus medial to the inferior orbital nerve (ION), limited posterior wall, or maxillary floor. MMA or modified endoscopic medial maxillectomy (MMM) will be needed for tumor surveillance. Sinus surgery to include MMA with or without MMM and SPA management and some angled instrumentation will be needed (see **Fig. 4**C). In zone 3, the tumor involves maxilla lateral to ION and up to the zygomatic recess. Nasolacrimal duct (NLD) or medial buttress may need resection. Surgery may require dacrocystorhinostomy (DCR), possible transseptal approach, possible sublabial maxillotomy,[108] or medial buttress removal. Open approaches are traditionally described for tumors in this location (sublabial Caldwell-Luc–type approach, open lateral rhinotomy, and midface degloving). Angled instrumentation is mandatory for ipsilateral surgery (see **Fig. 4**D). In zone 4, the tumor involves anterior maxillary wall without extension into premaxillary soft tissue. Surgery requires transseptal dissection with direct drilling to the anterior maxillary wall (mucosal side) or one of the previously described external approaches (see **Fig. 4**E). In zone 5, the tumor involves premaxillary tissue or skin. Surgery requires the open approach (see **Fig. 4**F).

Frontal recess and frontal sinus

Lesions involving the frontal recess or sinus require special consideration. As in other areas, access is required to resect the lesion, maintain sinus ventilation, and allow inspection of the area postoperatively. The minimum procedure required in this area is a Draf 2A dissection for lesions adjacent to the frontal recess to identify the drainage pathway and ensure it is not obstructed by the resection or repair. For lesions involving the frontal recess or the frontal sinus medial to the lamina papyracea, a Draf 2B or 3 procedure is required.[109] For lesions with attachment lateral to the level of the medial orbital wall, an open or adjunctive approach may be required, but several investigators have reported successful endoscopic removal of tumors in this area.[110–114] Although mucosa is preserved as far as possible, tumor resection may result in areas of exposed or drilled bone. In these cases, a wide opening should be made because resultant scarring and narrowing occurs, by an average of 33% for a Draf 3 procedure.[115] In most tumor cases, including inverted papilloma, fibro-osseous lesions, and malignancies, access to the bony walls with a drill will be required, as inverted papillomas have a bony attachment that can often be defined as an area of osteitis on preoperative CT scanning.[116–118] Although there are several published series of frontal sinus inverted papillomas treated endoscopically, the limits of endoscopic access are not clearly defined.[110–114] In the case of frontal osteoma, Chiu and colleagues[119] in 2005 recommended an open approach for any lesion with lateral extent beyond a sagittal plane at the level of the medial orbital wall or with anterior attachment. However, other investigators have subsequently described endoscopic removal of these more challenging lesions with good results.[120]

Becker and colleagues[121] described access to the frontal sinus after various frontal sinus procedures including Draf 3 using angled instruments and endoscopes. The ability to visualize an instrument at the lateral-most extent of the frontal sinus in this study was limited to 54% of cases. Access using a drill was not assessed, nor was the ability to access the orbital roof. We have performed a further cadaver study examining access to the bony walls of the frontal sinus with a 70° drill following Draf 3 procedure. In this study, access was achieved to the most lateral aspects of the anterior and posterior walls in 95% of sinuses. The orbital roof was divided into zones (**Fig. 5**). Access to zone 1 was reliably achieved, zone 2 in 57%, and zones 3 or 4 in 5% (Daniel Timperley and colleagues, unpublished data, 2010). Based on these findings our current algorithm for frontal sinus evaluation is summarized in **Table 9**.

THE END OF THE CASE

Optimizing the environment for postoperative healing and care is considered throughout the case. The importance of preservation of mucosa to reduce granulation and scar formation cannot be overstated. In addition, we emphasize the creation of a cavity that facilitates postoperative access for inspection, debridement, and patient irrigation.

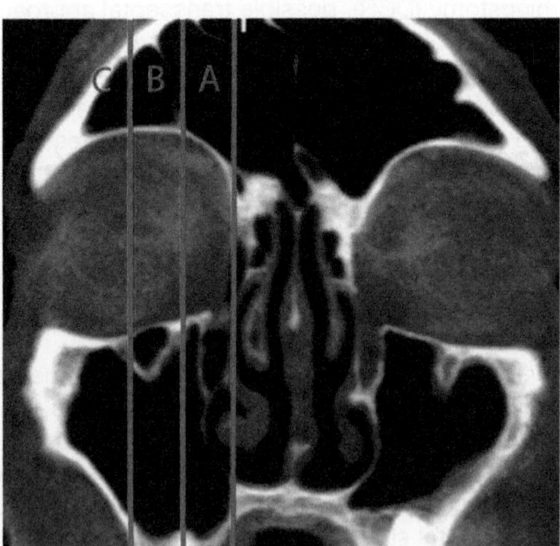

Fig. 5. Zones of the orbital roof. (*A*) Zone 1, the most medial quarter of the orbital roof. Endoscopic access is possible. (*B*) Zone 2, between the midorbital point and zone 1. Endoscopic access possible in 57%. (*C*) Zones 3 and 4, lateral to the midorbital point. Open approach required for lesions attached in this area.

Table 9
Frontal sinus evaluation algorithm

Degree of Frontal Extension	Area Involved	Procedure Required
Adjacent to frontal recess	Anterior ethmoid, middle turbinate, or medial orbital wall	Draf 2a for identification to ascertain whether resection, reconstruction, or packing will interfere with the frontal recess
Frontal recess	Frontal beak, intersinus septum, or frontal recess proper	Draf 2b/3 Reconstruction and short-term silastic stenting required in extensive bone exposure
Frontal sinus	Anterior/posterior walls	Draf 2b/3
	Orbital roof: medial quarter	Draf 2b/3
	Orbital roof: medial to midorbit	Draf 2b/3 Trephine/OPF may be required (43%)
	Orbital roof: beyond midorbital point	Trephine/OPF required

Abbreviation: OPF, osteoplastic flap.

The use of packing for postoperative hemostasis is unnecessary in most ESS cases.[122,123] However, it may be necessary in selected cases and may be used to prevent middle turbinate lateralization and promote healing. There are a wide variety of packing materials available that can be divided into absorbable and nonabsorbable types. Nonabsorbable materials include gauze, PVA sponge (Merocel, Medtronic Xomed, Jacksonville, FL, USA), and balloon devices. Their major drawbacks are patient discomfort, obstruction of the nasal airway, and bleeding on removal.[84,124] Less common complications include septal perforation, pack aspiration, toxic shock syndrome, alar necrosis, and obstructive sleep apnea.[125,126] Paraffin- and petroleum-based ointments are avoided if there is the possibility of an open orbital cavity because of the risk of foreign-body inflammatory reactions.[127–129] In addition, there may be loss of ciliated mucosa in the region of the pack.[130] Absorbable packing materials are summarized in **Table 7**. The ideal material would promote mucosal healing while providing sufficient structural support to prevent middle turbinate lateralization and would be completely removed by nasal irrigation. The authors' current practice is to place a short merocel tampon inside the cut finger of a surgical glove into the middle meatus, secured with a suture through the septum. The intention is solely to create a middle meatal spacer with no expectation that this will provide hemostasis. In our experience, the spacer does not obstruct the nasal airway or interfere with postoperative irrigation. Removal at 5 to 7 days is associated with minimal discomfort or bleeding in most cases. The spacer promotes a moist healing environment in the sinus cavity that is easily cleaned following removal.

SUMMARY

Optimal surgical outcomes depend on control of bleeding and adequate access, especially when extended endonasal approaches are used. This article reviews the multiple factors that may contribute to intraoperative bleeding and the current techniques that are available to optimize the surgical field. The access required for tumor resection, anterolaterally and in the frontal sinus, is assessed preoperatively by imaging and clinical examination. This method allows planning of a structured surgical approach to ensure that resection is not compromised by limited exposure.

REFERENCES

1. Rice DH, Schaefer SD. Endoscopic paranasal sinus surgery. 3rd edition. Philadelphia; London: Lippincott Williams & Wilkins; 2004.
2. Mason JD, Jones NS, Hughes RJ, et al. A systematic approach to the interpretation of computed tomography scans prior to endoscopic sinus surgery. J Laryngol Otol 1998;112(10):986–90.
3. Widdicombe J. Microvascular anatomy of the nose. Allergy 1997;52(Suppl 40): 7–11.
4. Corboz MR, Rivelli MA, Varty L, et al. Pharmacological characterization of postjunctional alpha-adrenoceptors in human nasal mucosa. Am J Rhinol 2005; 19(5):495–502.
5. Baraniuk JN. Neural regulation of mucosal function. Pulm Pharmacol Ther 2008; 21(3):442–8.
6. Wheater PR, Burkitt HG. Functional histology: a text and colour atlas. In: Deakin PJ, editor. 2nd edition. Edinburgh (UK): Churchill Livingstone; 1987. p. 146–8.
7. Sieskiewicz A, Olszewska E, Rogowski M, et al. Preoperative corticosteroid oral therapy and intraoperative bleeding during functional endoscopic sinus surgery in patients with severe nasal polyposis: a preliminary investigation. Ann Otol Rhinol Laryngol 2006;115(7):490–4.
8. Konkle BA. Bleeding and thrombosis. In: Fauci AS, Braunwald E, Kasper DL, et al, editors. Harrison's principles of internal medicine. 17th edition. McGraw-Hill; 2008. Chapter 59.
9. Soliman DE, Broadman LM, Soliman DE, et al. Coagulation defects. Anesthesiol Clin 2006;24(3):549–78.
10. Kaspar CK. Hereditary plasma clotting factor disorders and their management. In: W Fo, editor. Treatment of Hemophilia, vol. 4. 5th edition. Montreal (Canada): World Federation of Hemophilia; 2008. p. 1–17. Available at: http://www.wfh.org. Accessed April 5, 2010.
11. Sargi Z, Casiano R. Endoscopic sinus surgery in patients receiving anticoagulant or antiplatelet therapy. Am J Rhinol 2007;21(3):335–8.
12. Samama CM, Bastien O, Forestier F, et al. Antiplatelet agents in the perioperative period: expert recommendations of the French Society of Anesthesiology and Intensive Care (SFAR) 2001–summary statement [Guideline Practice Guideline]. Can J Anaesth 2002;49(6):S26–35.
13. Norred CL, Zamudio S, Palmer SK. Use of complementary and alternative medicines by surgical patients. AANA J 2000;68(1):13–8.
14. Kaye AD, Kucera I, Sabar R. Perioperative anesthesia clinical considerations of alternative medicines. Anesthesiol Clin North America 2004;22(1):125–39.
15. Hodges PJ, Kam PC. The peri-operative implications of herbal medicines. [review]. Anaesthesia 2002;57(9):889–99.
16. Ang-Lee MK, Moss J, Yuan CS. Herbal medicines and perioperative care. JAMA 2001;286(2):208–16.
17. Cobas M. Preoperative assessment of coagulation disorders. Int Anesthesiol Clin 2001;39(1):1–15.
18. Howells RC 2nd, Wax MK, Ramadan HH. Value of preoperative prothrombin time/partial thromboplastin time as a predictor of postoperative hemorrhage in pediatric patients undergoing tonsillectomy. Otolaryngol Head Neck Surg 1997;117(6):628–32.
19. Zwack GC, Derkay CS. The utility of preoperative hemostatic assessment in adenotonsillectomy. Int J Pediatr Otorhinolaryngol 1997;39(1):67–76.

20. Spiess BD. Coagulation monitoring in the perioperative period. Int Anesthesiol Clin 2004;42(2):55–71.
21. Kaplan A, Crosby GJ, Bhattacharyya N. Airway protection and the laryngeal mask airway in sinus and nasal surgery. Laryngoscope 2004;114(4):652–5.
22. Braude N, Clements EA, Hodges UM, et al. The pressor response and laryngeal mask insertion. A comparison with tracheal intubation. Anaesthesia 1989;44(7): 551–4.
23. Oczenski W, Krenn H, Dahaba AA, et al. Hemodynamic and catecholamine stress responses to insertion of the Combitube, laryngeal mask airway or tracheal intubation. Anesth Analg 1999;88(6):1389–94.
24. Atef A, Fawaz A. Comparison of laryngeal mask with endotracheal tube for anesthesia in endoscopic sinus surgery. Am J Rhinol 2008;22(6):653–7.
25. Nekhendzy V, Lemmens HJ, Vaughan WC, et al. The effect of deliberate hypercapnia and hypocapnia on intraoperative blood loss and quality of surgical field during functional endoscopic sinus surgery. Anesth Analg 2007;105:1404–9.
26. Ahn HJ, Chung SK, Dhong HJ, et al. Comparison of surgical conditions during propofol or sevoflurane anaesthesia for endoscopic sinus surgery. Br J Anaesth 2008;100(1):50–4.
27. Beule AG, Wilhelmi F, Kühnel TS, et al. Propofol versus sevoflurane: bleeding in endoscopic sinus surgery. Otolaryngol Head Neck Surg 2007;136:45–50.
28. Blackwell KE, Ross DA, Kapur P, et al. Propofol for maintenance of general anesthesia: a technique to limit blood loss during endoscopic sinus surgery. Am J Otolaryngol 1993;14(4):262–6.
29. Boezaart AP, van der Merwe J, Coetzee A. Comparison of sodium nitroprusside- and esmolol-induced controlled hypotension for functional endoscopic sinus surgery. Can J Anaesth 1995;42(5):373–6.
30. Cinçikas D, Ivaskevicius J. Application of controlled arterial hypotension in endoscopic rhinosurgery. Medicina (Kaunas) 2003;39(9):852–9.
31. Dogan IV, Ovalı E, Eti Z, et al. The in vitro effects of isoflurane, sevoflurane, and propofol on platelet aggregation. Anesth Analg 1999;88:432–6.
32. Durmus M, But AK, Dogan Z, et al. Effect of dexmedetomidine on bleeding during tympanoplasty or septorhinoplasty [Randomized Controlled Trial]. Eur J Anaesthesiol 2007;24(5):447–53.
33. Eberhart LHJ, Folz BJ, Wulf H, et al. Intravenous anesthesia provides optimal surgical conditions during microscopic and endoscopic sinus surgery. Laryngoscope 2003;113:1369–73.
34. Eberhart LH, Kussin A, Arndt C, et al. Effect of a balanced anaesthetic technique using desflurane and remifentanil on surgical conditions during microscopic and endoscopic sinus surgery. Rhinology 2007;45(1):72–8.
35. Elsharnouby NM, Elsharnouby MM. Magnesium sulphate as a technique of hypotensive anaesthesia [Randomized Controlled Trial]. Br J Anaesth 2006; 96(6):727–31.
36. Jacobi KE, Bohm BE, Rickauer AJ, et al. Moderate controlled hypotension with sodium nitroprusside does not improve surgical conditions or decrease blood loss in endoscopic sinus surgery. J Clin Anesth 2000;12:202–7.
37. Kaygusuz K, Yildirim A, Kol IO, et al. Hypotensive anaesthesia with remifentanil combined with desflurane or isoflurane in tympanoplasty or endoscopic sinus surgery: a randomised, controlled trial. J Laryngol Otol 2008;122(7):691–5.
38. Manola M, De Luca E, Moscillo L, et al. Using remifentanil and sufentanil in functional endoscopic sinus surgery to improve surgical conditions. ORL J Otorhinolaryngol Relat Spec 2005;67(2):83–6.

39. Nair S, Collins M, Hung P, et al. The effect of beta-blocker premedication on the surgical field during endoscopic sinus surgery. Laryngoscope 2004;114(6): 1042–6.
40. Okuyama K, Inomata S, Toyooka H. The effects of prostaglandin E1 or oral clonidine premedication on blood loss during paranasal sinus surgery. Can J Anaesth 2005;52(5):546–7.
41. Pavlin JD, Colley PS, Weymuller EA, et al. Propofol vs isoflurane for endoscopic sinus surgery. Am J Otolaryngol 1999;20:96–101.
42. Sivaci R, Yilmaz MD, Balci C, et al. Comparison of propofol and sevoflurane anesthesia by means of blood loss during endoscopic sinus surgery. Saudi Med J 2004;25(12):1995–8.
43. Tirelli G, Bigarini S, Russolo M, et al. Total intravenous anaesthesia in endoscopic sinus-nasal surgery. Acta Otorhinolaryngol Ital 2004;24(3):137–44.
44. Wormald PJ, van Renen G, Perks J, et al. The effect of the total intravenous anesthesia compared with inhalational anesthesia on the surgical field during endoscopic sinus surgery. Am J Rhinol 2005;19(5):514–20.
45. Wormald PJ, Athanasiadis T, Rees G, et al. An evaluation of effect of pterygopalatine fossa injection with local anesthetic and adrenalin in the control of nasal bleeding during endoscopic sinus surgery. Am J Rhinol 2005;19(3):288–92.
46. Kozek-Langenecker SA, Kozek-Langenecker SA. The effects of drugs used in anaesthesia on platelet membrane receptors and on platelet function [review]. Curr Drug Targets 2002;3(3):247–58.
47. Soonawalla ZF, Stratopoulos C, Stoneham M, et al. Role of the reverse-Trendelenberg patient position in maintaining low-CVP anaesthesia during liver resections. Langenbecks Arch Surg 2008;393(2):195–8.
48. Iwabuchi T, Sobata E, Suzuki M, et al. Dural sinus pressure as related to neurosurgical positions. Neurosurgery 1983;12(2):203–7.
49. Tankisi A. The effect of reverse Trendelenberg position on intracranial pressure cerebral perfusion pressure during craniotomy in patients with cerebral tumours and cerebral aneurysms. Dan Med Bull 2006;53:98.
50. Larsen JK, Haure P, Cold GE. Reverse Trendelenberg position reduces intracranial pressure during craniotomy. J Neurosurg Anesthesiol 2002;14(1):16–21.
51. Moraine JJ, Berre J, Melot C. Is cerebral perfusion pressure a major determinant of cerebral blood flow during head elevation in comatose patients with severe intracranial lesions? J Neurosurg 2000;92(4):606–14.
52. Gurr P, Callanan V, Baldwin D. Laser-Doppler blood flowmetry measurement of nasal mucosa blood flow after injection of the greater palatine canal. J Laryngol Otol 1996;110(2):124–8.
53. Ko MT, Chuang KC, Su CY. Multiple analyses of factors related to intraoperative blood loss and the role of reverse Trendelenburg position in endoscopic sinus surgery. Laryngoscope 2008;118:1687–91.
54. Cohen-Kerem R, Brown S, Villasenor LV, et al. Epinephrine/Lidocaine injection vs. saline during endoscopic sinus surgery. Laryngoscope 2008;118:1275–81.
55. van Hasselt CA, Low JM, Waldron J, et al. Plasma catecholamine levels following topical application versus infiltration of adrenaline for nasal surgery. Anaesth Intensive Care 1992;20(3):332–6.
56. Benjamin E, Wong DK, Choa D. 'Moffett's' solution: a review of the evidence and scientific basis for the topical preparation of the nose. Clin Otolaryngol Allied Sci 2004;29(6):582–7.
57. Kasemsuwan L, Griffiths MV. Lignocaine with adrenaline: is it as effective as cocaine in rhinological practice? Clin Otolaryngol Allied Sci 1996;21(2):127–9.

58. Latorre F, Klimek L. Does cocaine still have a role in nasal surgery? Drug Saf 1999;20(1):9–13.
59. Liao BS, Hilsinger RL Jr, Rasgon BM, et al. A preliminary study of cocaine absorption from the nasal mucosa. Laryngoscope 1999;109(1):98–102.
60. Yang JJ, Wang QP, Wang TY, et al. Marked hypotension induced by adrenaline contained in local anesthetic. Laryngoscope 2005;115(2):348–52.
61. Enlund M. Dose-dependent hypotension from epinephrine, or lidocaine, or both? [comment]. Acta Anaesthesiol Scand 2006;50(7):894 [author reply: 895].
62. Bharadwaj VK, Novotny GM. Greater palatine canal injection: an alternative to the posterior nasal packing and arterial ligation in epistaxis. J Otolaryngol 1986;15(2):94–100.
63. Weingarten CZ. Injection of the pterygopalatine fossa with glycerin for posterior epistaxis. Trans Am Acad Ophthalmol Otolaryngol 1972;76(4):932–7.
64. Williams WT, Ghorayeb BY. Incisive canal and pterygopalatine fossa injection for hemostasis in septorhinoplasty. Laryngoscope 1990;100(11):1245–7.
65. Kassam A, Snyderman CH, Carrau RL, et al. Endoneurosurgical hemostasis techniques: lessons learned from 400 cases. Neurosurg Focus 2005;19(1):E7.
66. Stangerup SE, Dommerby H, Lau T. Hot-water irrigation as a treatment of posterior epistaxis. Rhinology 1996;34(1):18–20.
67. Woodworth BA, Chandra RK, LeBenger JD, et al. A gelatin-thrombin matrix for hemostasis after endoscopic sinus surgery. Am J Otolaryngol 2009;30(1):49–53.
68. Gall RM, Witterick IJ, Shargill NS, et al. Control of bleeding in endoscopic sinus surgery: use of a novel gelatin-based hemostatic agent. J Otolaryngol 2002; 31(5):271–4.
69. Baumann A, Caversaccio M. Hemostasis in endoscopic sinus surgery using a specific gelatin-thrombin based agent (FloSeal). Rhinology 2003;41(4): 244–9.
70. Chandra RK, Conley DB, Kern RC. The effect of FloSeal on mucosal healing after endoscopic sinus surgery: a comparison with thrombin-soaked gelatin foam. Am J Rhinol 2003;17(1):51–5.
71. Chandra RK, Conley DB, Haines GK 3rd, et al. Long-term effects of FloSeal packing after endoscopic sinus surgery. Am J Rhinol 2005;19(3): 240–3.
72. Shrime MG, Tabaee A, Hsu AK, et al. Synechia formation after endoscopic sinus surgery and middle turbinate medialization with and without FloSeal. Am J Rhinol 2007;21(2):174–9.
73. Athanasiadis T, Beule AG, Wormald PJ. Effects of topical antifibrinolytics in endoscopic sinus surgery: a pilot randomized controlled trial. Am J Rhinol 2007;21(6):737–42.
74. Yaniv E, Shvero J, Hadar T. Hemostatic effect of tranexamic acid in elective nasal surgery. Am J Rhinol 2006;20:227–9.
75. Senghore N, Harris M. The effect of tranexamic acid (cyclokapron) on blood loss after third molar extraction under a day case general anaesthetic [Clinical Trial Randomized Controlled Trial]. Br Dent J 1999;186(12):634–6.
76. Seyednejad H, Imani M, Jamieson T, et al. Topical haemostatic agents. Br J Surg 2008;95(10):1197–225.
77. Sindwani R. Use of novel hemostatic powder MPH for endoscopic sinus surgery: initial impressions. Otolaryngol Head Neck Surg 2009;140(2):262–3.
78. Antisdel JL, Janney CG, Long JP, et al. Hemostatic agent microporous polysaccharide hemospheres (MPH) does not affect healing or intact sinus mucosa. Laryngoscope 2008;118(7):1265–9.

79. Kastl KG, Betz CS, Siedek V, et al. Control of bleeding following functional endoscopic sinus surgery using carboxy-methylated cellulose packing. Eur Arch Otorhinolaryngol 2009;266(8):1239–43.
80. Wagner WR, Pachence JM, Ristich J, et al. Comparative in vitro analysis of topical hemostatic agents. J Surg Res 1996;66(2):100–8.
81. Kastl KG, Betz CS, Siedek V, et al. Effect of carboxymethylcellulose nasal packing on wound healing after functional endoscopic sinus surgery. Am J Rhinol Allergy 2009;23(1):80–4.
82. Pomerantz J, Dutton JM. Platelet gel for endoscopic sinus surgery. Ann Otol Rhinol Laryngol 2005;114(9):699–704.
83. Sirlak M, Eryilmaz S, Yazicioglu L, et al. Comparative study of microfibrillar collagen hemostat (Colgel) and oxidized cellulose (Surgicel) in high transfusion-risk cardiac surgery [Clinical Trial Comparative Study Randomized Controlled Trial]. J Thorac Cardiovasc Surg 2003;126(3):666–70.
84. Chandra RK, Kern RC. Advantages and disadvantages of topical packing in endoscopic sinus surgery. Curr Opin Otolaryngol Head Neck Surg 2004; 12(1):21–6.
85. Valentine R, Athanasiadis T, Moratti S, et al. The efficacy of a novel chitosan gel on hemostasis after endoscopic sinus surgery in a sheep model of chronic rhinosinusitis. Am J Rhinol Allergy 2009;23(1):71–5.
86. Athanasiadis T, Beule AG, Robinson BH, et al. Effects of a novel chitosan gel on mucosal wound healing following endoscopic sinus surgery in a sheep model of chronic rhinosinusitis. Laryngoscope 2008;118(6):1088–94.
87. Maccabee MS, Trune DR, Hwang PH. Effects of topically applied biomaterials on paranasal sinus mucosal healing. Am J Rhinol 2003;17(4):203–7.
88. Proctor M, Proctor K, Shu XZ, et al. Composition of hyaluronan affects wound healing in the rabbit maxillary sinus. Am J Rhinol 2006;20(2):206–11.
89. Franklin JH, Wright ED. Randomized, controlled, study of absorbable nasal packing on outcomes of surgical treatment of rhinosinusitis with polyposis. Am J Rhinol 2007;21(2):214–7.
90. Frenkiel S, Desrosiers MY, Nachtigal D. Use of hylan B gel as a wound dressing after endoscopic sinus surgery. J Otolaryngol 2002;31(Suppl 1):S41–4.
91. Vaiman M, Eviatar E, Shlamkovich N, et al. Use of fibrin glue as a hemostatic in endoscopic sinus surgery. Ann Otol Rhinol Laryngol 2005;114(3):237–41.
92. Vaiman M, Martinovich U, Eviatar E, et al. Fibrin glue in initial treatment of epistaxis in hereditary haemorrhagic telangiectasia (Rendu-Osler-Weber disease). Blood Coagul Fibrinolysis 2004;15(4):359–63.
93. Vaiman M, Segal S, Eviatar E. Fibrin glue treatment for epistaxis. Rhinology 2002;40(2):88–91.
94. Vaiman M, Eviatar E, Segal S. Effectiveness of second-generation fibrin glue in endonasal operations. Otolaryngol Head Neck Surg 2002;126(4):388–91.
95. Gleich LL, Rebeiz EE, Pankratov MM, et al. Autologous fibrin tissue adhesive in endoscopic sinus surgery. Otolaryngol Head Neck Surg 1995;112(2): 238–41.
96. Laurent A, Wassef M, Chapot R, et al. Partition of calibrated tris-acryl gelatin microspheres in the arterial vasculature of embolized nasopharyngeal angiofibromas and paragangliomas. J Vasc Interv Radiol 2005;16(4):507–13.
97. Petruson K, Rodriguez-Catarino M, Petruson B, et al. Juvenile nasopharyngeal angiofibroma: long-term results in preoperative embolized and non-embolized patients. [Research Support, Non-US Government]. Acta Otolaryngol (Stockh) 2002;122(1):96–100.

98. Lefkowitz M, Giannotta SL, Hieshima G, et al. Embolization of neurosurgical lesions involving the ophthalmic artery [case reports]. Neurosurgery 1998; 43(6):1298–303.
99. Casasco A, Houdart E, Biondi A, et al. Major complications of percutaneous embolization of skull-base tumors [case reports]. AJNR Am J Neuroradiol 1999;20(1):179–81.
100. Schroth G, Haldemann AR, Mariani L, et al. Preoperative embolization of paragangliomas and angiofibromas. Measurement of intratumoral arteriovenous shunts. Arch Otolaryngol Head Neck Surg 1996;122(12):1320–5.
101. Simmen DB, Raghavan U, Briner HR, et al. The anatomy of the sphenopalatine artery for the endoscopic sinus surgeon. Am J Rhinol 2006;20(5):502–5.
102. Floreani SR, Nair SB, Switajewski MC, et al. Endoscopic anterior ethmoidal artery ligation: a cadaver study. Laryngoscope 2006;116(7):1263–7.
103. Pletcher SD, Metson R. Endoscopic ligation of the anterior ethmoid artery. Laryngoscope 2007;117(2):378–81.
104. Camp AA, Dutton JM, Caldarelli DD. Endoscopic transnasal transethmoid ligation of the anterior ethmoid artery. Am J Rhinol Allergy 2009;23(2):200–2.
105. Kocer N, Kizilkilic O, Albayram S, et al. Treatment of iatrogenic internal carotid artery laceration and carotid cavernous fistula with endovascular stent-graft placement [case reports]. AJNR Am J Neuroradiol 2002;23(3):442–6.
106. Aygun N, Zinreich SJ. Imaging for functional endoscopic sinus surgery. Otolaryngol Clin North Am 2006;39(3):403–16.
107. Branstetter BF, Weissman JL. Role of MR and CT in the paranasal sinuses. Otolaryngol Clin North Am 2005;38(6):1279–99, x.
108. James D, Crockard HA. Surgical access to the base of skull and upper cervical spine by extended maxillotomy. Neurosurgery 1991;29(3):411–6.
109. Harvey RJ, Sheahan PO, Schlosser RJ. Surgical management of benign sinonasal masses. Otolaryngol Clin North Am 2009;42:353–75.
110. Yoon BN, Batra PS, Citardi MJ, et al. Frontal sinus inverted papilloma: surgical strategy based on the site of attachment. Am J Rhinol Allergy 2009;23(3):337–41.
111. Zhang L, Han D, Wang C, et al. Endoscopic management of the inverted papilloma with attachment to the frontal sinus drainage pathway. Acta Otolaryngol 2008;128(5):561–8.
112. Wormald PJ, Ooi E, van Hasselt CA, et al. Endoscopic removal of sinonasal inverted papilloma including endoscopic medial maxillectomy. Laryngoscope 2003;113(5):867–73.
113. Sautter NB, Citardi MJ, Batra PS. Minimally invasive resection of frontal recess/sinus inverted papilloma. Am J Otolaryngol 2007;28(4):221–4.
114. Loehrl TA, Smith TL. Options in the management of inverting papilloma involving the frontal sinus. Oper Tech Otolaryngol Head Neck Surg 2004;15:32–6.
115. Tran KN, Beule AG, Singal D, et al. Frontal ostium restenosis after the endoscopic modified Lothrop procedure. Laryngoscope 2007;117(8):1457–62.
116. Yousuf K, Wright ED. Site of attachment of inverted papilloma predicted by CT findings of osteitis. Am J Rhinol 2007;21(1):32–6.
117. Lee DK, Chung SK, Dhong HJ, et al. Focal hyperostosis on CT of sinonasal inverted papilloma as a predictor of tumor origin. Am J Neuroradiol 2007;28(4): 618–21.
118. Chiu AG, Jackman AH, Antunes MB, et al. Radiographic and histologic analysis of the bone underlying inverted papillomas. Laryngoscope 2006;116(9):1617–20.
119. Chiu AG, Schipor I, Cohen NA. Surgical decisions in the management of frontal sinus osteomas. Am J Rhinol 2005;19:191–7.

120. Seiberling K, Floreani S, Robinson S, et al. Endoscopic management of frontal sinus osteomas revisited. Am J Rhinol Allergy 2009;23(3):331–6.
121. Becker SS, Bomeli SR, Gross CW, et al. Limits of endoscopic visualisation and instrumentation in the frontal sinus. Otolaryngol Head Neck Surg 2006;135(6): 917–21.
122. Orlandi RR, Lanza DC. Is nasal packing necessary following endoscopic sinus surgery? Laryngoscope 2004;114(9):1541–4.
123. Eliashar R, Gross M, Wohlgelernter J, et al. Packing in endoscopic sinus surgery: is it really required? Otolaryngol Head Neck Surg 2006;134(2):276–9.
124. Valentine R, Wormald PJ, Sindwani R. Advances in absorbable biomaterials and nasal packing. Otolaryngol Clin North Am 2009;42(5):813–28, ix.
125. Weber R, Hochapfel F, Draf W. Packing and stents in endonasal surgery. Rhinology 2000;38(2):49–62.
126. Weber R, Keerl R, Hochapfel F, et al. Packing in endonasal surgery. Am J Otolaryngol 2001;22(5):306–20.
127. Castro E, Seeley M, Kosmorsky G, et al. Orbital compartment syndrome caused by intraorbital bacitracin ointment after endoscopic sinus surgery. Am J Ophthalmol 2000;130(3):376–8.
128. Keefe MA, Bloom DC, Keefe KS, et al. Orbital paraffinoma as a complication of endoscopic sinus surgery. Otolaryngol Head Neck Surg 2002;127(6):575–7.
129. Rosner M, Kurtz S, Shelah M, et al. Orbital lipogranuloma after sinus surgery. Eur J Ophthalmol 2000;10(2):183–6.
130. Shaw CL, Dymock RB, Cowin A, et al. Effect of packing on nasal mucosa of sheep. J Laryngol Otol 2000;114(7):506–9.
131. Dinehart SM, Henry L. Dietary supplements: altered coagulation and effects on bruising. Dermatol Surg 2005;31(7 Pt 2):819–26.
132. Soucie JM, Evatt B, Jackson D. Occurrence of hemophilia in the United States. The Hemophilia Surveillance System Project Investigators. Am J Hematol 1998; 59(4):288–94.
133. Mitchell RN. Red blood cell and bleeding disorders. In: Kumar V, Abbas AK, Fausto N, Aster JC, editors. Robbins and Cotran pathologic basis of disease, professional edition. 8th edition. Philadelphia: Saunders Elsevier; 2009. p. 639–74.
134. Kumar S, Pruthi RK, Nichols WL. Acquired von Willebrand disease. Mayo Clin Proc 2002;77(2):181–7.
135. Parkinson RJ, Bendok BR, O'Shaughnessy BA, et al. Temporary and permanent occlusion of cervical and cerebral arteries. Neurosurg Clin North Am 2005;16: 249–56.
136. Parkinson RJ, Bendok BR, Getch CC, et al. Retrograde suction decompression of giant paraclinoid aneurysms using No. 7 French balloon containing guide catheter. Technical note. J Neurosurg 2006;105(3):479–81.
137. Ong CK, Lam DV, Ong MT, et al. Neuroapplication of amplatzer vascular plug for therapeutic sacrifice of major craniocerebral arteries: an initial clinical experience. Ann Acad Med Singapore 2009;38:763–8.

Preoperative Computed Tomography Evaluation in Sinus Surgery: A Template-Driven Approach

Samuel S. Becker, MD

KEYWORDS

- Computed tomographic evaluation • Preoperative evaluation
- Sinus surgery • Radiography of sinus
- Anatomic nasal abnormalities

With the increased availability of thin-cut computed tomography (CT) scans; and the ability to view anatomic variations in the coronal, axial, and sagittal planes, detailed knowledge of a patient's anatomy is available before surgery. This article presents a template-driven, methodical approach to CT evaluation of anatomic "danger zones" as well as other areas pertinent to planning for surgery on the paranasal sinuses.

PREOPERATIVE CHECKLIST OVERVIEW

When reviewing a patient's CT before surgery the author uses a methodical, step-by-step approach that involves 3 complete passes through all the sinuses. Anatomy is evaluated first by looking at each sinus: frontal, maxillary, ethmoid, and sphenoid, in all 3 CT views:

1. Coronal
2. Axial
3. Sagittal.

This procedure is followed by carefully scrolling through each CT view (coronal, axial, sagittal), and looking at every sinus on each view. Finally, the skull base is carefully evaluated for any defect. Typically, the author scrolls from anterior to posterior (coronal), from superior to inferior (axial), and from lateral to medial (sagittal). The direction of scrolling is not as important as the need to perform this evaluation in the same manner each time. A reference "checklist" is shown in **Box 1**. A methodical approach allows the

Becker Nose and Sinus Center, LLC, 2301 Evesham Road, Suite 404, Voorhees, NJ 08043, USA
E-mail address: sam.s.becker@gmail.com

Otolaryngol Clin N Am 43 (2010) 731–751
doi:10.1016/j.otc.2010.04.020 oto.theclinics.com

Box 1
CT checklist

Organized by sinus

Frontal

- Follow frontal sinus (FS) outflow tract
- Superior uncinate process attachment
- Frontal cells
- Anterior and posterior table dehiscence
- Orbital roof dehiscence
- Ethmo-frontal angle

Maxillary

- Uncinate process atelectasis/Silent sinus
- Nasolacrimal duct
- Haller/Infraorbital ethmoid cell
- Infraorbital nerve location
- Dehiscent maxillary sinus roof

Ethmoid

- Anterior ethmoid artery
- Medial skull base—Keros levels
- Skull base asymmetry
- Low/sloping skull base
- Ethmoid cell character—large cells versus tightly packed cells
- Skull base thickness; presence of polyps
- Lamina papyracea

Sphenoid

- Location of sphenoid ostium
- Onodi cells
- Bone over carotid
- Location of optic nerve

Is there a skull base defect in ethmoid (E), frontal (F), sphenoid (S) sinuses?

Organized by CT view

Axial (superior to inferior)

- F Follow FS outflow tract
  - Anterior + posterior table dehiscence
- E Ethmoid cell character—large cells versus tightly packed cells
  - Lamina papyracea
- S Location of sphenoid ostium
  - Bone over carotid
  - Location of optic nerve

Coronal (anterior to posterior)

- F Follow FS outflow tract
  - Superior uncinate process attachment
  - Frontal cells
  - Anterior and posterior table dehiscence
  - Orbital roof dehiscence
- M Uncinate process atelectasis/Silent sinus
  - Nasolacrimal duct
  - Haller/Infraorbital ethmoid cell
  - Infraorbital nerve location
  - Dehiscent maxillary sinus roof
- E Anterior ethmoid artery
  - Medial skull base—Keros levels
  - Skull base asymmetry
  - Low/sloping skull base
  - Ethmoid cell character—large cells versus tightly packed cells
  - Skull base thickness; presence of polyps
  - Lamina papyracea
- S Onodi cells
  - Location of Optic nerve

Sagittal

- F Follow FS outflow tract
  - Frontal cells
  - Anterior and posterior table dehiscence
  - Ethmo-frontal angle
- S Location of sphenoid ostium

surgeon to become increasingly familiar with the appearance of "normal" anatomy, and consequently more adept at recognizing anatomic variations.

FRONTAL SINUS

Precise knowledge of the anatomy of the frontal sinus outflow tract is imperative when manipulation of this area is to be performed. The axial CT scan is evaluated, scrolling from superior to inferior (**Fig. 1**). Typically, as the inferior aspects of the sinus are approached, the agger nasi and/or frontal cells can be appreciated on the CT defining the often labyrinthine drainage pathway. Most commonly, these cells push the drainage pathway medially, although variations occur frequently.[1]

Awareness of these cells, and the resultant drainage pathway, is reinforced with evaluation of the coronal plane, scrolling from anterior to posterior (**Fig. 2**). In most cases, these same frontal-area cells can be identified, thereby increasing the surgeon's 3-dimensional understanding of the drainage pathway location. Also of importance on the coronal views is the posteromedial location of the drainage opening within the frontal

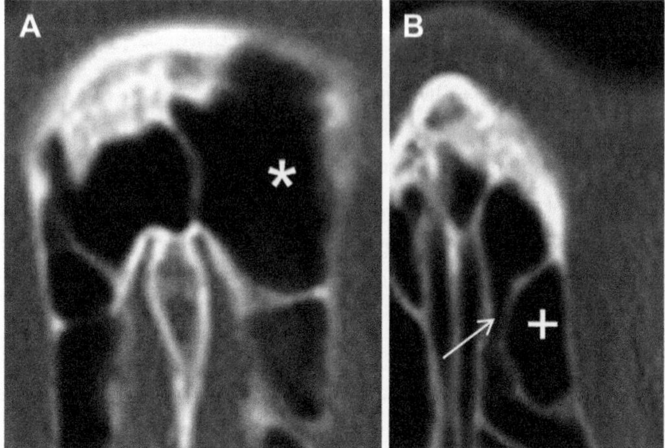

Fig. 1. Axial views of the left frontal sinus drainage pathway seen from superior (*A*) to inferior (*B*). In (*A*), only the frontal sinus proper (*asterisk*) is seen. In (*B*), the frontal sinus drainage pathway (*arrow*) can be appreciated medial to the agger nasi cell (*plus sign*).

sinus. Therefore, when the sinus is opened, enlargement is typically performed in an anterior and lateral direction. The anatomy of this drainage pathway may also be appreciated on sagittal films, typically viewed from lateral to medial (**Fig. 3**). Scrolling in the medial direction provides a view of the unobstructed pathway into the frontal sinus.

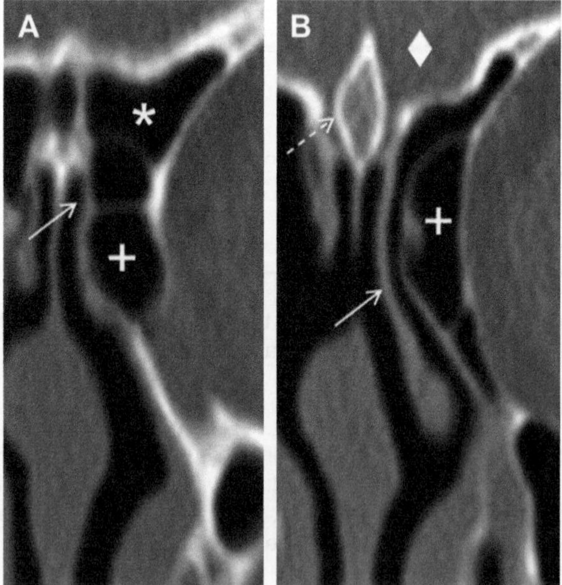

Fig. 2. Coronal views of the left frontal sinus drainage pathway seen from anterior (*A*) to posterior (*B*). In (*A*), the takeoff of the middle turbinate (*straight arrow*), frontal sinus floor (*asterisk*), and agger nasi (*plus sign*) and frontal cells can be appreciated. (*B*), just posterior, demonstrates how the sinus drains just lateral to the middle turbinate, and medial to the agger nasi cell. Surgical opening of the frontal sinus would typically follow along, and enlarge, this natural pathway. Note the close proximity to the crista galli (*dotted arrow*) and the intracranial contents (*diamond*).

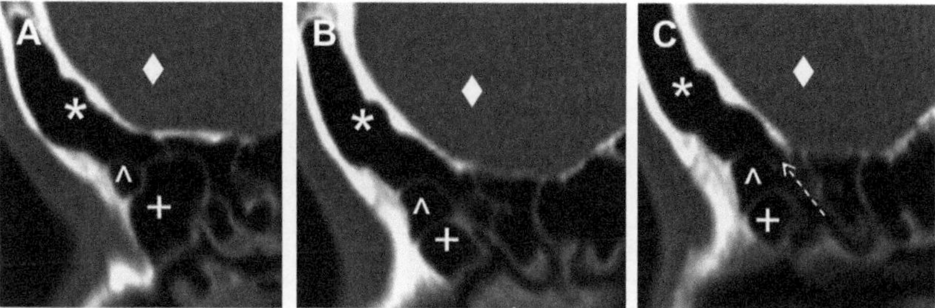

Fig. 3. Sagittal views of the frontal sinus drainage pathway seen from lateral (*A*) to medial (*B* and *C*). The entryway into the frontal sinus (*asterisk*) is most clear in the medial views (*dotted arrow*) seen just posterior to the agger nasi (*plus sign*) and frontal cell (*caret*). Similarly, the direction of surgical dissection in this area often proceeds from medial to lateral.

The varying sites of superior uncinate process attachment are well known. It is similarly well known that the site of attachment affects the frontal sinus drainage pathway and, consequently, the entrance into the frontal sinus during endoscopic surgery. Recent studies have delineated that the superior attachment of the uncinate is fluid at location, and may attach at locations between the traditional 3 sites: lamina, skull base, middle turbinate.[2] This site of attachment may be appreciated most easily on coronal images (**Fig. 4**).

Frontal cells can alter and obfuscate the drainage pathway of the frontal sinus.[3,4] Awareness of the impact of frontal cells on sinus drainage can be appreciated on CT scan. Typically, these cells are best appreciated on sagittal view, although coronal and axial films should also be reviewed because they allow for optimal understanding of the presence of these cells, and how the cells specifically alter the drainage of the frontal sinus. Type I frontal cells are single cells superior to the agger nasi cell that do not extend into the frontal sinus (**Fig. 5**). Type II frontal cells are 2 or more cells superior

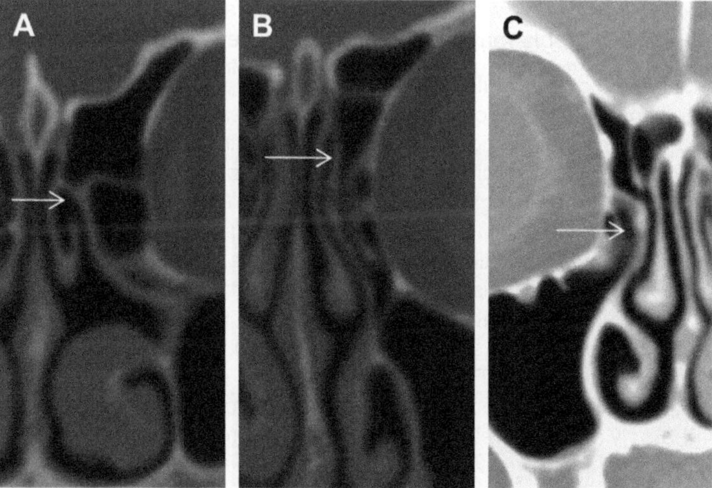

Fig. 4. Coronal views demonstrating some of the variable sites of superior attachment of the uncinate process. In (*A*), the uncinate attaches to the middle turbinate. In (*B*), the uncinate attaches superiorly. In (*C*), the uncinate attaches laterally, to the lamina papyracea.

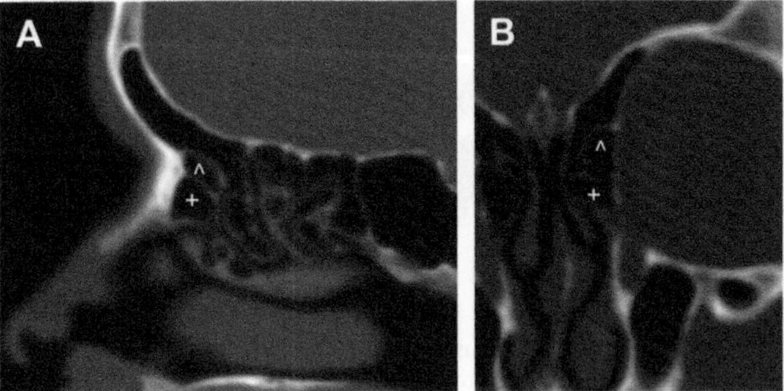

Fig. 5. Type I frontal cells (*caret*) are single cells located superior to the agger nasi cell (*plus sign*). They do not extend into the frontal sinus. Frontal cells are seen on sagittal view (*A*) and on coronal view (*B*).

to the agger nasi cell that do not extend into the frontal sinus. Type III cells extend into the sinus proper (**Fig. 6**), whereas Type IV cells have been defined as either entirely located within the frontal sinus, or as having more than 50% of their volume in the frontal sinus. As with frontal cells, supraorbital and suprabullar cells can also be appreciated on CT, although their impact on the drainage pathway is usually less severe.

During examination of the frontal sinus, the area is also carefully inspected for anterior and posterior table dehiscence. Dehiscence or malformation of the posterior table of the frontal sinus is easily appreciated on axial and sagittal films preoperatively (**Fig. 7**). While it may not always be necessary to repair a dehiscence, it is imperative that the surgeon be aware of any dehiscence prior to surgery because dehiscence may be associated with the presence of a meningo-encephalocele, or a cerebrospinal fluid (CSF) leak.[5] Failure to appreciate the exposure of the cranial contents from bony dehiscence may lead to an incomplete initial surgical plan, resulting in the need for a secondary procedure.

Anterior table dehiscence or malformation can also be easily recognized on axial and sagittal CT images. As with the posterior table, failure to appreciate an abnormality in the anterior table may lead to an incomplete primary surgical intervention and the later need for an unplanned secondary intervention. In many cases,

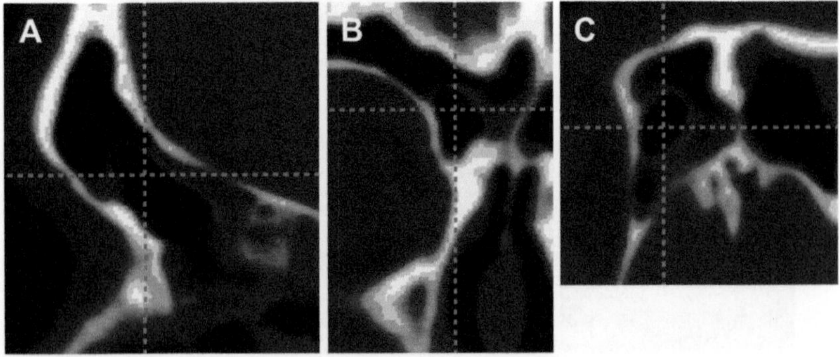

Fig. 6. Type III frontal cells extend into the frontal sinus proper. The cross-hairs on this image-guided scan are within a Type III cell, and can be seen on sagittal (*A*), coronal (*B*), and axial (*C*) views.

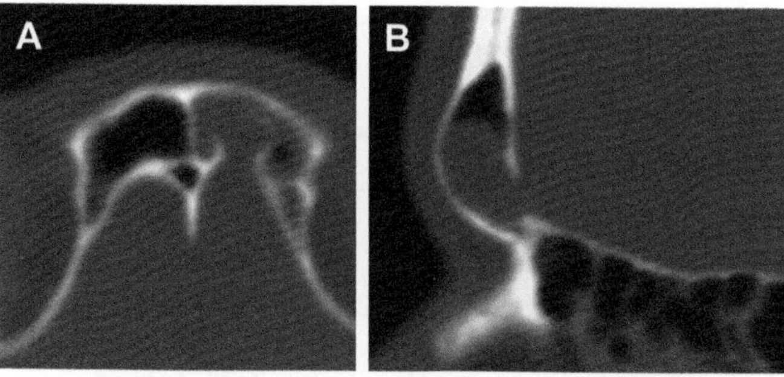

Fig. 7. Posterior table dehiscence with an associated meningo-encephalocele can be seen on axial (*A*) and sagittal (*B*) views.

appreciation of abnormalities prior to surgery may lead to a single, all-encompassing surgical plan that addresses the issues brought up by these abnormalities (**Fig. 8**).

After checking the anterior and posterior table, the orbital roof is evaluated for dehiscence. The frontal sinus often pneumatizes over and "rests" on the orbital roof (**Fig. 9**). Part of the orbital roof is, in fact, the floor of the frontal sinus. This intimate relationship may have surgical implications in the case of frontal sinus lesions. Mucoceles, acute infections, tumors, and other lesions may erode the orbital roof, increasing the vulnerability of the orbital contents. These changes can often be appreciated on preoperative CT, particularly in the axial and coronal planes (**Fig. 10**).

Finally, the entryway into the frontal sinus is evaluated by looking for the ethmo-frontal angle. As the ethmoid roof is followed anteriorly, it slopes upward along the posterior table of the frontal sinus. The ethmo-frontal angle (**Fig. 11**) is best appreciated on sagittal CT, and has been noted to range from 135° to 171°.[6] Moreover, this angle has asymmetry within any particular patient. Although knowledge of this angle has little impact on surgeons performing "frontal recess exploration," it may be of use to those instrumenting up within the frontal sinus proper.

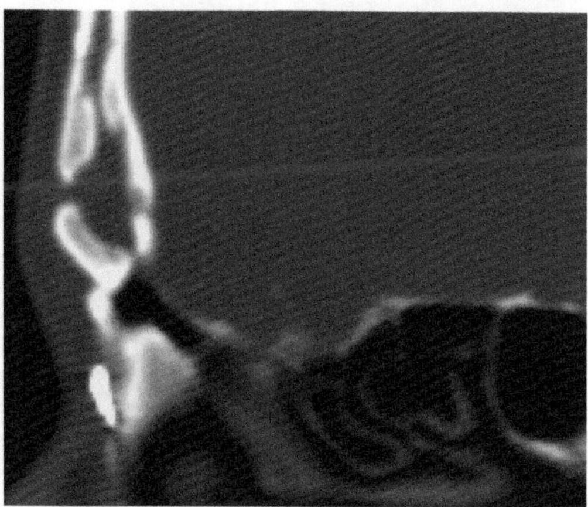

Fig. 8. An anterior table defect in sagittal view; this is also easily appreciated on axial view (not shown).

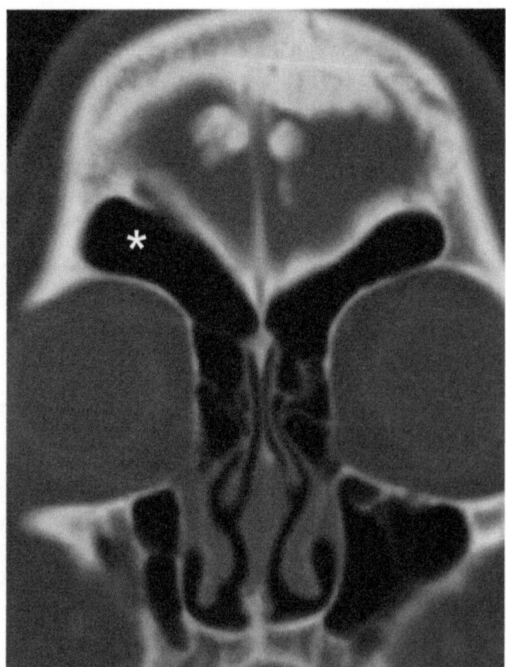

Fig. 9. Frontal sinus (*asterisk*) extends superior to the orbit, seen on coronal CT view.

MAXILLARY SINUS

Evaluation of the frontal sinus is followed by careful examination of the maxillary sinus. Typically, one begins by looking for uncinate process atelectasis. As the uncinate process extends superiorly from its attachment on the inferior turbinate, it passes medially to the maxillary sinus proper. In some cases, this "middle-third" of the

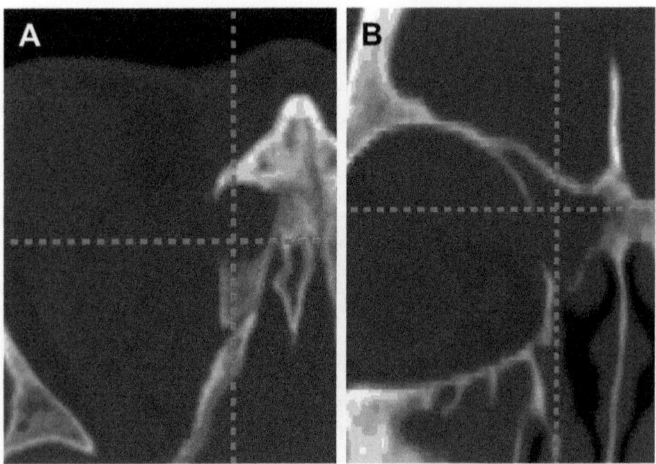

Fig. 10. Axial and coronal CT image-guided surgery images with cross-hairs in a mucocoele eroding into the orbit.

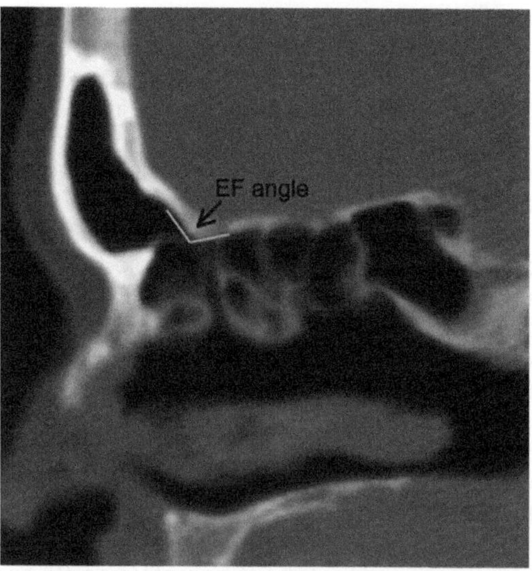

Fig. 11. Sagittal CT image demonstrates "ethmo-frontal angle" (EF) up into the frontal sinus.

uncinate may retract laterally toward the lateral wall of the sinus itself. This retraction, or "atelectatic" uncinate, may occur in varying degrees and can be viewed on axial and coronal images. In some cases (**Fig. 12**), the uncinate may be slightly retracted and lateralized, whereas in other cases a "silent sinus syndrome" may be present, involving severe uncinate retraction and enophthalmos along with retraction of medial

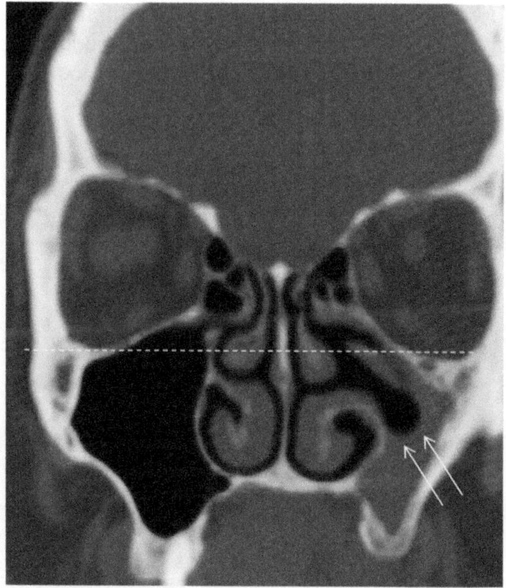

Fig. 12. Coronal CT reveals laterally retracted uncinate (*arrows*). There is slight enophthalmos; the left orbital floor drops below the horizontal line extended from the right orbital floor.

maxillary sinus walls.[7,8] In case of retraction, the uncinate process may be scarred against the lamina papyracea, and great care is required to avoid damage to the orbital contents.

Familiarization with the maxillary sinus anatomy continues with examination of the nasolacrimal duct. This duct, a conduit for tears to flow from the eye to the inferior meatus, is housed in a bony frame that passes just medial and anterior to the maxillary sinus, ending approximately 1 cm posterior to the anterior tip of the inferior turbinate. Endonasally, the duct can be appreciated by viewing the corresponding "maxillary line." Radiographically, the duct is easily recognizable by its distinct bony frame, seen on axial, sagittal, and coronal images (**Fig. 13**). In most cases of endoscopic sinus surgery, the duct is of little significance. However, on occasion over-aggressive resection of the uncinate process (particularly with a back-biter) may result in trauma to the duct and subsequent epiphora. Therefore, a glance at the nasolacrimal duct during the preoperative evaluation may be worthwhile to ensure that the bony frame is intact and protecting the duct.

Examination continues by looking for Haller (infraorbital ethmoid) cells. These cells are located along the maxillary sinus drainage pathway. Haller cells are clinically relevant insofar as they may narrow an already compromised infundibulum. These cells are easily recognizable on CT, particularly on coronal imaging, and vary in size from quite small to those which almost completely encompass the volume of the maxillary sinus proper (**Fig. 14**). When performing surgery on the maxillary sinus, the surgeon should be aware of the presence of Haller cells because they may obfuscate the natural maxillary sinus opening. In these instances, the surgeon should consider the use of angled endoscopes to ensure removal of the Haller cell. Failure to appreciate and remove a Haller cell may lead to maxillary sinus recirculation, and a "missed ostium sequence."[9] Haller cells can be best appreciated on axial and coronal imaging (**Fig. 15**).

Within the maxillary sinus proper, the location of the infraorbital nerve is noted. The infraorbital nerve courses anteriorly along the roof of the maxillary sinus in its bony canal toward its exit point at the infraorbital foramen. Although (like the nasolacrimal duct) it is not typically of concern during sinus surgery, its location should especially

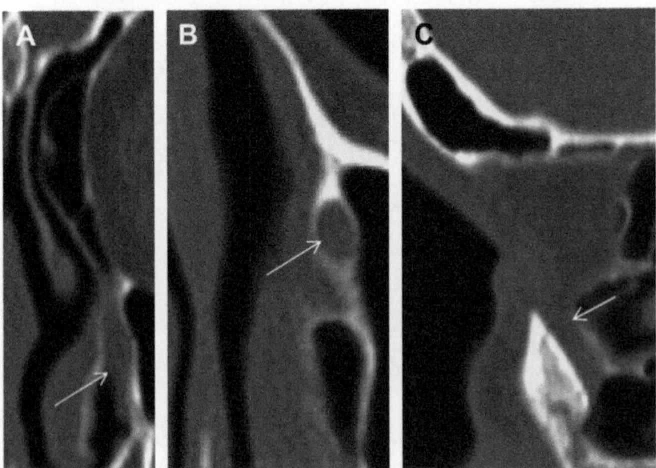

Fig. 13. The nasolacrimal duct (*arrows*) coursing through its bony channel on coronal, axial, and sagittal views.

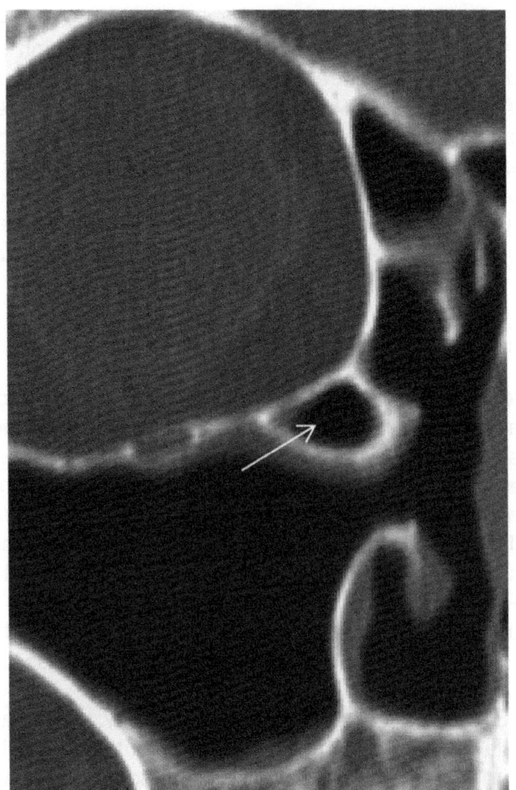

Fig. 14. Coronal CT of a patient who underwent prior surgery. A residual infraorbital ethmoid (or Haller) cell (*arrow*) is apparent by the right maxillary sinus.

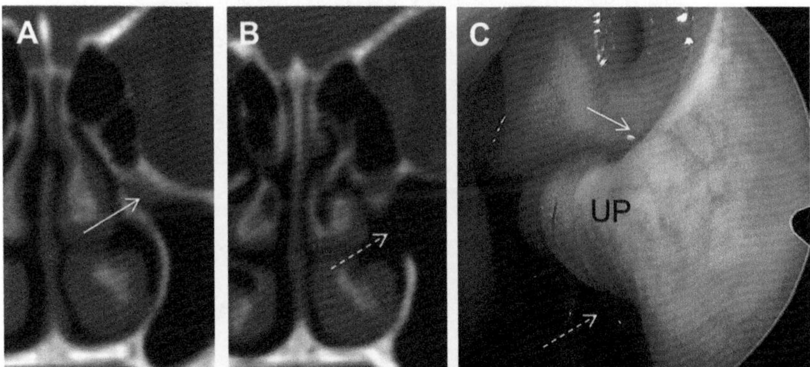

Fig. 15. Coronal images of the "missed ostium sequence." In (*A*), the natural sinus ostium (*solid arrow*) is just lateral to the uncinate process remnant. Image (*B*), just a few slices posterior to (*A*), reveals the surgical antrostomy (*dotted arrow*), which is distinct and unconnected to the natural ostium. Endoscopic view into the left nasal cavity (*C*) demonstrates recirculation from the natural ostium (*solid arrow*), over the uncinate process remnant, and into the surgical antrostomy (*dotted arrow*).

be noted when extended or anterior approaches into the maxillary sinus are planned. The nerve may be best appreciated on coronal view. Although the nerve is most commonly located in the lateral aspects of the maxillary sinus, it may course medially in some cases (**Fig. 16**). In cases of medial location, the nerve may be at greater risk for iatrogenic damage.

Evaluation of the maxillary sinus is completed by looking for any sign of a dehiscent maxillary sinus roof. Dehiscence in the roof of the maxillary sinus/floor of the orbit may be present, particularly in patients who have had prior sinus surgery or trauma. The maxillary sinus roof may be appreciated on preoperative CT, especially on the coronal views.

ETHMOID SINUS

After evaluating the maxillary sinus, attention is turned to the ethmoid sinus cavity. The anterior ethmoid artery, a branch of the ophthalmic artery off of the internal carotid, courses anteromedially as it leaves the orbit heading toward the intracranial area. Typically, the artery is housed in a bony canal as it courses along the skull base. Although this canal may be appreciated on axial CT views, the coronal view is most useful (**Fig. 17**). While several articles have researched the exact location of the artery in relationship to surrounding structures, these relationships, as well as whether or not the artery is "low-hanging," can be directly appreciated on the CT scan.[10,11] Accidental ligation of the artery may lead to retraction within the orbital cone and subsequent retrobulbar hemorrhage with increase in intraocular pressures and possible visual sequalae.

When using the CT scan to evaluate the ethmoid cavity, particular attention is paid to the lateral lamella of the cribriform plate. The height and angulation of this area between the cribriform plate and the fovea ethmoidalis is evaluated on coronal imaging with Keros' classification (**Fig. 18**).[12] This area of the ethmoid skull base is

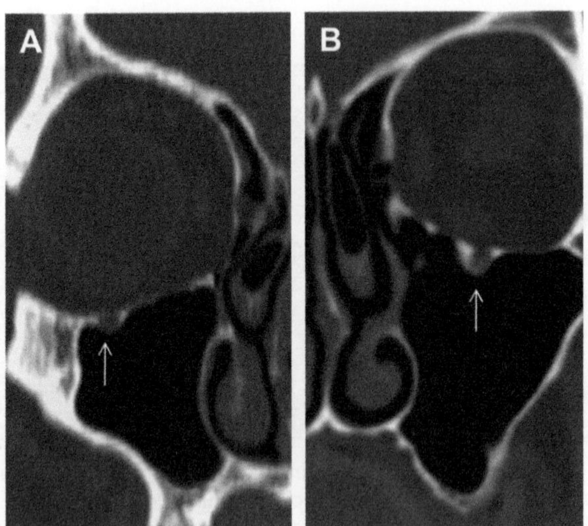

Fig. 16. Coronal views of the infraorbital nerve running through its bony canal along the roof of the maxillary sinus. In the patient shown in (*A*) the nerve courses more laterally than in the patient shown in (*B*).

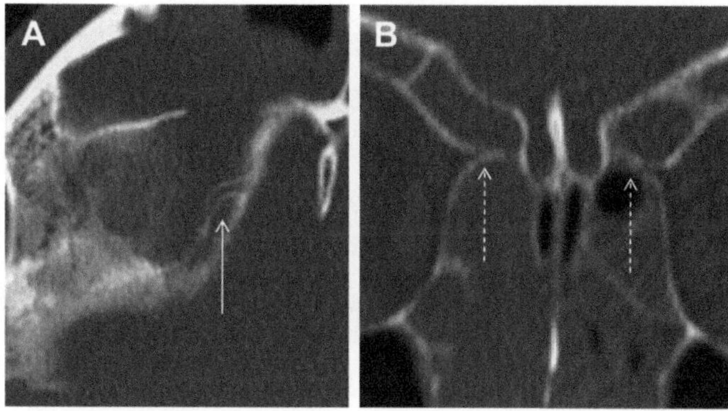

Fig. 17. (*A*) The anterior ethmoidal artery coursing through its bony canal as seen on axial view (*solid arrow*). (*B*) The artery on coronal imaging (*dotted arrows*). Note the low-hanging position of the arteries in (*B*).

also carefully examined on coronal imaging to look for skull base asymmetry (**Fig. 19**). The presence of a low or sloping skull base is also reviewed on coronal CT scans (**Fig. 20**).

The type and character of ethmoid cells may be appreciated on CT (**Fig. 21**). The ethmoid labyrinth may be characterized by a few large cells, or by a honeycomb of numerous small, tightly packed cells. The various formations may be appreciated on axial and coronal CT scans. Awareness of the ethmoid character can prepare the surgeon for simple removal of a few large cells as opposed to meticulous dissection of multiple, densely packed cells.

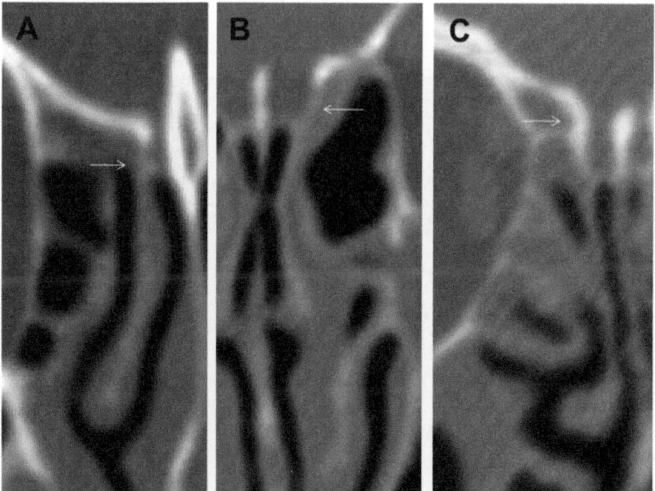

Fig. 18. (*A*) Keros I classification (*arrow*); a 1- to 3-mm vertical height between the cribriform plate and the fovea ethmoidalis. (*B*) Keros II classification (*arrow*); a 3- to 7-mm vertical height between the cribriform plate and the fovea ethmoidalis. (*C*) Keros III classification (*arrow*); a 7- to 16-mm vertical height between the cribriform plate and the fovea ethmoidalis. Note also the varying angulation of the lateral lamella.

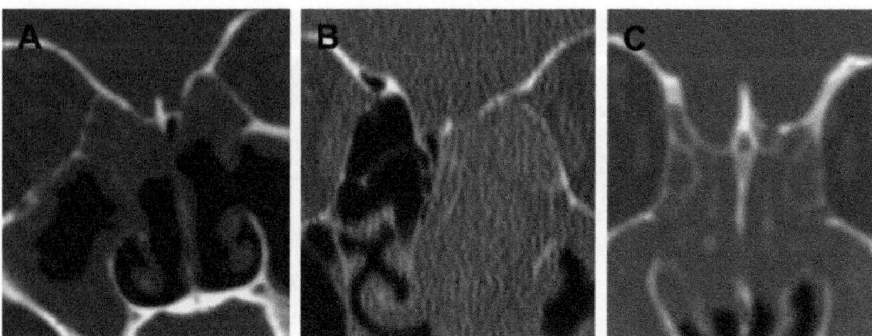

Fig. 19. (*A–C*) Significant skull base asymmetry on coronal views of 3 separate patients.

Variations in ethmoid skull base thickness can also be appreciated on coronal CT images (**Fig. 22**). In particular, sinonasal polyps may be associated with thinning of the skull base.

Images of the ethmoid cavity are evaluated for dehiscent or missing lamina papyracea that may occur as a result of polyps, mucoceles, and other sinonasal lesions, or from iatrogenic or traumatic sources. Coronal and axial images are best suited to evaluate this area (**Fig. 23**).

SPHENOID SINUS

The sphenoid ostium location can be evaluated on CT before surgery. The natural ostium of the sphenoid sinus is typically located just medial to the superior turbinate, approximately 1 to 1.5 cm superior to the choana; however, this location may vary. In some patients, the ostium may be quite superior or lateral. Easily identifiable on axial views, the ostium may also be appreciated on sagittal view for its superior dimensions (**Fig. 24**).

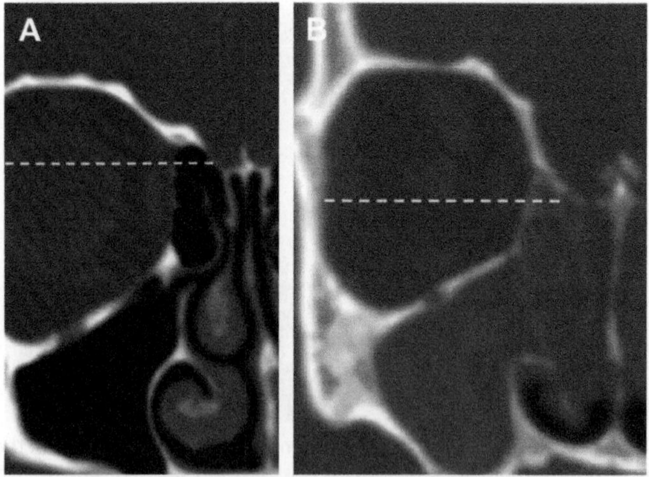

Fig. 20. (*A*) A normally situated skull base aligned with the upper one-third of the orbit, as illustrated by the dotted line drawn laterally from the skull base. (*B*) A low-lying skull base located inferior to this upper one-third of the orbit.

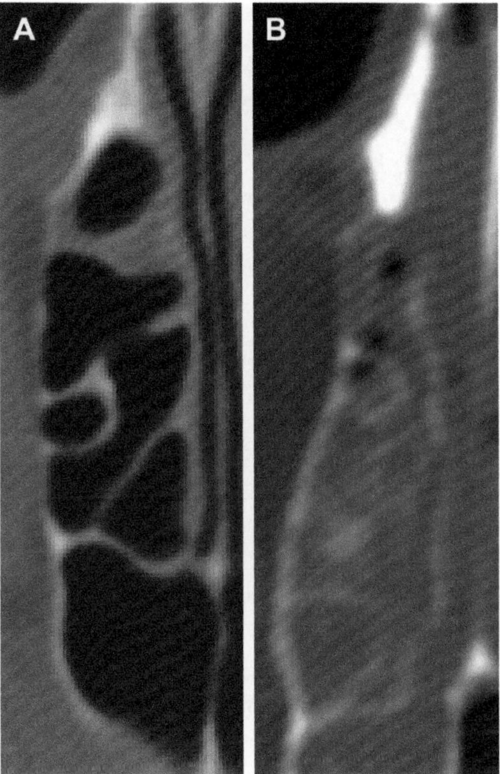

Fig. 21. (*A*) Axial view shows ethmoid cavity with 4 to 6 large ethmoid cells. (*B*) Axial view of a different patient shows ethmoid cavity with 8 to 10 smaller cells.

When examining the sphenoid, the surgeon should also evaluate the area for Onodi cells. Onodi cells, or spheno-ethmoidal cells, are ethmoid cells located superior and lateral to the sphenoid sinus. Because of their pneumatization patterns, Onodi cells may be intimately associated with the optic nerve and carotid artery. Because of their location in the sphenoid area, they may be mistaken for the sphenoid sinus intraoperatively. Fortunately, Onodi cells may be recognized on preoperative CT imaging. Most useful is the coronal view with its characteristic horizontal or oblique line separating the sphenoid and ethmoid cells (**Fig. 25**). Sagittal images may be used to confirm the sloping face of the sphenoid sinus, which represents the superolateral pneumatization of the ethmoid cell.

The carotid artery abuts the sphenoid sinus. Its anatomy and surrounding bony structure can be examined on CT scan, particularly on axial views (**Fig. 26**). There is, however, an imperfect correlation between the CT scan and anatomic findings in this area. In other words, a carotid artery whose bony covering is thinned or dehiscent may appear intact on CT. As the internal carotid artery courses toward the intracranial space, it runs adjacent to the sphenoid sinus. Recent cadaver studies have defined the anatomy of the paraclival and parasellar carotid in detail. On occasion, some studies estimate that up to 50% of the time the bony covering around the artery may be thinned or missing in its entirety. Other studies have reported aberrant carotid arteries that extend well within the sphenoid sinus itself, presenting as a sphenoid

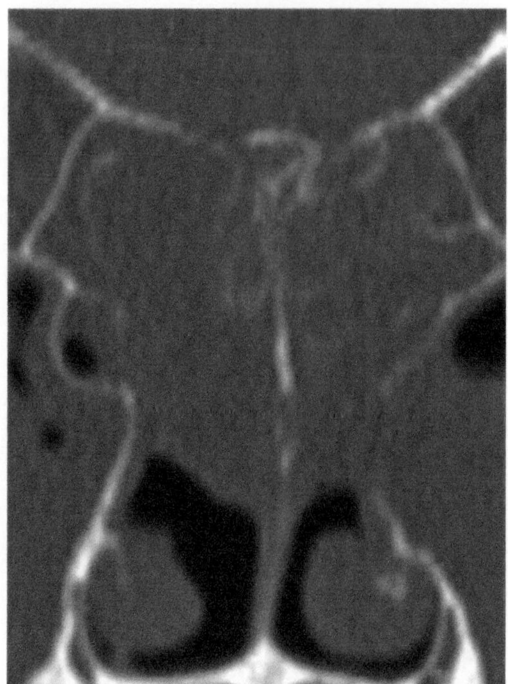

Fig. 22. Coronal CT image shows thinning of the skull base in a patient with sinonasal polyps.

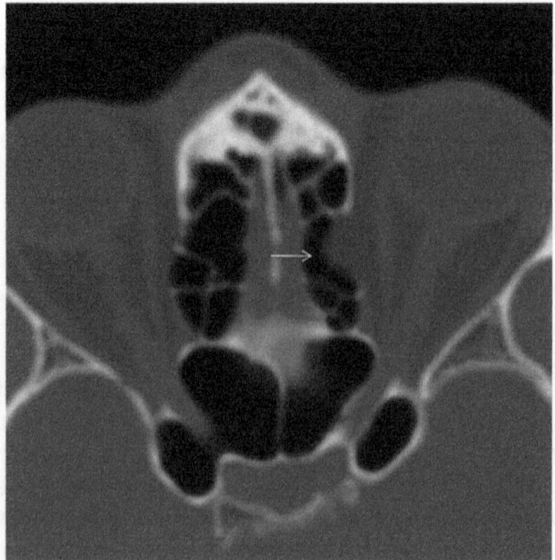

Fig. 23. Axial image shows a dehiscence (*arrow*) in the left lamina papyracea with a consequent bulging of the orbital contents into the sinonasal cavity. This patient reports no history of prior trauma or prior surgery.

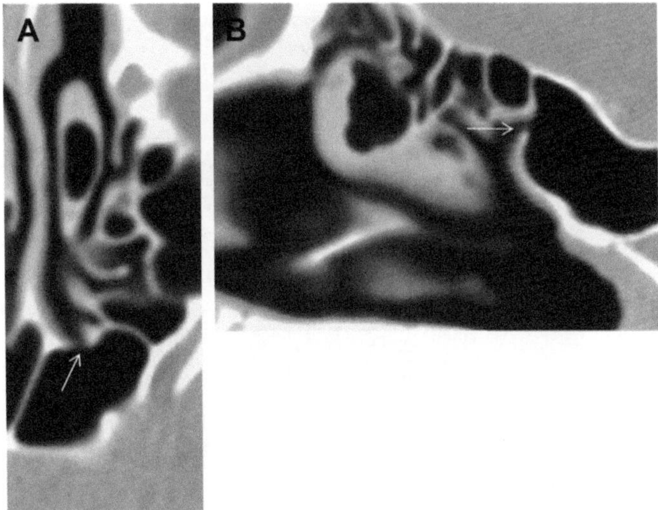

Fig. 24. Axial (*A*) and sagittal (*B*) images show the location of the sphenoid ostium (*arrow*).

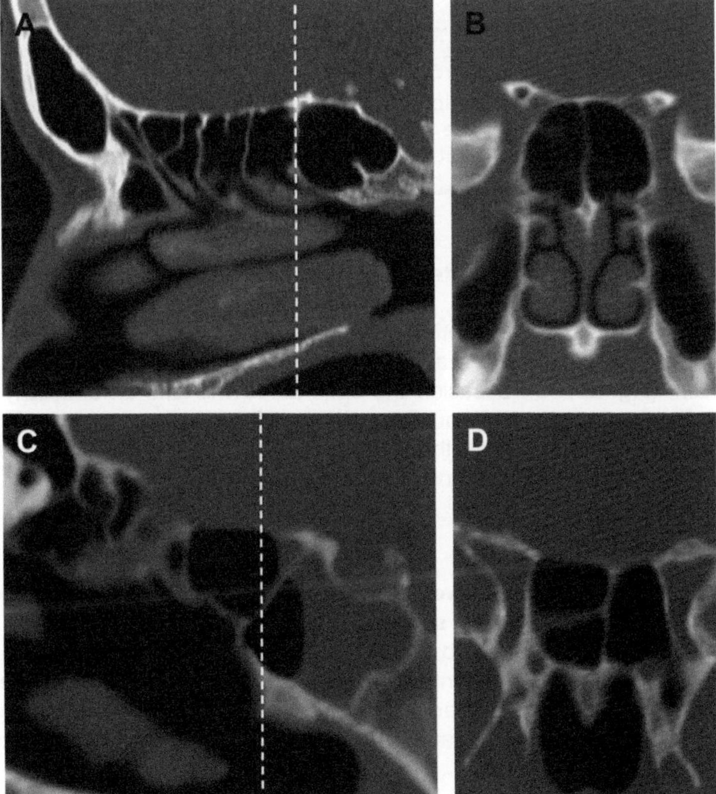

Fig. 25. Sagittal and coronal views of 2 separate patients. The first patient (*A*) does not have an Onodi cell. Consequently, when the coronal slice is taken (*vertical dotted line*), there is no horizontal or oblique partitioning of the sphenoid sinus on coronal view (*B*). On the other hand, in (*C*), a sagittal view of a patient with an Onodi cell, a coronal slice (*vertical dotted line*) reveals a horizontal partition of the superolaterally located Onodi cell (*D*).

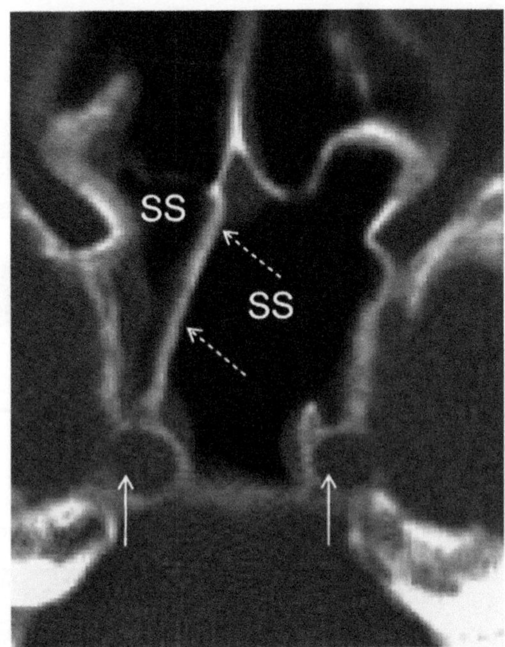

Fig. 26. Axial CT demonstrates relationship between carotid artery (*solid arrows*) and the adjacent sphenoid sinus. The course of the artery can be followed by scrolling through the axial films. Note the attachment of the intersphenoid sinus septum (*dotted arrows*) by the right carotid artery.

mass.[13] In such situations, the artery is at increased risk for iatrogenic (often catastrophic) injury.

As with the carotid artery, the optic nerve is in close proximity to the sphenoid sinus. The optic nerve courses from an anterolateral location, posteromedially toward the optic chiasm (**Fig. 27**). On occasion the optic nerve will take an unusually medial course, even coursing directly through the sinuses. The course can also be impacted by pneumatization patterns within the sinuses. The course of the nerve can be seen on CT, particularly the axial and coronal views (**Fig. 28**).

SKULL BASE DEFECT

After all sinuses have been reviewed on the CT scan, a final look is taken to detect any skull base defect by slowly scrolling through the axial, coronal, and sagittal images (**Fig. 29**). This process also serves as a bridge to the final review of the paranasal sinuses and skull base. During this review, the same checkpoints are evaluated. This time, however, instead of moving sinus to sinus, one moves from coronal to axial to sagittal CT scan, checking each scan for the appropriate landmarks (see **Box 1**).

REVIEW OF CT EVALUATION

After looking at each landmark of every sinus and then evaluating the skull base, a final pass is taken through all the sinuses (see **Box 1**). In this pass the axial, coronal, and

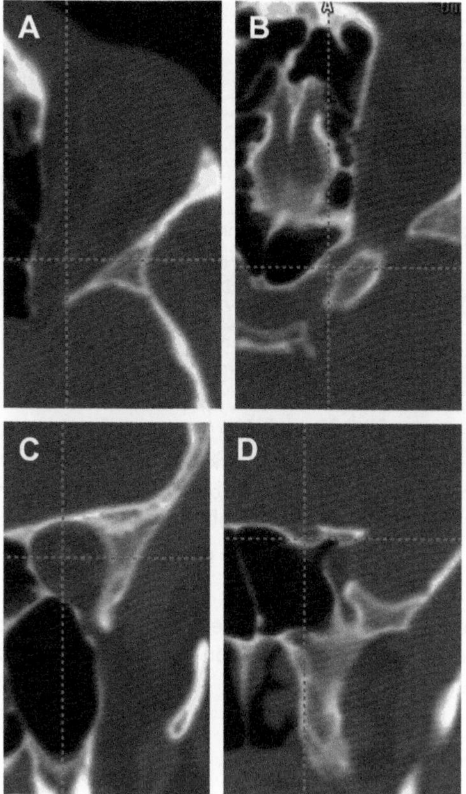

Fig. 27. Axial and coronal CT views demonstrate the course of the optic nerve in (*A*) (axial) and (*B*) (coronal). The cross-hairs are placed on the optic nerve in all images.

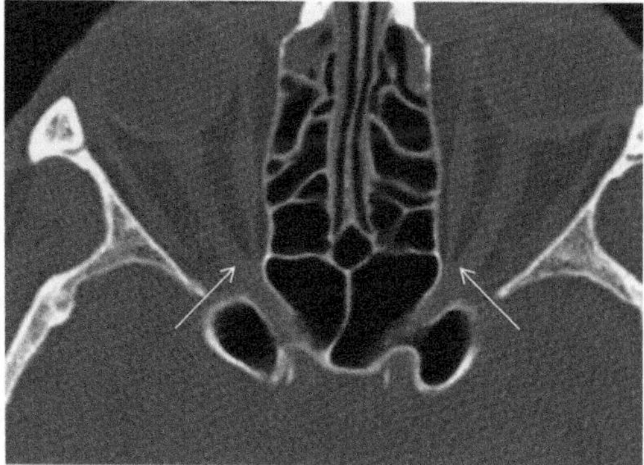

Fig. 28. The optic nerve (*arrows*) courses in a posteromedial direction, as seen on axial view. Pneumatization patterns in the sphenoid sinus and anterior clinoid area may lead to increased exposure of the optic nerve.

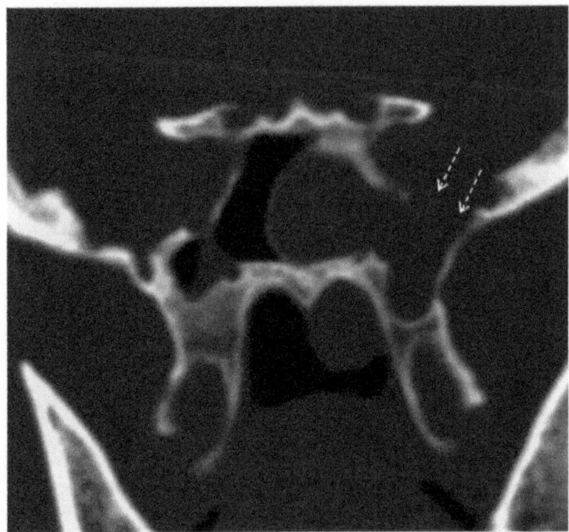

Fig. 29. A defect (*arrows*) in the lateral aspect of the left sphenoid sinus is seen on coronal view. An encephalocele is seen bulging through this defect.

sagittal films are viewed in that order in their entirety, looking for appropriate landmarks. This evaluation marks the completion of a 3-pass, template-driven review of preoperative CT scans.

REFERENCES

1. Wormald PJ. The agger nasi cell: the key to understanding the anatomy of the frontal recess. Otolaryngol Head Neck Surg 2003;129(5):497–507.
2. Yoon JH, Kim KS, Jung D, et al. Fontanelle and uncinate process in the lateral wall of the human nasal cavity. Laryngoscope 2000;110(2 Pt 1):281–5.
3. Bent JP, Cuilty-Siller C, Kuhn FA. The frontal cell as a cause of frontal sinus obstruction. Am J Rhinol 1994;8:185–91.
4. Meyer TK, Kocak M, Smith MM, et al. Coronal computed tomography analysis of frontal cells. Am J Rhinol 2003;17(3):163–8.
5. Becker SS, Russell PT. Intracranial abscess after anterior skull base defect: does pneumocephalus play a role? Rhinology 2009;47(3):287–92.
6. Becker SS, Beddow PA, Duncavage JA. Ethmo-frontal angle: a new anatomic and radiologic landmark for use in sinus surgery. Otolaryngol Head Neck Surg 2009;140(5):762–3.
7. Yousuf K, Velazquez-Villasenor L, Witterick I. Silent sinus syndrome: case series and literature review. J Otolaryngol Head Neck Surg 2009;38(5): E110–3.
8. Bossolesi P, Autelitano L, Brusati R, et al. The silent sinus syndrome: diagnosis and surgical treatment. Rhinology 2008;46(4):308–16.
9. Parsons DS, Stivers FE, Talbot AR. The missed ostium sequence and the surgical approach to revision functional endoscopic sinus surgery. Otolaryngol Clin North Am 1998;29(1):169–83.
10. McDonald SE, Robinson PJ, Nunez DA. Radiological anatomy of the anterior ethmoidal artery for functional endoscopic sinus surgery. J Laryngol Otol 2008; 122(3):264–7.

11. Riehm S, Penisson L, Charpiot A, et al. CT imaging of the anterior ethmoidal artery: anatomic correlation. J Radiol 2008;89(2):229–33.
12. Keros P. [On the practical value of difference in the level of the lamina cribrosa of the ethmoid]. Z Laryngol Rhinol Otol 1962;51:809–13 [in German].
13. Christmas DA, Mirante JP, Yanagisawa E. Endoscopic view of the carotid artery appearing as a sphenoid sinus mass. Ear Nose Throat J 2009;88(8):1028–9.

A Comprehensive Review of the Adverse Effects of Systemic Corticosteroids

David M. Poetker, MD, MA[a,b,*], Douglas D. Reh, MD[c]

KEYWORDS

- Steroid • Prednisone • Corticosteroids • Glucocorticoids
- Adverse effects • Complications • Steroid physiology • Review

Corticosteroids are commonly prescribed by practitioners in many medical specialties for the treatment of chronic inflammatory conditions. The use of corticosteroids in the treatment of chronic rhinosinusitis is well described and based on their antiinflammatory effects.[1] The duration of corticosteroid therapy in these conditions is often less than 1 month, in contrast to the treatment of chronic respiratory diseases (ie, asthma, chronic obstructive pulmonary disease) or autoimmune disorders (ie, rheumatoid arthritis, systemic lupus erythematosus, Crohn disease, and ulcerative colitis), which can last for years.

Although systemic corticosteroids provide an effective therapy for chronic sinusitis, they also have associated adverse effects that have been well studied and described.[1–3] The objective of this article is to present a comprehensive review of the physiology of systemic corticosteroids and the known side effects associated with their use.

MORPHOLOGIC CHANGES

Redistribution of adipose tissue is a common effect associated with prolonged corticosteroid treatment (**Table 1**). These changes are known as cushingoid changes, and

[a] Division of Rhinology and Sinus Surgery, Department of Otolaryngology and Communication Sciences, Medical College of Wisconsin, 9200 West Wisconsin Avenue, Milwaukee, WI 53226, USA

[b] Department of Surgery, VA Medical Center, 5000 West National Avenue, Milwaukee, WI 53295, USA

[c] Division of Rhinology and Sinus Surgery, Department of Otolaryngology-Head and Neck Surgery, Johns Hopkins Medical Institutions, 601 North Caroline Street, Baltimore, MD 21287, USA

* Corresponding author. Division of Rhinology and Sinus Surgery, Department of Otolaryngology and Communication Sciences, Medical College of Wisconsin, 9200 West Wisconsin Avenue, Milwaukee, WI 53226.

E-mail address: dpoetker@mcw.edu

Otolaryngol Clin N Am 43 (2010) 753–768
doi:10.1016/j.otc.2010.04.003
0030-6665/10/$ – see front matter. Published by Elsevier Inc.

Table 1
Summary of common complications following systemic corticosteroids

Complication	Signs/Symptoms	Comments
Morphologic changes	Cushingoid changes Truncal obesity Facial adipose tissue (moon facies) Dorsocervical adipose tissue (buffalo hump)	Variable reports about incidence and required dosage
Hyperglycemia	Increased blood sugar levels	Degree of increase in blood sugar level variable and not well characterized
Infection	Bacterial, fungal, and viral infections	Multiple effects on leukocytes Usually requires prolonged courses
Wound healing	Decrease monocytes/macrophages Delayed wound healing	Decrease phagocytosis and cytokine production Delay reepithelialization, decrease the fibroblast response, slow capillary proliferation, and inhibit collagen synthesis
Bone metabolism	Decrease bone density Avascular necrosis	Effect usually transient Can present months after use Reported after as few as 6 days Reported after as little as 290 mg prednisone (total dose)
Ophthalmic	Cataracts Glaucoma	Reported after as few as 2 months of use Usually requires months to years of use Up to 5% develop pressure increases within weeks
Skin changes	Dermal thinning, skin fragility, and ecchymosis Striae	Usually reversible with discontinuation Irreversible
Gastrointestinal	Peptic ulceration	No conclusive evidence to support associations Gastritis symptoms more common with steroid use

Adrenal suppression	Multiple systemic effects, blood pressure changes, water retention, lack of stress response	Individual variability in the dose that can lead to adrenal suppression Incidence of clinically evident adrenal insufficiency is believed to be much lower than the incidence based on objective measures
Myopathy	Type IIb muscle fiber atrophy	Usually involves the proximal limbs Usually resolves 1–4 months after steroid cessation
Cardiovascular	Increased blood pressure Myocardial infarction and cerebrovascular disease	Cause uncertain, usually transient Epidemiologic studies demonstrate increased risk Cause unclear
Psychiatric	Mild effects: agitation, anxiety, distractibility, fear, hypomania, indifference, insomnia, irritability, lethargy, mood lability, pressured speech, restlessness, and tearfulness	Incidence: 27.6% (range 13%–62%)
	Severe reactions: mania, depression (suicidal ideations), a mixed state, aggressiveness	Incidence: 5.7% (range 1.6%–50%) A past reaction is not predictive of a future reaction Past tolerance is not predictive of future tolerance Studies have not been able to correlate a history of psychiatric illness with a psychiatric reaction to prednisone Duration is variable Severe symptoms may take weeks to resolve More than 90% recover from these symptoms

include truncal obesity, facial adipose tissue referred to as moon facies, and dorsocervical adipose tissue referred to as buffalo hump.[4] The rate at which this occurs is variable. It has been reported to occur in 15% of patients in less than 3 months' time, with doses equivalent to 10 to 30 mg of prednisone per day.[4] A different study found that 13% of patients taking up to 12 mg of prednisone daily for more than 60 days developed moon facies, with up to 66% of the patients demonstrating this complication from corticosteroid use over 5 years.[5] A meta-analysis of randomized controlled trials found that these changes occur more frequently in patients receiving steroids than in patients receiving placebos.[6] Higher doses and longer duration of corticosteroid use seem to increase the frequency of adipose tissue redistribution. Patients taking daily prednisone demonstrated adipose redistribution or corticosteroid-induced lipodystrophy at incidences of 61%, 65%, and 69% at 3, 6, and 12 months, respectively, with mean doses of 32 mg, 19 mg, and 11 mg at the respective time points.[7] This study further demonstrated that the risk was higher in women, patients less than 50 years of age, and patients with either a high initial body mass index or a high calorie intake.

HYPERGLYCEMIA

Corticosteroids increase blood sugar levels by increasing hepatic gluconeogenesis and by decreasing glucose uptake in peripheral tissues.[8] Corticosteroids stimulate proteolysis, promote the release of gluconeogenesis-stimulating enzymes, and inhibit adipose and muscle tissue glucose uptake.[8] Furthermore, acute exposure to corticosteroids causes insulin resistance by decreasing the ability of adipocytes and hepatocytes to bind insulin. This effect can occur within 12 hours of beginning therapy, although it has been found to decrease with prolonged corticosteroid use.[8] Synthetic corticosteroids such as prednisone and dexamethasone are 4 and 30 times more potent, respectively, than natural corticosteroids such as hydrocortisone at decreasing carbohydrate tolerance.[8]

Correlations have also been made to steroid dose and the development of diabetes, with daily and cumulative dose likely independent risk factors.[4] Several studies have demonstrated a statistical correlation between hyperglycemia and exogenous corticosteroid use.[4,6,8,9] On cessation of corticosteroids, the inhibition of glucose uptake and metabolism in peripheral tissues usually returns to normal.[8] Despite their common use, the effect on blood glucose levels and the degree of hyperglycemia caused by steroids have not been clearly elucidated.

INFECTION

The mechanism by which corticosteroids decrease inflammation may also lead to immunosuppressive effects. Steroids decrease the peripheral concentration and function of leukocytes. Whereas circulating neutrophils increase as a result of enhanced release from bone marrow and reduced migration from blood vessels, the number of other leukocytes such as lymphocytes, monocytes, basophils, and eosinophils decrease. This decrease in peripheral leukocytes is a result of a migration from the vascular bed to lymphoid tissue.[10] Corticosteroids can further affect neutrophil function by reducing their adherence to vascular endothelium as well as their bactericidal activity.[11] Corticosteroids further inhibit the function of macrophages and other antigen-presenting cells by limiting chemotaxis, phagocytosis, and the release of cytokines such as tumor necrosis factor α and interleukin-1.[10,11] Corticosteroids have also been shown to decrease the expression of inflammatory mediators such as prostaglandin, leukotriene, and platelet-activating factor, and at higher doses have been shown to inhibit B-cell production of immunoglobulins.[10,11] The administration of corticosteroids on an alternate days has been shown to reduce their negative impact on leukocyte function.[11]

A meta-analysis by Stuck and colleagues[12] reviewed 71 clinical studies to assess for the relative risk of corticosteroids on the rate of infections. They found that the overall rate of infections was 8.0% in the control group and 12.7% in patients receiving corticosteroids, a statistically significant increase. Their review found that patients who received a daily dose of less than 10 mg per day or a cumulative dose of less than 700 mg of prednisone did not have an increased rate of infectious complications.[12]

A meta-analysis of more than 8700 patients by Conn and Poynard[6] found that bacterial sepsis occurred 1.5 times more frequently in patients using corticosteroids than in those using placebo ($P<.01$). The mean daily dose was the equivalent of 35 mg of prednisone and the mean total dose was 2200 mg of prednisone for these patients.[6] Although the disease processes for which the patients are being treated may themselves be independent risk factors for increased infection, few studies in the aforementioned meta-analyses included patients with autoimmune diseases, which are known risk factors for increased infections.[6,12]

Several studies have demonstrated that patients treated with glucocorticoids are at increased risk for developing invasive fungal infections, pneumocystosis, and viral infections, especially in patients who have undergone bone marrow transplantation.[4,13–17] O'Donnell and colleagues[13] retrospectively reviewed 331 allogeneic bone marrow recipients and found that the major risk factor for candidemia or aspergillosis was prednisone treatment (0.5–1 mg/kg/d). None of the 36 cases of systemic fungal infections were in the paranasal sinuses. Several studies from the Fred Hutchinson Cancer Research Center and University of Washington demonstrate an increased risk of invasive mold infections (including *Aspergillus* and Zygomycetes) as well as an increased risk of death from these infections in bone marrow transplant patients receiving high-dose corticosteroids ($\geq$2 mg/kg/d prednisone or methylprednisolone).[14,16,17]

WOUND HEALING

Wound healing occurs in an orderly fashion. The initial response to a surgical injury is an inflammatory reaction in which the wound is invaded by polymorphonuclear leukocytes and lymphocytes. These cells are then replaced by macrophages from circulating blood monocytes. The presence of the macrophages is essential for normal wound healing. Within 48 hours, reepithelialization and angiogenesis occur as part of the proliferation phase, which includes extensive capillary budding and proliferation of fibroblasts in the wound site. Collagen deposition begins within 4 or 5 days, and is responsible for the initial wound strength. Collagen deposition is followed by the formation of covalent bonds and scar remodeling, which leads to additional wound strength and maturation.[18]

Corticosteroids inhibit the natural wound-healing process in several ways. First, they decrease the circulating monocytes, thus decreasing the influx of macrophages.[18,19] Studies suggest that the reduced number of macrophages may decrease phagocytosis as well as growth factor/cytokine production.[20,21] In addition, corticosteroids can delay reepithelialization, decrease the fibroblast response, slow capillary proliferation, and inhibit collagen synthesis and wound maturation,[18,20,22] ultimately leading to delayed wound healing and decreased tensile strength.[22]

Several topical and systemic agents such as epidermal growth factor, transforming growth factor β, platelet-derived growth factor, and tetrachlorodecaoxygen have been shown to counteract the effect of corticosteroids on wound healing.[18] Systemic agents such as vitamin A and insulinlike growth factor 1 also may counter the impact of corticosteroids on wound healing.[21]

BONE METABOLISM

The role of steroids in bone loss is well described and may occur through several different mechanisms. First, they cause a negative calcium balance via an anti–vitamin D effect by reducing intestinal calcium absorption and increasing urinary calcium excretion. This negative calcium balance stimulates parathyroid hormone production, which increases osteoclast activity, accelerates bone absorption, and releases calcium into the circulation at the expense of bone mass. In addition, steroids inhibit osteoblast activity, negatively affecting trabecular bone formation. This effect places bones, such as vertebral bodies, femoral necks, and distal radii, at increased risk for fracture.[23,24]

Corticosteroids also suppress the production of adrenal androgens, decreasing their beneficial effect on bone formation. Prednisone doses higher than 20 mg per day decrease the production of gonadotropin-releasing hormone, which decreases the production of luteinizing hormone, leading to a secondary hypogonadism state. This secondary hypogonadism decreases testosterone production, further decreasing bone formation and increasing bone resorption.[24]

Corticosteroids have been found to cause apoptosis of osteoblasts and osteocytes. This effect has been shown to occur within 1 month of use; however, it slows after 6 to 12 months.[25] A reduction in bone formation based on markers of bone metabolism has been demonstrated with as little as 5 mg of prednisone daily for as short as 2 weeks.[25,26] van Staa and colleagues[26] found a dose-related reduction in osteocalcin levels, a marker of bone formation, within the first 24 hours of prednisone therapy. This effect was rapidly reversible with cessation of prednisone therapy.

Paglia and colleagues[27] studied bone resorption and formation in 14 elderly men who were placed on courses of prednisone for less than 30 days at a mean cumulative dose of 338 mg of prednisone. The investigators found statistical differences in the steroid group, with significant increases in markers of bone turnover and decreases in markers of bone formation. In addition, osteocalcin levels were inversely correlated with the cumulative dose of prednisone.[27] A second study measured the dose-related changes in serum osteocalcin in patients with asthma on a 12-day course of oral prednisolone with doses increasing every 4 days.[28] They found that after 4 days of 5 mg daily, there were no significant differences in osteocalcin levels; however, a significant decrease was noted after 10 mg, and the levels continued to decrease after daily doses of 20 mg.[28]

The clinical significance of these changes in markers of bone metabolism as they relate to changes in bone mineral density has been debated. A study performed by Laan and colleagues[29] compared bone mineral densities in patients treated with or without corticosteroids for their rheumatoid arthritis. The investigators found that postmenopausal women taking a mean daily dose of 6.8 mg of prednisone (mean cumulative dose was 22.5 g) for a mean duration of 7.9 years (range 1.1–31.9) had a statistically significant decrease in trabecular bone mineral density, cortical bone mineral density, and a statistically significant increase in vertebral deformities compared with patients not using prednisone. Male patients taking a mean daily dose of 7.1 mg of prednisone for a mean duration of 4.2 years (range 0.9–9.2) had no statistically significant difference in bone mineral density or vertebral deformities compared with patients not using prednisone.[29] Although these data conflict with earlier studies, the investigators used quantitative computed tomography, which is more accurate than traditional bone density studies in assessing bone mineral densities. Limitations of this study include insufficient premenopausal women to include for statistical analysis, a relatively small sample size, and the fact that patients receiving prednisone had clinically more severe rheumatoid arthritis, which itself is a risk factor for reduced bone mineral density.

Data are conflicting as to whether daily dose or cumulative dose has a more significant clinical effect on bone density. A meta-analysis by van Staa and colleagues[26] demonstrated a stronger correlation between cumulative steroid dose on bone mineral density than daily dose. Fracture risks have also been shown to increase based on dose, duration, age, gender, and body weight.[4] Several studies have demonstrated that supplemental calcium and vitamin D, as well as bisphosphonates can help reduce the corticosteroid-induced loss of bone mineral density.[4]

Corticosteroid use has also been associated with avascular necrosis or osteonecrosis. This complication has been correlated with cumulative dose, and has been seen primarily in the head of the femur, although other weight-bearing and non–weight-bearing bones can be affected.[23] The exact cause is not fully understood, but is thought to include embolic events in the blood supply, a hyperviscous state of the blood, cellular cytotoxic factors, hypertrophy of marrow fat cells, which increases the pressure in the femoral head, resulting in decreased blood flow, or generation of bone edema, all leading to impaired perfusion of the bone.[23,30,31]

A retrospective review of patients treated for osteonecrosis of the femoral head in an orthopedic clinic identified 15 patients who had been treated with a single course of glucocorticoids over a 3-year period, before presentation.[32] All patients were male; 13 had received prednisone, 2 dexamethasone. The mean age was 32.2 years (range 20–41 years), the mean cumulative dose was 850 mg of prednisone (range 290–3300 mg), and the mean duration of therapy was 20.5 days (range 6–39 days). The patient who presented after the lowest cumulative dose of prednisone, 290 mg in 7 days, was one of the latest presenters. He presented with pain 23 months after corticosteroid treatment for poison ivy. The mean time from treatment to symptoms in the study was 16.6 months (range 6–33 months).[32] Another retrospective series of 1352 patients treated with corticosteroids for neurosurgical issues identified 4 cases of avascular necrosis, a risk of 0.03%. The mean age was 26 years (range 21–31 years), the mean cumulative dose was equivalent to 673 mg of prednisone (range 389–990 mg of prednisone equivalents), and the mean duration was 20 days (15–27 days).[33] The time for onset of symptoms in this group ranged from 4 to 27 months, with a mean of 14.5 months.

OPHTHALMIC

Corticosteroids can have extensive ophthalmic effects, depending on the route of administration. Systemic administration of corticosteroids can lead to cataract formation, increased intraocular pressure, myopia, exophthalmos, papilledema, central serous chorioretinopathy, and subconjunctival hemorrhages.[34] The most commonly encountered ophthalmologic side effects include cataract formation and increased intraocular pressure or glaucoma. The correlation between corticosteroids and posterior subcapsular cataracts was first described in the 1960s, with the incidence dependent on dose and duration of corticosteroid use. Although studies have shown that doses as low as 5 mg of oral prednisone taken for as little as 2 months can lead to cataracts, most report doses of 10 mg or more daily for at least 1 year before the onset of cataract formation.[34] Many causes of steroid-induced cataract formation have been proposed. One theory suggests that steroid molecules bond covalently with the lysine residues of the lens, leading to opacities. Another proposed mechanism states that corticosteroids inhibit the sodium-potassium pump in the lens, leading to an accumulation of water and coagulation of lens proteins.[34]

Increased intraocular pressure can lead to visual field loss, optic disk cupping, and optic nerve atrophy. The correlation between increased intraocular pressure and glaucoma was first identified in the early 1950s.[34] Corticosteroids cause significant increases in intraocular pressure in approximately 5% of patients within the first few weeks of therapy.[24] Eventually, between 18% and 36% of the population will develop at least a moderate (5 mm Hg or greater) increase in pressure with prolonged steroid treatment.[24] Factors associated with a greater risk of increased intraocular pressure induced by corticosteroids include open-angle glaucoma, diabetes mellitus, high myopia, rheumatoid arthritis, hypertension, migraine headaches, and first-degree relatives with open-angle glaucoma.[24,34] The route of administration seems to play an important role; topical ophthalmic and systemic administration have a high correlation with the incidence of glaucoma. The exact mechanism by which corticosteroids cause glaucoma is unknown. One theory suggests that corticosteroids may have a negative effect on the trabecular meshwork by causing the buildup of proteins such as glycosaminoglycans, fibronectin, elastin, laminin, and collagens or by preventing the appropriate expression of prostaglandins, collagenase, plasminogen activator, and stromelysin, enzymes that help break down outflow obstructions.[24,34] When the trabecular meshwork does not allow for proper drainage, fluid is retained and pressures increase.

SKIN CHANGES

Cutaneous complications caused by corticosteroids include Cushing syndrome, skin atrophy, striae, ecchymoses, and changes in mechanical properties of the skin. Less commonly, pustular acne, tinea incognito, and Stevens-Johnson syndrome may occur.[24] Corticosteroids cause a reduction in mitotic activity of the keratinocytes in the germinal layer and flattening of the rete ridges. They may also cause a loss of ground substance and reduction of fibroblast size. These changes ultimately cause thinning of the dermis and increase the fragility of the skin. In some cases, a steroid effect on microvascular endothelial cell development causes telangiectasia formation, whereas the loss of ground substance decreases the structural support for vessels and increases their dilation, leading to ecchymosis.[24] Atrophy and ecchymoses are often reversible on the discontinuation of corticosteroids, but striae are not. Striae are visible linear scars that occur as a result of inflammation and edema of the dermis. Collagen and elastin are then deposited along these lines of mechanical stress, causing scar tissue formation.[24]

The frequency with which these complications occur is not entirely understood; however, they seem to be more common with systemic corticosteroids than topical or inhaled corticosteroids. One study demonstrated cutaneous changes in 37 of 80 (46%) patients on a mean dose of 31 mg of prednisone over 3 months. These changes included hirsutism, spontaneous bruising, and altered wound healing. Of the patients with hirsutism, all were female, and the risk tended to increase with age.[35] A second study demonstrated almost a 5-fold increase in ecchymoses with corticosteroid use; another study found a 4-fold increase in the frequency of Cushing syndrome, acne, and hirsutism.[5]

GASTROINTESTINAL

Despite the commonly held perception that steroid use increases the risk of peptic ulcer disease, several large meta-analyses of randomized, placebo-controlled trials have failed to show this association.[5] Specifically, Conn and Blitzer[36] performed a meta-analysis of 26 placebo-controlled, randomized clinical trials and found no correlation between corticosteroid use and peptic ulcer disease. This study was followed by a meta-analysis of 71 similar placebo-controlled, randomized clinical trials by Messer and colleagues.[37] This study demonstrated a 2-fold increase in peptic ulcer disease with corticosteroid use. Messer's data were reviewed by Conn and Poynard who could not find a statistically significant association. They performed a follow-up meta-analysis of 93 randomized, double-blind, placebo-controlled trials and found no statistically significant association between ulcer development and prednisone use.[6] These studies did find that patients using prednisone complained of peptic ulcer–type symptoms more frequently than the control patients. The investigators suggest that this could be due to superficial ulcers that were not deep enough to be detected by barium studies in the pre-endoscopic era.[6] The lack of association between corticosteroids and peptic ulcer disease was confirmed by Piper and colleagues.[38]

In addition to gastric issues, pancreatitis has been reported with the use of corticosteroids.[4] The exact incidence and the mechanism by which the corticosteroids cause pancreatitis is unknown.

ADRENAL SUPPRESSION

In the normal, nonstressed adult, the adrenal gland secretes 10 to 20 mg of cortisol per day, which translates to approximately 5 to 7 mg of prednisone per day.[10,39] Exogenous steroids increase the circulating corticosteroid levels, which can lead to a negative feedback on the hypothalamic-pituitary-adrenal (HPA) axis at the levels of the hypothalamus and the pituitary gland. This effect can lead to a decrease in production of corticotropin-releasing hormone from the hypothalamus and corticotropin or adrenocorticotropic hormone from the pituitary gland.[40] Decreased production of adrenocorticotropic hormone then leads to decreased cortisol secretion from the adrenal cortex.

There seems to be inconsistency in the dose of exogenous corticosteroids that can lead to adrenal suppression. This inconsistency is believed to be due to individual variability, as well as the specific synthetic corticosteroid administered, with some having a more dramatic effect than others.[4,41] Post mortem studies have shown atrophy of adrenal glands following as few as 5 days of corticosteroid therapy.[4] A retrospective review of rheumatologic patients identified no definitive cases of adrenal suppression with prednisone doses less than 5 mg per day, even if that dose is taken for many months.[42] The study previously referenced by Wilson's group demonstrated no significant decreases in plasma cortisol levels following a 4-day course of 5 mg of prednisolone daily.[28] When the doses were increased to 10 mg and then to 20 mg per day, each for 4 days, there was a significant decrease in plasma cortisol levels.[28]

Other studies have demonstrated that short courses for less than 30 days, with doses ranging from 15 to 50 mg of prednisone per day, can result in significant adrenal suppression in patients.[4] This suppression can then last for many weeks after the course is completed. Longer-term, lower-dose synthetic corticosteroids can also lead to adrenal insufficiency, requiring months for adrenal recovery.[4] The incidence of clinically evident adrenal insufficiency is unknown but it is believed to be much lower than the incidence based on objective measures.[4]

MYOPATHY

Muscle weakness associated with corticosteroid use is believed to be caused by type IIb muscle fiber atrophy.[4,5,43] Corticosteroids interfere with skeletal muscle oxidative phosphorylation, protein synthesis, muscle membrane excitability, and carbohydrate metabolism.[4,43] The onset is usually asymptomatic with the muscles of the proximal limbs affected first.[44] Rarely are the distal limb muscles, sphincters, or facial muscles affected, and smooth muscle does not seem to be involved at all. Patients often notice difficulty with tasks such as climbing stairs. This effect gradually resolves over 1 to 4 months after cessation of the corticosteroids and affected muscles regain their strength.[44] This effect has been shown to be dose dependent, with the corticosteroid effect lasting from days to months after the cessation of therapy.[4]

One study demonstrated a 64% incidence of muscle weakness on formal muscle testing in patients with asthma taking more than 40 mg of prednisone daily and a 12% incidence in those taking less than 40 mg of prednisone daily.[44] Although myopathy was worse in patients using more than 40 mg daily, doses as low as 10 mg daily, dosing every other day, and recurrent bursts of prednisone all caused evidence of muscle weakness in some patients.[44] These results are consistent with a case-control study that demonstrated a 6.7-fold increase in reported frequency of muscle weakness in patients with lung disease taking corticosteroids for longer than 6 months.[45] The latter study demonstrated increased risk of muscle weakness with increased daily and cumulative doses of prednisolone.[45] Other studies have contradicted these results. Picado and colleagues[46] demonstrated no significant difference in respiratory or skeletal muscle force, endurance, or histologic appearance in patients with asthma taking an average daily dose of approximately 12 mg of prednisone (mean duration approximately 8 years) compared with those not using oral prednisone.

CARDIOVASCULAR

Corticosteroids have been associated with increases in blood pressure, although the mechanisms have not been clearly elucidated. One debated theory is that mineralocorticoids increase plasma volume by binding to mineralocorticoid receptors in the renal distal tubular epithelial cells, resulting in increased sodium reabsorption and water retention with subsequent extracellular volume expansion.[4,5,47] The incidence of secondary hypertension due to corticosteroids has not been adequately described. One study did look at individuals taking mean daily doses of prednisone between 6.7 mg and 8.4 mg, and found no association with the development of hypertension.[5] The Conn and Poynard meta-analysis demonstrated a statistically significant increase in hypertension in those patients treated with corticosteroids.[6]

Two large observational studies from the United Kingdom analyzed the correlation between systemic corticosteroids and cardiovascular disease.[48,49] Both studies demonstrated significant increases in the risk of myocardial infarction and cardiovascular disease with the use of systemic corticosteroids. This risk increased in both studies based on average daily dose; however, only the Wei study demonstrated an increased risk with a higher cumulative dose. Only 1 of the 2 studies demonstrated an increased risk of cerebrovascular disease with the use of corticosteroids; the second reported a slight decrease in the risk of cerebrovascular disease.[48,49] This risk was found to be associated with cumulative dose, and seemed to be higher in patients with increased baseline risk such as cardiac or pulmonary disease.

PSYCHIATRIC

Corticosteroids cause cognitive as well as psychiatric disturbances. Cognitive deficits, such as memory disturbances, may emerge as early as 4 days after starting steroids, and appear to be dose dependent and reversible on termination of the medication.[50] The most common psychiatric manifestations include agitation, anxiety, distractibility, fear, hypomania, indifference, insomnia, irritability, lethargy, mood lability, pressured speech, restlessness, and tearfulness. Most psychiatric side effects occur within the first week of therapy and the time of onset has not been correlated with dose.[51] Although these effects can cause significant detriment to an individual's daily quality of life, they are not considered severe reactions. Severe reactions include mania, depression, or a mixed state.[50] Most individuals developing psychiatric manifestations on short courses report euphoria or hypomania, whereas those on long-term therapy tend to develop depressive symptoms.[50]

There is a dramatic variability in the incidence of steroid-induced psychiatric side effects reported in the literature, reflective of the unpredictability of these reactions, the wide range of steroid doses, and inconsistencies in effect definitions. A meta-analysis reported an incidence of 27.6% (range 13%–62%) of individuals who experienced mild to moderate psychiatric complications from corticosteroid use, whereas only 5.7% (range 1.6%–50%) reported severe complications.[52]

Corticosteroid dose was found to be the most significant risk factor associated with psychiatric reactions, with 1 series of 676 patients reporting a 3.1% incidence. Of the patients with acute psychiatric reactions, 62% demonstrated inappropriate euphoria, 9.5% were severely depressed, and 28.6% were maniacal.[53] When psychiatric symptoms were analyzed based on prednisone dose, there was a 1.3% incidence in those patients receiving a daily prednisone dose less than or equal to 40 mg, a 4.6% incidence in those receiving 41 to 80 mg of prednisone, and an 18.4% incidence in those receiving more than 80 mg.[53] The investigators found that reduction of the dose resulted in resolution of symptoms in all cases. A past reaction is not predictive of a future reaction, nor is past tolerance of prednisone predictive of future tolerance.[50] Additional studies have not been able to correlate a history of psychiatric illness with a psychiatric reaction to prednisone.[51]

The association between corticosteroids and psychiatric side effects was supported by the meta-analysis of Conn and Poynard. They reported that with a mean daily dose of 35 mg of prednisone, psychiatric side effects occurred 2 times more often than in those receiving placebo (P<.02).[6] A smaller prospective study found similar results, with more than half of the 80 patients demonstrating neuropsychiatric disorders during their 3-month course of prednisone (>30 mg per day).[35] Most of these reactions occurred early in the course of therapy, and most involved irritability and anxiety. However, 6 patients had severe episodes, 5 of whom required hospitalization. Of the 6, 3 had severe manic episodes, 2 had severe depression with suicidal thoughts, and 1 had aggressiveness.[35] Of these 6, only 1 patient had a history of minor depression.

Duration of the psychiatric disturbance is variable with delirium resolving within days, whereas severe symptoms such as depression or mania may take up to 6 weeks to resolve.[50] More than 90% of individuals with psychiatric reactions to corticosteroids recover from these symptoms.[51] Patient education about potential psychiatric side effects is crucial for early reporting and management.

TOPICAL PREPARATIONS

Topical use of corticosteroids is a common practice among otolaryngologists. These topical preparations can include more potent corticosteroids such as betamethasone and dexamethasone, each with several times the glucocorticoid potency of prednisone, as well as higher concentrations of commonly used topical steroids such as budesonide.[54] Regardless of the specific preparation, the goal is to deliver a high dose of corticosteroid to the tissues without the systemic side effects.

The systemic effects of these medications are determined by their bioavailability after topical administration as well as the degree to which they are metabolized by the first pass effect in the liver. It is commonly believed that approximately 30% of the topically applied nasal steroid sprays stay in the nasal cavity and can thus be absorbed.[55] The exact amount that becomes systemically absorbed is difficult to ascertain. The remaining 70% is distributed to the oropharynx and swallowed, either directly or through the mucociliary clearance of the sinonasal epithelium. The ingested drug gets absorbed by the gastric mucosa and passes to the liver where the amount metabolized by the liver varies by agent. Traditional topical medications such as mometasone furoate and fluticasone propionate have exceptionally small bioavailabilities, each less than 1%, whereas beclomethasone dipropionate has a much higher bioavailability of 44%.[56] Budesonide, when used intranasally, has approximately 34% bioavailability.[57] Dexamethasone and betamethasone are believed to have even higher bioavailabilities.

The effect of topical intranasal sprays on the HPA axis has been studied extensively.[58–61] There have been more than a dozen studies measuring adrenal suppression in adults and children as young as 2 years of age that have demonstrated no effect on the HPA axis from the aforementioned intranasal corticosteroid sprays.[59]

There are at least half a dozen case reports in the literature discussing adrenal suppression and/or Cushing syndrome with the use of more potent topical preparations such as betamethasone or dexamethasone drops.[62–66] It was hypothesized that dexamethasone may have a high rate of direct absorption through the nasal and respiratory mucosa in addition to the uptake in the gastrointestinal tract.[66] Many of these cases were believed to be caused by medication overdosing, which can occur as a result of inconsistent dosing and delivery from the use of drops.[67]

Two recent studies have investigated the effect of budesonide nasal irrigations on the HPA axis. Sachanandani and colleagues[68] assessed the adrenal function of 9 patients before and after 30 days of topical budesonide. Patients were asked to mix 0.25 mg of budesonide with 5 mL of saline, then administer 5 mL of the mixture into their nasal cavity. Using the cosyntropin stimulation test, the investigators were unable to identify any evidence of adrenal suppression. Similarly, Welch and colleagues[69] demonstrated no evidence of adrenal suppression using serum cortisol and 24-hour urinary cortisol in 10 patients irrigating their sinuses with 0.5 mg of budesonide mixed into 240 mL of saline solution twice daily.

There have been at least 2 reports of significant growth retardation that correlated with the use of the betamethasone drops intranasally.[64] Both patients demonstrated a return to normal growth velocity once the betamethasone use was stopped. However, the patients were not observed long enough to determine their adult stature.[64]

SUMMARY

This article presents a comprehensive review of the side effects of exogenous corticosteroids and their relative frequencies. Otolaryngologists commonly prescribe corticosteroids to treat various conditions and diseases. For this reason, it is essential that the specific effects of these drugs, including their relative frequencies, severities, and associated doses, are better understood. It is also imperative that the informed consent process includes the more significant and more common reactions described here. Unfortunately, there exists a paucity of data on the adverse effects associated with shorter courses and smaller doses of corticosteroids. Further prospective studies analyzing these effects are necessary.

REFERENCES

1. Nadel DM. The use of systemic steroids in otolaryngology. Ear Nose Throat J 1996;75:502–5 509–10, 511-2 passim.
2. Wright ED, Agrawal S. Impact of perioperative systemic steroids on surgical outcomes in patients with chronic rhinosinusitis with polyposis: evaluation with the novel perioperative sinus endoscopy (POSE) scoring system. Laryngoscope 2007;117(Suppl 115):1–28.
3. Cope D, Bova R. Steroids in otolaryngology. Laryngoscope 2008;118:1556–60.
4. Fardet L, Kassar A, Cabane J, et al. Corticosteroid-induced adverse events in adults: frequency, screening and prevention. Drug Saf 2007;30:861–81.
5. McEvoy CE, Niewoehner DE. Adverse effects of corticosteroid therapy for COPD. Chest 1997;111:732–43.
6. Conn HO, Poynard T. Corticosteroids and peptic ulcer: metaanalysis of adverse events during steroid therapy. J Intern Med 1994;236:619–32.
7. Fardet L, Cabane J, Lebbé C, et al. Incidence and risk factors for corticosteroid-induced lipodystrophy: a prospective study. J Am Acad Dermatol 2007;57: 604–9.
8. Hirsch IB, Paauw DS. Diabetes management in special situations. Endocrinol Metab Clin North Am 1997;26:631–45.
9. Greenstone MA, Shaw AB. Alternate day corticosteroid causes alternate day hyperglycemia. Postgrad Med J 1987;63:761–4.
10. Chrousos GP. Adrenocorticosteroids & adrenocortical antagonists. In: Katzung BG, editor. Basic & clinical pharmacology. 10th edition. New York (NY): McGraw-Hill; 2007. p. 635–52.
11. Segal BH, Sneller MC. Infectious complications of immunosuppressive therapy in patients with rheumatic diseases. Rheum Dis Clin North Am 1997;23:219–37.
12. Stuck AE, Minder CE, Frey FJ. Risk of infectious complications in patients taking glucocorticosteroids. Rev Infect Dis 1989;11:954–63.
13. O'Donell MR, Schmidt GM, Teftmeier BR, et al. Prediction of systemic fungal infection in allogeneic marrow recipients: impact of amphotericin prophylaxis in high-risk patients. J Clin Oncol 1994;12:827–34.
14. Fukada T, Boeckh M, Carter RA, et al. Risks and outcomes of invasive fungal infections in recipients of allogeneic hematopoietic stem cell transplants after nonmyeloablative conditioning. Blood 2003;102:827–33.
15. Lionakis MS, Kontoyiannis DP. Glucocorticoids and invasive fungal infections. Lancet 2003;362:1828–38.
16. Upton A, Kirby KA, Carpenter P, et al. Invasive aspergillosis following hematopoietic cell transplantation: outcomes and prognostic factors associated with mortality. Clin Infect Dis 2007;44:531–40.
17. Marr KA, Carter RA, Boeckh M, et al. Invasive aspergillosis in allogeneic stem cell transplant recipients: changes in epidemiology and risk factors. Blood 2002;100: 4358–66.
18. Atkinson JB, Kosi M, Srikanth MS, et al. Growth hormone reverses impaired wound healing in protein-malnourished rats treated with corticosteroids. J Pediatr Surg 1992;27:1026–8.

19. Nguyen H, Lim J, Dresner ML, et al. Effect of local corticosteroids on early inflammatory function in surgical wound of rats. J Foot Surg 1998;37:313–8.
20. Goforth P, Gudas CJ. Effects of steroids on wound healing: a review of the literature. J Foot Surg 1980;19:22–8.
21. Suh DY, Hunt TK, Spencer EM. Insulin-like growth factor-I reverses the impairment of wound healing induced by corticosteroids in rats. Endocrinology 1992; 131:2399–403.
22. Lenco W, McKnight M, MacDonald AS. Effects of cortisone acetate, methylprednisolone and medroxyprogesterone on wound contracture and epithelialization in rabbits. Ann Surg 1975;181:67–73.
23. Keenan GF. Management of complications of glucocorticoid therapy. Clin Chest Med 1997;18:507–20.
24. Allen DB, Bielory L, Derendorf H, et al. Inhaled corticosteroids: past lessons and future issues. J Allergy Clin Immunol 2003;112:S1–40.
25. Ton FN, Gunawardene SC, Lee H, et al. Effects of low-dose prednisone on bone metabolism. J Bone Miner Res 2005;20:464–70.
26. van Staa TP, Leufkens HGM, Cooper C. The epidemiology of corticosteroid-induced osteoporosis: a meta-analysis. Osteoporos Int 2002;13:777–87.
27. Paglia F, Dionisis S, De Geronimo S, et al. Biomarkers of bone turnover after a short period of steroid therapy in elderly men. Clin Chem 2001;47:1314–6.
28. Wilson AM, McFarlane LC, Lipworth BJ. Systemic bioactivity profiles of oral prednisolone and nebulized budesonide in adult asthmatics. Chest 1998; 114:1022–7.
29. Laan RFJM, Van Riel PLCM, Van Erning LJTO, et al. Vertebral osteoporosis in rheumatoid arthritis patients: effects of low dose prednisone therapy. Br J Rheumatol 1992;31:91–6.
30. Cui Q, Wang G-J, Balian G. Steroid-induced adipogenesis in a pluripotential cell line from bone marrow. J Bone Joint Surg Am 1997;79:1054–63.
31. Mirzai R, Chang C, Greenspan A, et al. The pathogenesis of osteonecrosis and the relationship to corticosteroids. J Asthma 1999;36:77–95.
32. McKee MD, Waddell JP, Kudo PA, et al. Osteonecrosis of the femoral head in men following short-course corticosteroid therapy: a report of 15 cases. CMAJ 2001; 164:205–6.
33. Wong GK, Poon WS, Chiu KH. Steroid-induced avascular necrosis of the hip in neurosurgical patients: epidemiological study. ANZ J Surg 2005;75:409–10.
34. Carnahan MC, Goldstein DA. Ocular complications of topical, peri-ocular, and systemic corticosteroids. Curr Opin Ophthalmol 2000;11:478–83.
35. Fardet L, Flahault A, Kettaneh A, et al. Corticosteroid-induced clinical adverse events: frequency, risk factors and patient's opinion. Br J Dermatol 2007;157: 142–8.
36. Conn HO, Blitzer BL. Nonassociation of adrenocorticosteroid therapy and peptic ulcer. N Engl J Med 1976;294:434–79.
37. Messer J, Reitman D, Sacks H, et al. Association of adrenocorticosteroid therapy and peptic ulcer disease. N Engl J Med 1983;309:21–4.
38. Piper J, Ray W, Daugherty J, et al. Corticosteroid use and peptic ulcer disease: role of nonsteroidal anti-inflammatory drugs. Ann Intern Med 1991;114:735–40.
39. Asare K. Diagnosis and treatment of adrenal insufficiency in the critically ill patient. Pharmacotherapy 2007;27:1512–38.
40. Ganong WF. The adrenal medulla & adrenal cortex. In: Ganong WF, editor. Review of medical physiology. 22nd edition. New York (NY): McGraw-Hill; 2007. p. 356–81.

41. Downie WW, Dixon JS, Lowe JR, et al. Adrenocortical suppression by synthetic corticosteroid drugs: a comparative study of prednisolone and betamethasone. Br J Clin Pharmacol 1978;6:397–9.
42. LaRochelle GE, LaRochelle AG, Ratner RE, et al. Recovery of the hypothalamic-pituitary-adrenal axis in patients with rheumatic diseases receiving low-dose prednisone. Am J Med 1993;95:258–64.
43. Polsonetti BW, Joy SD, Laos LF. Steroid-induced myopathy in the ICU. Ann Pharmacother 2002;36:1741–4.
44. Bowyer SL, LaMothe MP, Hollister JR. Steroid myopathy: incidence and detection in a population with asthma. J Allergy Clin Immunol 1985;76:234–42.
45. Walsh LJ, Wong CA, Oborne J, et al. Adverse effects of oral corticosteroids in relation to dose in patients with lung disease. Thorax 2001;56:279–84.
46. Picado C, Fiz JA, Montserrat JM, et al. Respiratory and skeletal muscle function in steroid-dependent bronchia asthma. Am Rev Respir Dis 1990;141:14–20.
47. Nussberger J. Investigating mineralocorticoid hypertension. J Hypertens 2003; 21:S25–30.
48. Wei L, MacDonald TM, Walker BR. Taking glucocorticoids by prescription is associated with subsequent cardiovascular disease. Ann Intern Med 2004;141: 764–70.
49. Souverein PC, Berard A, Van Staa TP, et al. Use of oral glucocorticoids and risk of cardiovascular and cerebrovascular disease in a population based case-control study. Heart 2004;90:859–65.
50. Warrington TP, Bostwick JM. Psychiatric adverse effects of corticosteroids. Mayo Clin Proc 2006;81:1361–7.
51. Kershner P, Wang-Cheng R. Psychiatric side effects of steroid therapy. Psychosomatics 1989;30:135–9.
52. Lewis DA, Smith RE. Steroid-induced psychiatric syndromes. J Affect Disord 1983;5:319–32.
53. The Boston Collaborative Drug Surveillance Program Acute adverse reactions to prednisone in relation to dosage. Clin Pharmacol Ther 1972;13:694–8.
54. Schimmer BP, Parker KL. Adrenocorticotropic hormone; adrenocortical steroids and their synthetic analogs; inhibitors of the synthesis and actions of adrenocortical hormones. In: Brunron LL, Lazo JS, Parker KL, editors. Goodman & Gilman's the Pharmacological basis of therapeutics, 11th edition.
55. Lipworth BJ, Jackson CM. Safety of inhaled and intranasal corticosteroids: lessons for the new millennium. Drug Saf 2000;23:11–33.
56. Daley-Yates PT, Kunka RL, Yin Y, et al. Bioavailability of fluticasone propionate and mometasone furoate aqueous nasal sprays. Eur J Clin Pharmacol 2004;60: 265–8.
57. Demoly P. Safety of intranasal corticosteroids in acute rhinosinusitis. Am J Otolaryngol 2008;29:403–13.
58. Bachert C, Lukat KF, Lange B. Effect of intranasal fluticasone propionate and triamcinolone acetonide on basal and dynamic measures of hypothalamic-pituitary-adrenal-axis activity in healthy volunteers. Clin Exp Allergy 2004;34: 85–90.
59. Galant SP, Melamed IR, Nayak AS, et al. Lack of effect of fluticasone propionate aqueous nasal spray on the hypothalamic-pituitary-adrenal axis in 2- and 3-year-old patients. Pediatrics 2003;112:96–100.
60. Wilson AM, Sims EJ, McFarlane LC, et al. Effects of intranasal corticosteroids on adrenal, bone, and blood markers of systemic activity in allergic rhinitis. J Allergy Clin Immunol 1998;102:598–604.

61. Salib RJ, Howarth PH. Safety and tolerability profiles of intranasal antihistamines and intranasal corticosteroids in the treatment of allergic rhinitis. Drug Saf 2003; 26:863–93.
62. Gill G, Swift A, Jones A, et al. Severe adrenal suppression by steroid nasal drops. J R Soc Med 2001;94:350–1.
63. Stevens DJ. Cushing's syndrome due to the abuse of betamethasone nasal drops. J Laryngol Otol 1988;102:219–21.
64. Daman Willems CE, Dinwiddie R, Grant DB, et al. Temporary inhibition of growth and adrenal suppression associated with the use of steroid nose drops. Eur J Pediatr 1994;153:632–4.
65. Findlay CA, Macdonald JF, Wallace AM, et al. Childhood Cushing's syndrome induced by betamethasone nose drops and repeat prescriptions. BMJ 1998; 317:739–40.
66. Kimmerle R, Rolla AR. Iatrogenic Cushing's syndrome due to dexamethasone nasal drops. Am J Med 1985;79:535–7.
67. Gallagher G, Mackay I. Doctors and drops. Br Med J 1991;303:761.
68. Sachanandani NS, Piccirillo JF, Kramper MA, et al. The effect of nasally administered budesonide respules on adrenal cortex function in patients with chronic rhinosinusitis. Ach Otolaryngol Head Neck Surg 2009;135:303–7.
69. Welch KC, Thaler ER, Doghramji LL, et al. The effects serum and urinary cortisol levels of topical intranasal irrigations with budesonide added to saline in patients with recurrent polyposis after endoscopic sinus surgery. Am J Rhinol Allergy 2010;24:26–8.

Postoperative Prevention and Treatment of Complications After Sinus Surgery

Bruce K. Tan, MD, Rakesh K. Chandra, MD*

KEYWORDS

- Endoscopic Sinus Surgery • Postsurgical • Complications
- Outcomes • Chronic rhinosinusitis

In the past 25 years, there has been widespread adoption of functional endoscopic sinus surgical (FESS) techniques among otolaryngologists. In addition to the management of medically refractory chronic rhinosinusitis (CRS), these same techniques are currently applied to the management of acute complications of acute rhinosinusitis, resection of intranasal tumors, occuloplastic procedures, and approaches to the anterior skull base.[1,2] Since its initial description by Messerklinger, and throughout its subsequent evolution, the underlying surgical philosophy of FESS has utilized endoscopic visualization to identify obstructed or inflamed natural drainage pathways of the paranasal sinuses and restore drainage and ventilation of these sinuses using meticulous mucosal-sparing techniques. These techniques have resulted in an effective therapy for CRS with intermediate and long-term symptomatic improvement reported by over 90% of patients undergoing FESS.[3] Despite excellent surgical technique, however, postoperative complications and disease recurrence requiring revision surgery are reported in 18% of patients in long-term follow up.[4]

Even following technically precise surgery, postoperative complications such as bleeding and excessive crusting can arise both in the immediate postoperative period, while other complications such as synechia formation, middle turbinate lateralization ,and infection may manifest within weeks of surgery.[5,6] Underlying host factors, anatomy, surgical technique, and post-operative care ultimately dictate long-term complications such as ostial stenosis and disease recurrence. Hence, it is critical

Financial Disclosure: None.

Department of Otolaryngology – Head and Neck Surgery, Northwestern University, Feinberg School of Medicine, 676 North Street Clair, Suite 1325, Chicago, IL 60611, USA
* Corresponding author.
E-mail address: rchandra@nmff.org

Otolaryngol Clin N Am 43 (2010) 769–779
doi:10.1016/j.otc.2010.04.004
oto.theclinics.com

for the otolaryngologist to carefully evaluate post-FESS patients using postoperative course, nasal endoscopy, and even computed tomography scanning for the occurrence of such complications, since early recognition of such complications may facilitate outpatient interventions to stave off subsequent complications.

As the popularity of FESS has grown, there is an increasing interest in interventions and therapies targeted at optimizing outcomes. These interventions frequently are grounded in, and simultaneously limited, by the understanding about the pathogenesis of the inflammation associated with chronic rhinosinusitis. Traditionally, theories on the pathogenesis of CRS include obstruction of the osteomeatal complex, impaired mucociliary clearance, osteitis, atopy, and microbial resistance, including biofilm formation. These potential pathogenic mechanisms form the underpinnings of most current therapies for CRS, including antimicrobials, antihistamines, leukotriene antagonists, topical and systemic corticosteroids, and nasal rinses. More recently, research into host factors such as an aberrant host response to ubiquitous environmental mould and *Staphylococcus aureus* colonization and host barrier dysfunction have inspired clinical trials of therapeutics aimed at eliminating these potential agents in post-FESS patients.[7] In a separate line of research, clinical trials have been conducted on various biomaterials and biological agents that may facilitate wound healing and reduce scarring in the post-FESS patient. This article reviews the available literature examining the role of operative or postoperative management strategies for reducing postoperative complications.

PREVENTION OF POST-FESS COMPLICATIONS USING INTRAOPERATIVE MEASURES

Prevention of postoperative complications begins in the operating room itself, immediately following dissection of the cavity.

Nasal Packing

Nonabsorbable nasal packing traditionally has been the method of controlling ongoing bleeding after surgery to the paranasal sinuses and reduction of clot in the surgical bed. Additional theoretical benefits of nasal packing include preventing adhesion formation, middle turbinate lateralization, and restenosis after surgery. Unfortunately, the presence of nasal packing and its subsequent removal is frequently uncomfortable and is often rated by patients as the most unpleasant aspect of the FESS surgical experience.[8] This has spurred development of absorbable hemostatic nasal packing materials that obviate the need for removal but need to degrade in an appropriate time frame without inducing an inflammatory reaction. Orlandi and Lanza have argued that the routine placement of hemostatic nasal packing for hemostasis is unnecessary, with 87% of their series of 165 patients not requiring any hemostatic agent packed in their nose without any increase in postoperative bleeding.[9] A comprehensive review of the data and types of nasal packing in the literature, recently was published; however, the authors have selected a few specific studies in this article to highlight some of the more salient studies on nasal packing in the post-FESS patient.

Nonabsorbable packing

An excellent randomized, blinded controlled clinical trial was performed on the effect of middle meatus Merocel packing for 5 days in 61 patients after FESS. Contrary to the experience of the authors of this article, patients with Merocel packing did not experience any differences in the mean scores for nasal pain, headache, nasal congestion or postoperative bleeding.[10] The primary benefit this study found from the placement of nasal packing was the reduction of synechia or adhesions that was seen in none of the 31 patients with nasal packing but 10 of those who did not receive nasal packing.

In a separate study, Lee demonstrated thee use of silicone elastomer sheeting as a middle turbinate spacer in cases of a floppy middle turbinate following FESS and showed a reduction in synechiae formation from 44% to 6% in the treated side.[11]

Absorbable packing

One of the absorbable hemostatic agents studied extensively in post-FESS patients is the Floseal matrix consisting of bovine-derived gelatin particles and human thrombin (Floseal, Baxter, Deerfield, IL, USA). A prospective uncontrolled study on 18 patients on using Floseal as a means of controlling bleeding post-FESS found it effective in providing postoperative hemostasis, with only one patient requiring additional post-surgical intervention for bleeding.[12] Another study compared their prospective experience with Floseal on 50 patients with 50 controls receiving Merocel packing and found equal efficacy in postoperative hemostasis but less patient discomfort.[13] However, a randomized study performed by the authors' group on Floseal compared with thrombin-soaked gelatin foam and an additional larger retrospective study performed by a separate investigator, demonstrate an increased propensity of patients in the Floseal group to form early granulation tissue and subsequent adhesions.[14–16]

Other groups have reported a prospective study utilizing microporous hemispheres, controlled-porosity spherical particles manufactured from bioinert plant polysaccharide, for use in the post-FESS setting with no differences noted in the immediate postoperative period when compared with the untreated control side.[17] However, they did not report the presence of adhesion formation as one of their measured outcomes. Dissolvable carboxymethyl cellulose (CMC) foam was reported in a recent prospective study of 60 patients to reduce adhesion formation. Specifically, adhesions were observed in 35.7% of those receiving cotton gauze wrapped in latex glove fingers versus 6.7% in patients receiving CMC foam, with decreased levels of localized pain in the latter cohort.[18] It was unclear from the methods whether the decision to place CMC-foam was randomized. A study examining hyaluronic acid nasal packs (Merogel, Medtronic, Jacksonville, FL, USA) failed to demonstrate any benefit of the spacer on bleeding, synechia formation, or edema when compared with the unpacked side.[19]

Together, these studies demonstrate that the routine use of nasal packing, whether absorbable or nonabsorbable, has little effect on postoperative bleeding but more importantly, plays a more important role in postoperative healing. Definitive reductions in synechiae appear to be reported in studies involving nonabsorbable packs or splints, while the data regarding absorbable materials is more equivocal, and further studies and new materials will need to be developed for this purpose.

Middle Turbinate Stabilization

In addition to the operative placement of nasal packing, other intraoperative techniques to promote post-FESS healing include techniques to encourage the middle turbinate to heal in the medialized position, maintaining the patency of the ostia lateral to the middle turbinate. Published techniques include suture stabilization of the middle turbinate to the septum, metal clips, biological glue, and a controlled synechiae (Bolgerization).[20–23]

Mitomycin C

Mitomycin C is a DNA cross-linking antineoplastic agent that has been used in ophthalmologic surgery to reduce scar tissue. Several groups have examined the application of mitomycin C via a middle meatal pledget at the end of surgery to reduce the formation of lateral synechiae. Chung applied mitomycin C at 0.4 mg/mL unilaterally in 55 patients and found a nonsignificant decrease of unilateral adhesions on the side receiving mitomycin C but also excluded the patients who formed bilateral adhesions from this analysis.[24] Similarly, separate studies by Anand and Kim of similar design and mitomycin C concentration also failed to find significant benefit of mitomycin C in their studies.[25] Conversely Konstantinidis applied mitomycin C to the middle meatus both at the conclusion of FESS and once in the postoperative period and was able to demonstrate a reduction in adhesions (4 of 30 moderate on the control side vs none on the treated side) and ostial stenosis.[26] Together, these studies suggest that there may be a role mitomycin C in postoperative synechiae prevention; however, the effect probably is relatively small.

Frontal Sinus Stents

The use of indwelling stents has been described for the middle meatus, but in clinical practice, stenting generally is applied to the frontal sinus, where there has been significant debate about several related issues, including type of material, duration, and the basic need for stenting. A recent review has summarized the data behind frontal sinus stenting, but unfortunately to date, there are no controlled studies examining the effect of frontal sinus stenting.[27,28] Weber retrospectively reviewed a series of 12 patients with refractory disease who had received frontal sinus stents for more than 6 months and found a patency rate of 70% and advocated for the placement of stents for that duration. Orlandi recently reviewed a series of nine patients on whom the frontal sinusotomy was felt to be tenuous, with a diameter less than 5 mm, and a Rains frontal sinus stent was placed. He has followed these patients for a mean duration of 33 months and has had to remove only one of these stents for infection.[29]

PREVENTION OF POSTOPERATIVE COMPLICATIONS USING POSTOPERATIVE TECHNIQUES

Debridement

Throughout the development of FESS, debridement of the postoperative surgical cavity has been advocated for optimizing surgical outcomes. Several randomized controlled trials have directly examined the effect of postsurgical debridements on the outcome of surgery. Bugten has published short- and long-term follow-up to a prospectively enrolled study of 60 patients randomized to postoperative debridement or not. Each patient underwent debridements at 6 days and 2 weeks after surgery, and the study found that patients who received endoscopic debridement showed a more rapid resolution of the sensation of nasal congestion and reduced the number of middle meatal adhesions (11 adhesions vs 29 in control) when examined 12 weeks postoperatively.[30] Lee randomized his patients into three groups receiving postoperative debridement ranging from twice weekly to every other week and concluded that once weekly debridement for 4 weeks was optimal for reducing patient discomfort from debridement or nasal crusting.[31]

Postoperative Nasal Irrigation

The use of nasal irrigation in the postoperative period has been investigated, with several studies varying the use of nasal irrigation, the nature and tonicity of nasal irrigation, and even positioning during nasal irrigation. Freeman randomized his post-FESS nasal polyp patients to unilateral saline irrigation and found symptomatic improvements in his patients but few differences in crusting or edema.[32] A rather exhaustive randomized study that included extensive postoperative biopsies on 80 patients who were randomized to receive either sulfurous-arsenical-ferruginous thermal water from the (Levico Spa, Trento, Italy) or isotonic sodium chloride solution for 6 months demonstrated a reduction in tissue eosinophilia in the group receiving spa water.[32] Unfortunately, the authors did not report any endoscopic or clinical parameters in their paper. A controlled study examined hypertonic nasal saline spray, isotonic nasal spray, and no spray on a group of 60 patients in the post-FESS period and found that hypertonic nasal sprays had a detrimental effect of increasing the amount of nasal discharge and postoperative pain, but the study found no beneficial effect of either nasal saline spray.[33] Nasal irrigation and douching techniques were not examined by this study.

Several other studies relevant to the discussion of irrigation in the post-FESS patient are Wormald's study, in which the distribution of a nasal saline irrigation containing Technetium 99 m sulfur colloid was examined following nasal irrigation using a metered nasal spray, nebulization, and nasal douching with the head on the floor.[34] This study found nasal douching to be most effective in distributing irrigant solution into the frontal recess and maxillary sinus. All techniques studied were unable to access the sphenoid sinus or frontal sinus well. In a separate study by the same group, a higher volume of irrigant (200 cc) was better able to penetrate the frontal sinus. The effect of tonicity of the nasal solution was shown to only transiently affect ciliary beat frequency in a study of either 0.9% saline spray or 3.0% saline spray. There has been no clinical trial demonstrating a sustained improved effect of hypertonic nasal irrigation or spray in the clinical setting.[35]

In a cautionary note, Welch recently published a study of the irrigation bottles used by patients after FESS and found that bacteria could be cultured from the irrigation bottles in 29% of studied patients including *Pseudomonas aeruginosa*, *Acinetobacter baumannii,* and *Klebsiella pneumoniae,* although fortunately no clinically significant postoperative infections were noted. Frequent changing and sterilization of nasal irrigation bottles is advocated.[36]

POSTOPERATIVE MEASURES TO PREVENT RECURRENCE OR RECALCITRANT DISEASE

Systemic Antibiotics

In chronic sinusitis, culture-directed antibiotics often are recommended as a cornerstone of treatment of post-FESS patients, although the significance of isolated bacteria continues to be controversial. In a study of cultured bacteria, Nadel found that cultures obtained from patients with chronic sinusitis, particularly those with prior sinus surgery, exhibited higher levels of *P aeruginosa* when compared with normal controls.[37] Additionally, rates of culturable *S aureus* were similar, but growth was heavier, in patients with chronic sinusitis. In a separate study, Al-Shemari obtained cultures from asymptomatic post-FESS sinus cavities and found that bacterial organisms were recovered in 97% of subjects (mean 1.5 organisms per patient).[38] The flora predominantly consisted of coagulase-negative staphylococci (69%) and diphtheroids (25%). *S aureus* was recovered in 31% of subjects and *P aeruginosa* in 3% only. As such, the presence of cultured bacteria from post-FESS patients and the clinical significance of bacterial colonization obtained from post-FESS cavities remains unclear. More recently, several investigators have described the presence of biofilms in post-FESS cavities, and a retrospective pathologic study by Psaltis using confocal microscopy to detect biofilm formation found that bacterial biofilms were found in 20 (50%) of the 40 CRS patients.[39] Patients with biofilms also had significantly worse preoperative radiological scores and, postoperatively, had statistically worse postoperative symptoms and mucosal outcomes. Whether these biofilms are the cause of the increased disease burden or merely reflective of the underlying host epithelial barrier defect is still under investigation.[40]

Despite widespread use of systemic antibiotics in the treatment of CRS, there are only two recent randomized controlled trials using macrolides specifically for treating chronic sinusitis. Wallwork performed a double-blind randomized controlled trial with either 150 mg roxithromycin daily for 3 months or placebo and found statistically significant results in their sino-nasal outcome test (SNOT)-20 scores, nasal endoscopy, and saccharine transit times, although they did not report what proportion of their patients may have had prior FESS.[41] Evidently, further trials in the role of systemic antibiotics in managing CRS and post-FESS CRS patients are needed.

Topical Antibiotics

In cystic fibrosis patients, Moss reported a substantial reduction (22% vs 72%) in a small nonrandomized trial of 32 patients receiving non-FESS sinus surgery who got monthly antral lavages of tobramycin solution when compared with controls treated with the usual postoperative protocol.[42] Desrosiers, however, performed a randomized double-blind trial of tobramycin solution versus saline solution delivered via a large particle nebulizer in 20 noncystic fibrosis patients who had failed FESS and found no benefit from the nebulized tobramycin versus control in both nasal symptoms and endoscopic evaluation.[43] Recently, Uren reported an uncontrolled prospective open-label pilot study on 16 patients with surgically recalcitrant CRS who had positive endoscopically guided cultures for *S aureus* and were treated with twice-daily nasal lavage containing 0.05% Mupirocin in a lactated ringer for 3 weeks.[44] Fifteen patients reportedly had improved endoscopic findings, while 12 patients noted overall symptom improvement.

Topical Antifungals

A controversial topic in the management of chronic sinusitis involves the utility of topical amphotericin B with conflicting studies demonstrating variable efficacy of this intervention. In 2005, Ponikau published a randomized-controlled, double-blind trial of 24 patients who received either 20 mL amphotericin B (250 μg/mL) or placebo to each nostril twice daily for 6 months.[45] This study demonstrated efficacy in reducing mucosal inflammation seen on a standardized coronal CT scan using a methodology pioneered by this group. No differences were demonstrated using SNOT-20 scores or nasal endoscopy. A larger, multicenter trial then was performed by Ebbens on 116 randomized patients utilizing clinical endpoints and showed no benefit of topical amphotericin B.[46] Additionally, Weschta conversely found that patients receiving topical amphotericin B became more symptomatic.[47]

Topical Corticosteroids

While the pathophysiology of chronic sinusitis with and without polyps continues to be debated, one of the few consensus articles regarding the treatment of chronic sinusitis advocates the use of topical corticosteroids. In the pre-FESS era, several studies demonstrated conflicting results regarding the efficacy of topical nasal steroids following nasal polypectomy.[48,49] More recently, Dijkstra performed a randomized, double-blind controlled trial randomizing 162 patients with nasal polyposis to fluticasone propionate at a dose of 400 μg twice daily, 800 μg twice daily, or placebo for 1 year following FESS.[50] This study utilized nasal endoscopy and symptomatic visual analog scores (VAS) to evaluate patients for a period of 1 year but withdrew patients from randomization for any signs of progressive or persistent disease, poor medication compliance, or adverse effects. They found an overall recurrence rate of between 39% and 55% between groups, with no differences between treatment arms. There was not formal grading system reported for defining recurrence, however, and patients were not treated in an intent-to-treat manner. In a contrast,

Rowe-Jones randomized 199 patients with and without nasal polyps to receiving fluticasone propionate aqueous nasal spray 200 μg twice daily or placebo, commencing 6 weeks after FESS with a 5-year follow-up. The change in overall symptom VAS was significantly better in the fluticasone group at 5 years.[51] Additionally, significantly more rescue medications consisting of prednisolone and an antibiotic were prescribed to the placebo group. More recently, Jorissen reported a randomized trial of 99 patients with CRS with and without nasal polyps who were randomized to receive 6 months' treatment with mometasone furoate nasal spray (MFNS) 200 μg twice daily or placebo in a double-blind manner approximately beginning 2 weeks after FESS. Using an endoscopic score taking into account inflammation, edema, and polyps, they found significant improvement in the group receiving mometasone.[52]

Several groups additionally have reported the off-label use of topically applied steroids via nasal nebulization or local instillation for the treatment of refractory postsurgical rhinosinusitis. Lavigne performed a randomized, double-blind controlled study of 26 persistently symptomatic, dust mite allergic, postsurgical patients who had daily self-administered instillation via irrigation catheter of 256 μg of budesonide or placebo for 3 weeks.[53] He found significant improvement in a compound score derived from endoscopic grade and self-reported VAS outcome in the group receiving budesonide. Similarly, Kanowitz reported an uncontrolled series of postoperative patients who were persistently symptomatic despite maximal medical therapy consisting of systemic steroids for 3 weeks, culture-directed antibiotics, and nasal steroids.[54] They received budesonide via a mucosal atomization device and found improvements in patient symptoms, reduction in the need for prednisone, and nasal endoscopy scores.

For the prevention of ostial stenosis in patients with postoperative frontal recess nasal polyposis and edema, Citardi reported results from an uncontrolled series of local instillations of 84 μg beclomethasone into the frontal sinus and found complete resolution of the frontal recess polyposis and edema in 21 of 31 frontal recesses.[55] Similarly, Delgaudio utilized off-label use of topical ophthalmic dexamethasone, prednisolone drops administered intranasally, and found an overall improvement in ostial stenosis.[56]

Use of Other Adjunctive Treatments in Postoperative Patients with Aspirin Sensitivity Triad Disease (Samter's Triad)

For patients with Samter's triad, the use of aspirin desensitization was examined on a group of 65 patients initiating aspirin therapy. Compared to the patients' medical history prior to aspirin desensitization, the authors reported that in the years after initiating therapy, patients had a reduction in the number of sinus infections and nasal polypectomies.[57] This study was limited by the retrospective nature of the examination of the patients' prior medical history and possible bias on the timing of referral for aspirin desensitization. In more recent study, 14 Samter's triad patients were assigned to either 100 mg or 300 mg of aspirin for maintenance following aspirin challenge. In all seven of the patients receiving 100 mg of daily aspirin, recurrent nasal polyps were observed, while none of the seven patients receiving the 300 mg aspirin dose had recurrent nasal polyps.[58] In a separate study, Lee found no additional benefit of administering 650 mg maintenance daily aspirin therapy over 325 mg daily aspirin therapy on the recurrence of sinonasal symptoms.[59] Another small retrospective study examined Samter's patients and found improvements in overall symptomatic improvement following initiation of antileukotriene therapy.[60]

FUTURE DIRECTIONS AND CONCLUSIONS

Based on the available research discussed earlier, there is paucity of well-established and effective adjunctive therapies that can substantially alter postoperative outcomes following FESS. Currently, ongoing efforts are being made to develop novel absorbable biomaterials that are able to prevent synechia formation and other absorbable delivery systems that can elute medications such as corticosteroids. Bleier recently reported on a biodegradable matrix of chitosan that could reversibly bind to dexamethasone that was trialed on rabbits with an encouraging pharmacologic elution profile.[61] Other lines of research focus on agents such as retinoids that can facilitate wound healing and reciliation of disrupted sinonasal mucosa.[62] Separate efforts are focusing on the potential role of biofilms in the pathogenesis of persistent sinusitis following FESS and are targeting therapies that help to disrupt the biofilm matrix that protects these bacteria from the host immune system.[40,63] Finally, as the understanding of chronic sinusitis continues to expand, new targets for drug therapy will be identified and enable practitioners to better prevent recurrence following FESS.[7]

SUMMARY

Although FESS is overall an effective means of treating chronic sinusitis, iatrogenic complications occur in 5% to 30% of patients, and recurrence is reported in about 18% of patients. Effective therapies in the operating room for reducing this postsurgical complication rate include the use of middle meatal packing and in certain cases frontal sinus stents. In the postoperative period, attention to debridement is effective in reducing the formation of adhesions, and irrigation may play a beneficial role with little adverse impact. Prevention of recurrence following FESS involves the use of topical corticosteroids, particularly in the setting of nasal polyps. Although the use of topical antimicrobials and antifungals has had some encouraging results, the data at this point do not advocate the routine use of these medications for preventing recurrence. Aspirin desensitization may be beneficial in managing nasal polyposis in addition to asthma in Samter's triad patients. Further research into measures to optimize post-FESS outcomes is needed.

REFERENCES

1. Thomas M, Yawn BP, Price D, et al. EPOS primary care guidelines: European position paper on the primary care diagnosis and management of rhinosinusitis and nasal polyps 2007—a summary. Prim Care Respir J 2008;17:79–89.
2. Welch KC, Stankiewicz JA. A contemporary review of endoscopic sinus surgery: techniques, tools, and outcomes. Laryngoscope 2009;119:2258–68.
3. Soler ZM, Mace J, Smith TL. Symptom-based presentation of chronic rhinosinusitis and symptom-specific outcomes after endoscopic sinus surgery. Am J Rhinol 2008;22:297–301.
4. Senior BA, Kennedy DW, Tanabodee J, et al. Long-term results of functional endoscopic sinus surgery. Laryngoscope 1998;108:151–7.
5. Cohen NA, Kennedy DW. Revision endoscopic sinus surgery. Otolaryngol Clin North Am 2006;39:417–35, vii.
6. Kuhn FA, Citardi MJ. Advances in postoperative care following functional endoscopic sinus surgery. Otolaryngol Clin North Am 1997;30:479–90.
7. Tan BK, Schleimer RP, Kern RC. Perspectives on the etiology of chronic rhinosinusitis. Curr Opin Otolaryngol Head Neck Surg 2010;18:21–6.

8. Valentine R, Wormald PJ, Sindwani R. Advances in absorbable biomaterials and nasal packing. Otolaryngol Clin North Am 2009;42:813–28.
9. Orlandi RR, Lanza DC. Is nasal packing necessary following endoscopic sinus surgery? Laryngoscope 2004;114:1541–4.
10. Bugten V, Nordgard S, Skogvoll E, et al. Effects of nonabsorbable packing in middle meatus after sinus surgery. Laryngoscope 2006;116:83–8.
11. Lee JY, Lee SW. Preventing lateral synechia formation after endoscopic sinus surgery with a silastic sheet. Arch Otolaryngol Head Neck Surg 2007;133: 776–9.
12. Gall RM, Witterick IJ, Shargill NS, et al. Control of bleeding in endoscopic sinus surgery: use of a novel gelatin-based hemostatic agent. J Otolaryngol 2002;31: 271–4.
13. Baumann A, Caversaccio M. Hemostasis in endoscopic sinus surgery using a specific gelatin–thrombin-based agent (FloSeal). Rhinology 2003;41:244–9.
14. Chandra RK, Conley DB, Haines GK 3rd, et al. Long-term effects of FloSeal packing after endoscopic sinus surgery. Am J Rhinol 2005;19:240–3.
15. Chandra RK, Conley DB, Kern RC. The effect of FloSeal on mucosal healing after endoscopic sinus surgery: a comparison with thrombin-soaked gelatin foam. Am J Rhinol 2003;17:51–5.
16. Shrime MG, Tabaee A, Hsu AK, et al. Synechia formation after endoscopic sinus surgery and middle turbinate medialization with and without FloSeal. Am J Rhinol 2007;21:174–9.
17. Antisdel JL, West-Denning JL, Sindwani R. Effect of microporous polysaccharide hemispheres (MPH) on bleeding after endoscopic sinus surgery: randomized controlled study. Otolaryngol Head Neck Surg 2009;141:353–7.
18. Szczygielski K, Rapiejko P, Wojdas A, et al. Use of CMC foam sinus dressing in FESS. Eur Arch Otorhinolaryngol 2010;267:537–40.
19. Wormald PJ, Boustred RN, Le T, et al. A prospective single-blind randomized controlled study of use of hyaluronic acid nasal packs in patients after endoscopic sinus surgery. Am J Rhinol 2006;20:7–10.
20. Bolger WE, Kuhn FA, Kennedy DW. Middle turbinate stabilization after functional endoscopic sinus surgery: the controlled synechiae technique. Laryngoscope 1999;109:1852–3.
21. Friedman M, Schalch P. Middle turbinate medialization with bovine serum albumin tissue adhesive (BioGlue). Laryngoscope 2008;118:335–8.
22. Moukarzel N, Nehme A, Mansour S, et al. Middle turbinate medialization technique in functional endoscopic sinus surgery. J Otolaryngol 2000;29:144–7.
23. Thornton RS. Middle turbinate stabilization technique in endoscopic sinus surgery. Arch Otolaryngol Head Neck Surg 1996;122:869–72.
24. Chung JH, Cosenza MJ, Rahbar R, et al. Mitomycin C for the prevention of adhesion formation after endoscopic sinus surgery: a randomized, controlled study. Otolaryngol Head Neck Surg 2002;126:468–74.
25. Anand VK, Tabaee A, Kacker A, et al. The role of mitomycin C in preventing synechia and stenosis after endoscopic sinus surgery. Am J Rhinol 2004;18:311–4.
26. Konstantinidis I, Tsakiropoulou E, Vital I, et al. Intra- and postoperative application of Mitomycin C in the middle meatus reduces adhesions and antrostomy stenosis after FESS. Rhinology 2008;46:107–11.
27. Bednarski KA, Kuhn FA. Stents and drug-eluting stents. Otolaryngol Clin North Am 2009;42:857–66.
28. Weber R, Mai R, Hosemann W, et al. The success of 6-month stenting in endonasal frontal sinus surgery. Ear Nose Throat J 2000;79:930–2 ,934, 937–8 passim.

29. Orlandi RR, Knight J. Prolonged stenting of the frontal sinus. Laryngoscope 2009; 119:190–2.
30. Bugten V, Nordgard S, Steinsvag S. The effects of debridement after endoscopic sinus surgery. Laryngoscope 2006;116:2037–43.
31. Lee JY, Byun JY. Relationship between the frequency of postoperative debridement and patient discomfort, healing period, surgical outcomes, and compliance after endoscopic sinus surgery. Laryngoscope 2008;118:1868–72.
32. Freeman SR, Sivayoham ES, Jepson K, et al. A preliminary randomised controlled trial evaluating the efficacy of saline douching following endoscopic sinus surgery. Clin Otolaryngol 2008;33:462–5.
33. Pinto JM, Elwany S, Baroody FM, et al. Effects of saline sprays on symptoms after endoscopic sinus surgery. Am J Rhinol 2006;20:191–6.
34. Wormald PJ, Cain T, Oates L, et al. A comparative study of three methods of nasal irrigation. Laryngoscope 2004;114:2224 7.
35. Unal M, Gorur K, Ozcan C. Ringer-lactate solution versus isotonic saline solution on mucociliary function after nasal septal surgery. J Laryngol Otol 2001;115:796–7.
36. Welch KC, Cohen MB, Doghramji LL, et al. Clinical correlation between irrigation bottle contamination and clinical outcomes in postfunctional endoscopic sinus surgery patients. Am J Rhinol Allergy 2009;23:401–4.
37. Nadel DM, Lanza DC, Kennedy DW. Endoscopically guided cultures in chronic sinusitis. Am J Rhinol 1998;12:233–41.
38. Al-Shemari H, Abou-Hamad W, Libman M, et al. Bacteriology of the sinus cavities of asymptomatic individuals after endoscopic sinus surgery. J Otolaryngol 2007; 36:43–8.
39. Psaltis AJ, Weitzel EK, Ha KR, et al. The effect of bacterial biofilms on postsinus surgical outcomes. Am J Rhinol 2008;22:1–6.
40. Kilty SJ, Desrosiers MY. Are biofilms the answer in the pathophysiology and treatment of chronic rhinosinusitis? Immunol Allergy Clin North Am 2009;29:645–56.
41. Wallwork B, Coman W, Mackay-Sim A, et al. A double-blind, randomized, placebo-controlled trial of macrolide in the treatment of chronic rhinosinusitis. Laryngoscope 2006;116:189–93.
42. Moss RB, King VV. Management of sinusitis in cystic fibrosis by endoscopic surgery and serial antimicrobial lavage. Reduction in recurrence requiring surgery. Arch Otolaryngol Head Neck Surg 1995;121:566–72.
43. Desrosiers MY, Salas-Prato M. Treatment of chronic rhinosinusitis refractory to other treatments with topical antibiotic therapy delivered by means of a large-particle nebulizer: results of a controlled trial. Otolaryngol Head Neck Surg 2001;125:265–9.
44. Uren B, Psaltis A, Wormald PJ. Nasal lavage with mupirocin for the treatment of surgically recalcitrant chronic rhinosinusitis. Laryngoscope 2008;118:1677–80.
45. Ponikau JU, Sherris DA, Weaver A, et al. Treatment of chronic rhinosinusitis with intranasal amphotericin B: a randomized, placebo-controlled, double-blind pilot trial. J Allergy Clin Immunol 2005;115:125–31.
46. Ebbens FA, Scadding GK, Badia L, et al. Amphotericin B nasal lavages: not a solution for patients with chronic rhinosinusitis. J Allergy Clin Immunol 2006; 118:1149–56.
47. Weschta M, Rimek D, Formanek M, et al. Topical antifungal treatment of chronic rhinosinusitis with nasal polyps: a randomized, double-blind clinical trial. J Allergy Clin Immunol 2004;113:1122–8.

48. Dingsor G, Kramer J, Olsholt R, et al. Flunisolide nasal spray 0.025% in the prophylactic treatment of nasal polyposis after polypectomy. A randomized, double-blind, parallel, placebo-controlled study. Rhinology 1985;23:49–58.
49. Hartwig S, Linden M, Laurent C, et al. Budesonide nasal spray as prophylactic treatment after polypectomy (a double-blind clinical trial). J Laryngol Otol 1988; 102:148–51.
50. Dijkstra MD, Ebbens FA, Poublon RM, et al. Fluticasone propionate aqueous nasal spray does not influence the recurrence rate of chronic rhinosinusitis and nasal polyps 1 year after functional endoscopic sinus surgery. Clin Exp Allergy 2004;34:1395–400.
51. Rowe-Jones JM, Medcalf M, Durham SR, et al. Functional endoscopic sinus surgery: 5-year follow-up and results of a prospective, randomised, stratified, double-blind, placebo-controlled study of postoperative fluticasone propionate aqueous nasal spray. Rhinology 2005;43:2–10.
52. Jorissen M, Bachert C. Effect of corticosteroids on wound healing after endoscopic sinus surgery. Rhinology 2009;47:280–6.
53. Lavigne F, Cameron L, Renzi PM, et al. Intrasinus administration of topical budesonide to allergic patients with chronic rhinosinusitis following surgery. Laryngoscope 2002;112:858–64.
54. Kanowitz SJ, Batra PS, Citardi MJ. Topical budesonide via mucosal atomization device in refractory postoperative chronic rhinosinusitis. Otolaryngol Head Neck Surg 2008;139:131–6.
55. Citardi MJ, Kuhn FA. Endoscopically guided frontal sinus beclomethasone instillation for refractory frontal sinus/recess mucosal edema and polyposis. Am J Rhinol 1998;12:179–82.
56. DelGaudio JM, Wise SK. Topical steroid drops for the treatment of sinus ostia stenosis in the postoperative period. Am J Rhinol 2006;20:563–7.
57. Stevenson DD, Hankammer MA, Mathison DA, et al. Aspirin desensitization treatment of aspirin-sensitive patients with rhinosinusitis-asthma: long-term outcomes. J Allergy Clin Immunol 1996;98:751–8.
58. Rozsasi A, Polzehl D, Deutschle T, et al. Long-term treatment with aspirin desensitization: a prospective clinical trial comparing 100 and 300 mg aspirin daily. Allergy 2008;63:1228–34.
59. Lee JY, Simon RA, Stevenson DD. Selection of aspirin dosages for aspirin desensitization treatment in patients with aspirin-exacerbated respiratory disease. J Allergy Clin Immunol 2007;119:157–64.
60. Ulualp SO, Sterman BM, Toohill RJ. Antileukotriene therapy for the relief of sinus symptoms in aspirin triad disease. Ear Nose Throat J 1999;78:604–6, 608, 613 passim.
61. Bleier BS, Paulson DP, O'Malley BW, et al. Chitosan glycerophosphate-based semirigid dexamethasone eluting biodegradable stent. Am J Rhinol Allergy 2009;23:76–9.
62. Erickson VR, Antunes M, Chen B, et al. The effects of retinoic acid on ciliary function of regenerated sinus mucosa. Am J Rhinol 2008;22:334–6.
63. Cohen M, Kofonow J, Nayak JV, et al. Biofilms in chronic rhinosinusitis: a review. Am J Rhinol Allergy 2009;23:255–60.

Prevention and Management of Lacrimal Duct Injury

Noam A. Cohen, MD, PhD[a,*], Marcelo B. Antunes, MD[b], Kenneth E. Morgenstern, MD[c]

KEYWORDS

• Chronic rhinosinusitis • CT • Dacryocystorhinostomy
• Functional endoscopic sinus surgery • Lacrimal duct injury

Since its introduction in the 1980s, functional endoscopic sinus surgery (FESS) has been widely accepted as the treatment for medically recalcitrant chronic rhinosinusitis (CRS) and complicated acute rhinosinusitis. It provides excellent visualization of the sinonasal structures and, when combined with frameless stereotactic surgical navigation (image-guidance system), is an effective and safe treatment modality. However, complications occur with inadvertent violation of the orbit and cranial vault. The prevention and management of lacrimal duct injury (LDI) after FESS has been neglected in the literature, and relevant anatomy and treatment strategies are discussed in this article.

ANATOMY

The tear film drains to the nasal cavities through the nasolacrimal system. Once produced by the lacrimal gland in the superior lateral lid, the tears flow medially and drain through the inferior and superior puncta, which are minute orifices, approximately 0.3 mm in diameter, located in the medial most aspect of the upper and lower lid. These orifices quickly narrow to form the superior and inferior canaliculus, which travel vertically, in the superior and inferior direction respectively for about 2 mm, and then turn 90° medially, extending for approximately 8 mm within the fibers of the orbicularis oculi muscle.

In approximately 90% of the people, the horizontal portion of the superior and inferior canaliculus merge into the common canaliculus that drains into the lacrimal sac.

[a] Division of Rhinology, Department of Otorhinolaryngology–Head and Neck Surgery, Hospital of the University of Pennsylvania, University of Pennsylvania School of Medicine, 5th floor Ravdin Building, 3400 Spruce Street, Philadelphia, PA 19104, USA
[b] Department of Otorhinolaryngology–Head and Neck Surgery, University of Pennsylvania School of Medicine, Philadelphia, PA 19104, USA
[c] Morgenstern Center for Orbital and Facial Plastic Surgery, 123 Bloomingdale Avenue, Wayne, PA 19087, USA
* Corresponding author.
E-mail address: cohenn@uphs.upenn.edu

Otolaryngol Clin N Am 43 (2010) 781–788
doi:10.1016/j.otc.2010.04.005
0030-6665/10/$ – see front matter. Published by Elsevier Inc.

The lacrimal sac lies in the lacrimal fossa, which is a depression in the anteromedial aspect of the bony orbit at the junction of the frontal process of the maxilla anteriorly and the lacrimal bone posteriorly. The lacrimal sac is approximately 10 to 15 mm in vertical height and continues inferiorly as the nasolacrimal duct. The duct resides in a bony canal that is composed by the maxilla anteriorly and the lacrimal bone posteriorly and terminates in the inferior meatus as the valve of Hasner, located approximately 35 mm posterior to the insertion of the inferior turbinate head. Endonasally, the nasolacrimal system corresponds to the maxillary line, which is the curvilinear eminence that projects from the anterior attachment of the middle turbinate superiorly to the root of the inferior turbinate inferiorly (**Fig. 1**).

The lacrimal sac and duct have an intimate relationship with the structures on the lateral nasal wall. The uncinate process attaches to the lateral nasal wall at the suture between the maxilla and the lacrimal bone and extends posteriorly. Calhoun and colleagues[1] found that the nasolacrimal duct and sac lie 1 to 8 mm anterior to the root of the uncinate process and that the distance from the natural ostium of the maxillary sinus to the lacrimal drainage system ranges from 0.5 to 18 mm. In this region, the lacrimal bone can be particularly thin, or even absent in 20% of individuals.[2] Hartikainen and colleagues[3] reported that the mean thickness of lacrimal bone was less than 100 μm, and that this thickness was greater than 300 μm in only 4% of patients.

Furthermore, the pneumatization of the agger nasi cell is variable and can extend anteriorly, pneumatizing the lacrimal bone and the frontal process of the maxilla in up to 54% of individuals. Under these circumstances, the bone overlying the nasolacrimal sac and duct can be thin, posing a risk for injury when dissecting on this area.[4]

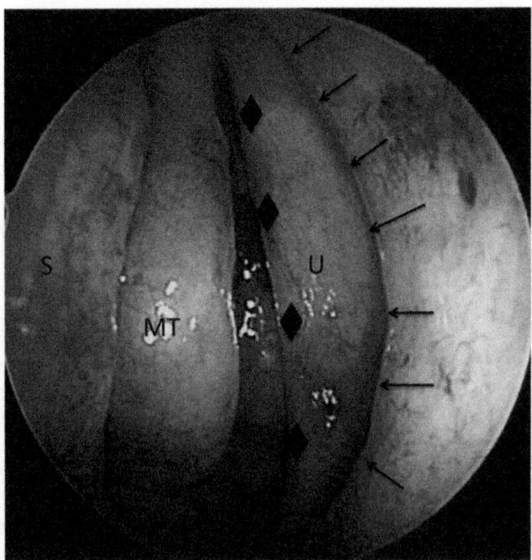

Fig. 1. Endoscopic appearance of the left maxillary line. The maxillary line is found running in a curvilinear fashion along the lateral nasal wall from the insertion of the middle turbinate (MT) superiorly to the insertion of the inferior turbinate. In this view of the left nasal cavity, the maxillary line is highlighted by the short arrows, whereas the free margin of the uncinate process (U) is demarcated by the diamonds. S, septum.

PREVENTION

Surgery of the osteomeatal complex begins with an uncinectomy. The best way to prevent LDI is to have a comprehensive understanding of the relationship of the duct to the uncinate process and anterior medial maxillary sinus.

Uncinectomy can be performed using several techniques. The anterior to posterior approach uses a sickle knife to incise along the maxillary line in a posterolateral trajectory, liberating the uncinate from its attachment and exposing the infundibulum. The uncinate is then grasped with a Blakesley forceps and rotated medially/inferiorly to remove the uncinate from the superior and then inferior attachments. If the initial incision is made anterior to the root of the uncinate, one can easily violate the duct.

The posterior to anterior approach for removing the uncinate process uses backbiting forceps. This procedure is performed in a retrograde manner, introducing the forceps in the middle meatus, turning the blade laterally, and inserting behind the free margin of the uncinate to rest in the infundibulum. The forceps is then closed and in this manner and the uncinate process is removed piecemeal from posterior to anterior. The dissection is terminated when the "hard bone" of the lacrimal bone is encountered. However, because in many individuals this bone is not always hard, but rather thin or absent, the surgeon cannot rely solely on "palpation of hard bone" to stop the dissection. At that point, an injury is likely to have already occurred.

One tool that can significantly improve visualization of this area is the angled endoscope. Using a 30° or 45° endoscope can help visualize the true ostia of the maxillary sinus and determine the limit of the anterior dissection. The authors advocate that the safest way to perform an uncinectomy and avoid LDI is to use the ball-tipped ostium seeker to palpate the infundibulum and fracture the uncinate medially, as initially described by Parsons and colleagues.[5] At that point, the backbiting forceps is introduced in the inferior portion of the uncinate and used to remove the uncinate from the inferior attachment anteriorly to its root or until the maxillary ostium is visualized. An upbiting 90° Blakesley forceps is then introduced and, through a push–pull maneuver, the superior and anterior attachments are disrupted and the uncinate removed. Alternatively, once the uncinate process has been delivered medially with the ball-tipped seeker, a microdebrider can be used to remove the freed component of the uncinate, taking care to remove the retained attachments with either a backbiting forceps or the 90° Blakesley forceps.

The proximity of the natural ostia to the nasolacrimal duct should also be appreciated. Thus, when enlargement of the natural ostium is clinically indicated, one should only enlarge toward the posterior fontanelle, leaving the natural anterior margin of the anterior fontanelle, as the anterior limit of the surgical antrostomy. If using the backbiting forceps to enlarge anteriorly, one can easily injure the nasolacrimal duct. Thus, by enlarging the ostia only posteriorly, not only is an intact rim of mucosa preserved, minimizing the degree of postsurgical stenosis, but also injury to the duct can be avoided.

CLINICAL EVALUATION

Bolger and colleagues[4] reported a 15% occult incidence of LDI during FESS that included ethmoidectomy and maxillary antrostomy (7 of 46 procedures), whereas Saengpanich and colleagues[6] reported an incidence of 3% (1 of 32 procedures) when using the microscope to perform the same procedures. In both studies, no patients experienced symptomatic sequelae, such as epiphora or dacryocystitis. The study by Bolger and colleagues[4] followed up the patients with evidence of intraoperative LDI and determined that, although the duct was violated, a patent drainage system had been created into the middle meatus or the duct spontaneously healed. These studies showed that intraoperative injury to the lacrimal drainage system is common with FESS, but that clinical sequelae is rare and thus observation alone is appropriate treatment after injury.[4]

Although rare, epiphora does occur after injury, with an incidence of 0.1% to 1.7%.[4,7–10] Serdahl and colleagues[11] reported eight cases of epiphora after FESS. Of these patients, six presented with their symptoms immediately after surgery, whereas the remaining two developed epiphora in the first 2 weeks after surgery. These findings suggest that if patients are going to develop clinical sequelae of LDI, the symptoms manifest within a short time after surgery. Follow-up of these patients is recommended for several months, because the epiphora may resolve as postoperative intranasal inflammation resolves.

Every patient presenting with epiphora should have a complete ophthalmologic examination. Even in patients experiencing symptoms after FESS, in whom the cause is presumably surgical trauma, other causes should be excluded.

EVALUATION OF EPIPHORA

Epiphora is usually evaluated with tests that document excessive tearing. Schirmer's test is used to quantify tear production. It is used to differentiate obstruction from hypersecretion and can be performed with or without local anesthesia. To perform the test, a strip of filter paper is placed at the junction of the middle and lateral thirds of the lower eyelids and the tear production is measured along the length of the filter paper. A normal result would show 10 to 15 mm of capillary action in 5 minutes. More than 30 mm indicates lacrimal outflow obstruction.

The fluorescein dye disappearance test relies on the fact that the normal turnover of the lacrimal film coating the cornea is 10 minutes. To perform this test, fluorescein is placed on the inferior fornix and the yellow film is observed for 5 to 10 min. The dye should quickly disappear, whereas persistent dye after 10 minutes indicates abnormal outflow. In addition to patient history, both tests document epiphora and indicate that the lacrimal draining system is insufficient. However, these tests do not determine the site of obstruction.

Other office-based tests that can be used to further clarify the site obstruction are the lacrimal irrigation test and the Jones tests. In the lacrimal irrigation test, a 23- or 27-gauge cannula is passed through the puncta and irrigation is performed. With a patent or partially patent system, the solution should pass into the nose. Reflux though the same canaliculus indicates obstruction, where reflux through the other canaliculus indicates common canaliculus obstruction. Distension of the nasolacrimal sac or reflux of mucus or purulence indicates nasolacrimal duct obstruction.

In the Jones I test, as in the fluorescein dye disappearance test, fluorescein is placed in the conjunctival sac. The difference is that fluorescein is then recovered from the nasal cavity though a cotton-tip applicator that is placed in the inferior meatus. When recovery of fluorescein in the inferior meatus is achieved the test is positive, whereas failure to recover the dye results in a negative test.

The Jones II test is performed after a negative Jones I test, and is similar to the lacrimal irrigation test. The inferior canaliculus is cannulated and irrigated with clear saline and, again, the solution is recovered from the nose. Presence of fluorescein in the solution (positive result) indicates that the dye entered the lacrimal sac, and indicates a functional and anatomically intact canalicular system, with the lower system partially open but not functional. Recovery of clear fluid without fluorescein (negative result) indicates a dysfunctional canalicular system.

Radiologic tests not only aid in the diagnosis of epiphora but also can be helpful in surgical planning. The dacryocystogram, or contrast fluoroscopic study, affords a good anatomic study of the sac and duct and tends to yield the most information. If the dimensions are larger than the contralateral side or than expected according to anatomic standards, dilation of the sac secondary to partial or total obstruction can be assumed. Another detail that should be evaluated is the contour of the sac, with an irregular contour indicating inflammation. The dacryocystogram is helpful in surgical planning to determine the level of obstruction. When the obstruction is at the level of the canaliculus, a dacryocystorhinostomy (DCR) will not solve the problem. A CT scan in conjunction with a dacryocystogram can yield valuable information regarding the anatomy of the nasolacrimal draining system.

Lacrimal scintigraphy is usually performed with technetuim-99. A drop is placed in the conjunctiva and images are acquired 5 to 10 minutes later. This relatively sensitive method can identify functional obstruction, but does not provide the anatomic detail afforded by a dacryocystogram.

MANAGEMENT

Epiphora secondary to nasolacrimal obstruction is treated with a DCR, which can be performed through an open or endonasal approach.

Endonasal approaches to correct nasolacrimal obstruction date back to the late 1800s, but because of limited visualization, the endonasal approaches lost their popularity and were replaced by the external approaches, described by Toti[12] in Italy in the early 1900s. With the advent of endoscopes in the nose, the technique was revisited in the late 1980s with McDonogh[13,14] in South Africa.

A critical component to surgical success is proper patient selection. The most important variable to be determined Is the level of obstruction. Ideally, it should be at or distal to the junction of lacrimal sac and duct, with a more proximal obstruction being more unfavorable.

Endoscopic DCR is usually performed under general anesthesia. The first step of the procedure is to localize the lacrimal sac in the nose, with the landmarks being the insertion of the middle turbinate and the maxillary line (see **Fig. 1**). The maxillary line corresponds to the junction of the lacrimal bone and the frontal process of the maxilla. The lacrimal sac usually lies anterior to this line. The sac can also be localized by passing a 20-gauge fiber-optic endoilluminator through the canaliculus and observing the transillumination in the nose with an endoscope. Once the outline of the sac is identified, a mucosal flap is elevated. However, the use of mucosal flaps to line the surgical drainage path does not seem to be necessary for successful outcomes, as shown in a recent study by Ramakrishnan and colleagues.[15] Despite whether mucosal flaps are incorporated, an incision is made anterior to the sac site to ensure good bony exposure.

An anatomic study by Wormald and colleagues[16] showed that the sac extends, on average, 8 mm above the insertion of the middle turbinate, suggesting that the mucosal incision should be extended up superiorly to ensure adequate exposure. The bone is removed, usually using a high-speed drill or a Kerrison punch forceps. Adequate bone removal is critical to ensure an appropriate opening of the sac wall, and should be 6 to 8 mm. Once the bone window is removed and the medial wall of the sac is exposed, a surgical assistant should tent the mucosa medially with the lacrimal probe to allow the surgeon to incise the mucosa with a sickle knife, thereby opening the sac. The rest of the mucosa is removed with either a through-cut forceps or a microdebrider. Mucosal flaps can be used to line the tract, as described by Tsirbas and Wormald,[17] with the nasal mucosa and mucosa of the lacrimal sac cut and opposed so no bone is exposed. Once adequate resection is performed and an adequate DCR achieved, bicanalicular intubation is performed with Crawford tubes, which consist of two malleable stainless olive-tipped probes covered with a thin coating of silastic that forms an intervening silastic band. The probes are placed through the superior and inferior canaliculus, with subsequent retrieval in the nose through the rhinostomy site under direct endoscopic visualization. The probes are removed and the silastic band tied loosely, assuring that the medial canthus is not under tension.

Application of mitomycin C to the rhinostomy site to decrease stenosis has been described. Only one prospective randomized study evaluated the efficacy of adding mitomycin C in conjunction with silicone stenting without formal DCR. The study concluded that mitomycin C did not improve outcomes in patients experiencing epiphora for 6 months or less. However, in patients whose epiphora lasted more than 6 months, mitomycin C seemed to have some benefit.[18] If used, mitomycin C is usually applied with a cotton-tipped applicator at a concentration of 0.2 to 0.4 mg/mL for 2 to 5 minutes, with subsequent copious irrigation through the nasolacrimal system.

Postoperatively, patients are placed on a combination of antibiotic and steroid eye drops for 2 weeks and nasal saline irrigations twice a day. The timeframe for removal of the lacrimal stents varies, typically between 6 and 12 weeks. The success rates in the literature for endoscopic DCR range from 87% to 98%.[15,17,19–24] Most of these studies confirm the reported 90% to 95% success rate of the open approach, some authors consider the gold standard for treatment. As with most techniques, a learning curve is evident, as shown in a study by Onerci and colleagues,[25] who showed that the success rate was 94% in experienced hands versus 58% in inexperienced surgeons.

Complications of DCR can be categorized as minor or major. Minor complications include ecchymosis, cheek emphysema, orbital fat exposure, and stenosis, whereas major complications include bleeding into the orbit, medial rectus injury, lacerations to the inferior canaliculus, and cerebrospinal fluid leak.[26] The most common complication is persistent or recurrent epiphora secondary to stenosis of the rhinostomy or intranasal synechiae. Thus, frequent and meticulous postoperative evaluation with debridement is necessary to assure success.

SUMMARY

Due to the proximity of the lacrimal duct and sac to the uncinate process, occult injury to the lacrimal drainage system is common during uncinectomy and maxillary antrostomy. Fortunately, these injuries do not often progress to develop clinical symptoms as most either heal on their own, or drain into the middle meatus. In the event that injury to the lacrimal drainage system does become clinical evident, symptoms will present within the first two weeks following surgery. These symptoms may resolve over the ensuing weeks as the intranasal inflammation resolves. In cases of persistent epiphora, determination of the level of obstruction is critical for proper intervention. This can be achieved with several office-based studies as well as radiographic studies. If the obstruction is in the lacrimal duct, dacryocystorhinostomy is a highly successful surgical procedure. However, complications do occur with inadvertent violation of the orbit and cranial vault the subject of substantial publications while lacrimal duct injury (LDI) following FESS has been relatively neglected.

REFERENCES

1. Calhoun KH, Rotzler WH, Stiernberg CM. Surgical anatomy of the lateral nasal wall. Otolaryngol Head Neck Surg 1990;102:156–60.

2. Unlu HH, Goktan C, Aslan A, et al. Injury to the lacrimal apparatus after endoscopic sinus surgery: surgical implications from active transport dacryocystography. Otolaryngol Head Neck Surg 2001;124:308–12.
3. Hartikainen J, Seppa H, Grenman R. External DCR. Ophthalmology 1996;103:200.
4. Bolger WE, Parsons DS, Mair EA, et al. Lacrimal drainage system injury in functional endoscopic sinus surgery. Incidence, analysis, and prevention. Arch Otolaryngol Head Neck Surg 1992;118:1179–84.
5. Parsons DS, Stivers FE, Talbot AR. The missed ostium sequence and the surgical approach to revision functional endoscopic sinus surgery. Otolaryngol Clin North Am 1996;29:169–83.
6. Saengpanich S, Kerekhanjanarong V, Chochaipanichnon L, et al. Nasolacrimal duct injury from microscopic sinus surgery: preliminary report. J Med Assoc Thai 2001;84:562–5.
7. Freedman HM, Kern EB. Complications of intranasal ethmoidectomy: a review of 1,000 consecutive operations. Laryngoscope 1979;89:421–34.
8. Kennedy DW, Zinreich SJ, Shaalan H, et al. Endoscopic middle meatal antrostomy: theory, technique, and patency. Laryngoscope 1987;97:1–9.
9. Davis WE, Templer JW, Lamear WR, et al. Middle meatus anstrostomy: patency rates and risk factors. Otolaryngol Head Neck Surg 1991;104:467–72.
10. Unlu HH, Govsa F, Mutlu C, et al. Anatomical guidelines for intranasal surgery of the lacrimal drainage system. Rhinology 1997;35:11–5.
11. Serdahl CL, Berris CE, Chole RA. Nasolacrimal duct obstruction after endoscopic sinus surgery. Arch Ophthalmol 1990;108:391–2.
12. Toti A. Nuovo metodo conservative di cura radicalle dellesupporazioni chronicle del sacco lacrimale. Clin Mod Firenze 1904;10:385–9.
13. McDonogh M. Endoscopic transnasal dacryocystorhinostomy. Results in 21 patients. S Afr J Surg 1992;30:107–10.
14. McDonogh M, Meiring JH. Endoscopic transnasal dacryocystorhinostomy. J Laryngol Otol 1989;103:585–7.
15. Ramakrishnan VR, Hink EM, Durairaj VD, et al. Outcomes after endoscopic dacryocystorhinostomy without mucosal flap preservation. Am J Rhinol 2007;21:753–7.
16. Wormald PJ, Kew J, Van Hasselt A. Intranasal anatomy of the nasolacrimal sac in endoscopic dacryocystorhinostomy. Otolaryngol Head Neck Surg 2000;123:307–10.
17. Tsirbas A, Wormald PJ. Mechanical endonasal dacryocystorhinostomy with mucosal flaps. Br J Ophthalmol 2003;87:43–7.
18. Tabatabaie SZ, Heirati A, Rajabi MT, et al. Silicone intubation with intraoperative mitomycin C for nasolacrimal duct obstruction in adults: a prospective, randomized, double-masked study. Ophthal Plast Reconstr Surg 2007;23:455–8.
19. Tripathi A, Lesser TH, O'Donnell NP, et al. Local anaesthetic endonasal endoscopic laser dacryocystorhinostomy: analysis of patients' acceptability and various factors affecting the success of this procedure. Eye (Lond) 2002;16:146–9.
20. Massegur H, Trias E, Adema JM. Endoscopic dacryocystorhinostomy: modified technique. Otolaryngol Head Neck Surg 2004;130:39–46.
21. Fayet B, Racy E, Assouline M. Complications of standardized endonasal dacryocystorhinostomy with unciformectomy. Ophthalmology 2004;111:837–45.
22. Durvasula VS, Gatland DJ. Endoscopic dacryocystorhinostomy: long-term results and evolution of surgical technique. J Laryngol Otol 2004;118:628–32.

23. Wormald PJ, Tsirbas A. Investigation and endoscopic treatment for functional and anatomical obstruction of the nasolacrimal duct system. Clin Otolaryngol Allied Sci 2004;29:352–6.
24. Javate R, Pamintuan F. Endoscopic radiofrequency-assisted dacryocystorhinostomy with double stent: a personal experience. Orbit 2005;24:15–22.
25. Onerci M, Orhan M, Ogretmenoglu O, et al. Long-term results and reasons for failure of intranasal endoscopic dacryocystorhinostomy. Acta Otolaryngol 2000; 120:319–22.
26. Badilla J, Dolman PJ. Cerebrospinal fluid leaks complicating orbital or oculoplastic surgery. Arch Ophthalmol 2007;125:1631–4.

Prevention and Management of Orbital Hematoma

Vijay R. Ramakrishnan, MD[a], James N. Palmer, MD[b,*]

KEYWORDS

• Orbital hemorrhage • Orbital hematoma • Lateral canthotomy

Orbital hematoma is defined as a collection of blood inside the orbit, and the major adverse sequelae that develop arise because the orbit is a bony cone with tight fascial attachments holding the globe at its anterior edge. Therefore, the occurrence of orbital bleeding and hematoma formation can cause the pressure in the globe to increase rapidly, causing damage to sensitive structures inside the orbit. Orbital hematoma is best grouped into categories of spontaneous, traumatic, or iatrogenic. The iatrogenic category is a feared complication of endoscopic sinus surgery (ESS), blepharoplasty, or reconstructive trauma surgery. Awareness, diagnosis, and management of this complication is essential for every head and neck surgeon when operating near or in the orbit. Orbital complications of ESS occur in fewer than 0.4% of cases.[1,2] Known contributing factors to orbital complications during ESS are surgeon disorientation, bleeding, scarring from prior surgery, and preexisting medial wall abnormality. Some surgeons believe orbital complications occur more frequently on the right side for right-handed surgeons because of the loss of orientation performing surgical dissection towards oneself.

The most commonly described mechanism for orbital hemorrhage during ESS is transection of the anterior ethmoid artery and subsequent retraction of the bleeding artery into the orbit. Increased intraorbital pressure or vasospasm of the central retinal artery then causes blindness from retinal or optic nerve ischemia. Animal models of central retinal artery ischemia suggest that irreversible blindness may occur within 100 minutes. However, clinical reports of permanent blindness have occurred within 1 hour. Early diagnosis and therapy are essential, because permanent sequelae, such as vision loss, are reversible or preventable. This article first reviews the surgical anatomy and strategies for preventing orbital hemorrhage, and then reviews immediate evaluation and treatment strategies for this dreaded complication of ESS.

[a] Department of Otolaryngology, University of Colorado Denver, Denver, CO, USA
[b] Division of Rhinology, Department of ORL:HNS, University of Pennsylvania, 5 Ravdin, 3400 Spruce Street, Philadelphia, PA 19104, USA
* Corresponding author.
E-mail address: james.palmer@uphs.upenn.edu

Otolaryngol Clin N Am 43 (2010) 789–800
doi:10.1016/j.otc.2010.04.006 oto.theclinics.com

SURGICAL ANATOMY

The orbit is a conical shaped cavity roughly 4 x 5 cm in size. Seven bones contribute to the orbit: maxillary, lacrimal, ethmoid, frontal, zygomatic, sphenoid, and palatine (**Fig. 1**). The thickness of these bones along the orbit is variable, but the medial and inferior walls are the thinnest, less than 1 mm in certain places. Natural dehiscences are uncommon in the medial orbital wall, also known as the *lamina papyracea*. The orbit is surrounded by bony walls on all sides except anteriorly, where fascial planes hold the globe in position. The globe is supported by the extraocular muscles, which are suspended by several ligaments to the bony orbit. Increased intraorbital pressure therefore causes proptosis, but the amount of globe protrusion is limited by these tendons and ligaments. As pressures approach mean arterial pressure, decreased arterial perfusion of the retina and optic nerve occur, and venous outflow may also be impaired. To release the globe anteriorly for temporary pressure relief, division of the medial or lateral canthal connections is required.

The arterial supply of the orbit and neighboring ethmoid region comes from the internal carotid artery distribution (**Fig. 2**). The anterior and posterior ethmoid arteries arise from the internal carotid artery through the ophthalmic branch, therefore embolization is not recommended because of the risk for blindness, embolus, and stroke. If needed, these arteries may be ligated through transcutaneous or transconjunctival approaches to the medial orbit. In certain cases, endoscopic transethmoid ligation is possible. The anterior ethmoidal foramen is found on the medial orbital wall 24 mm back from the anterior orbital margin. The posterior ethmoidal foramen is located another 12 mm posteriorly, and the optic foramen another 6 mm posteriorly. The optic foramen typically transmits the ophthalmic artery on the inferolateral aspect of the optic nerve, but it may enter on the inferomedial side in rare cases. When viewed from the lateral aspect, the axial plane containing the anterior and posterior ethmoid

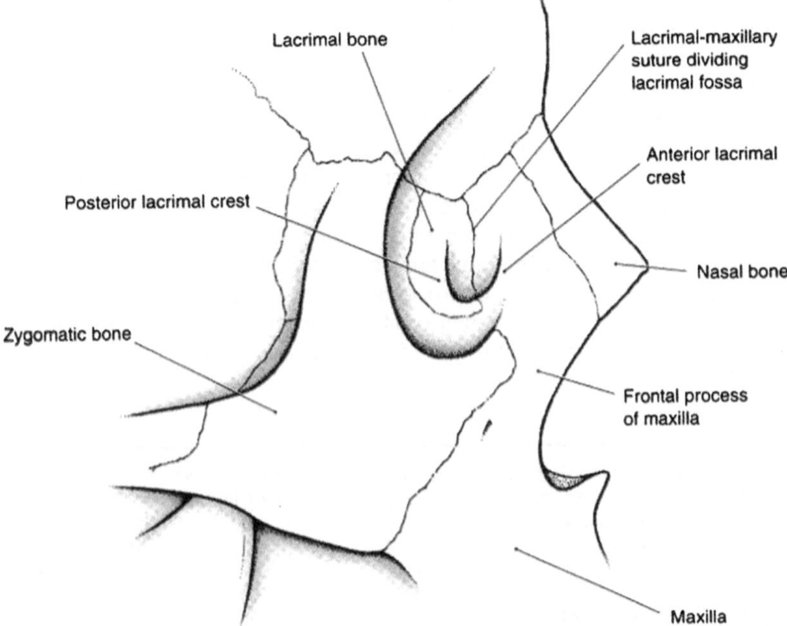

Fig. 1. External bony relationships of the orbit.

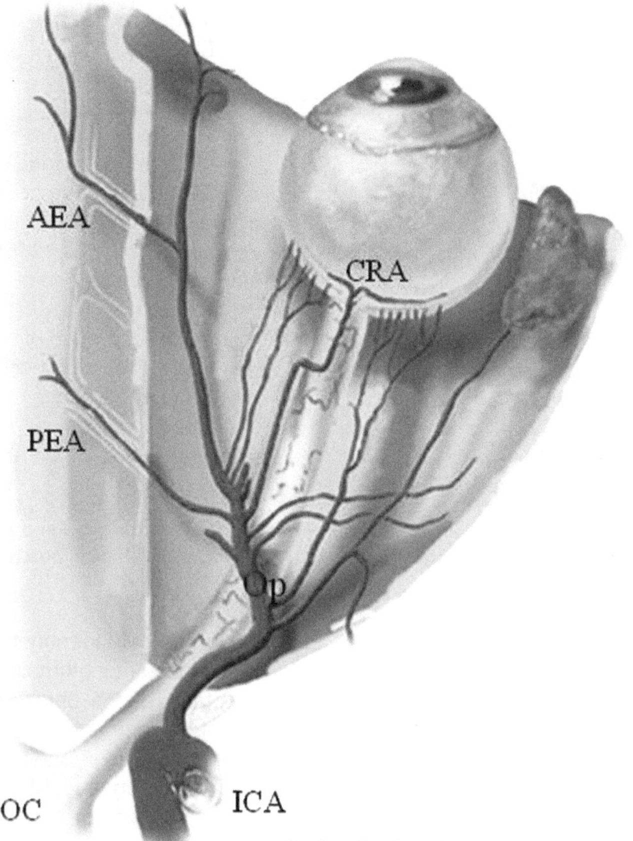

Fig. 2. Arteries of the orbit from the internal carotid artery. AEA, anterior ethmoid artery; CRA, central retinal artery; ICA, internal carotid artery; OC, optic chiasm; Op, ophthalmic artery; PEA, posterior ethmoid artery.

arteries corresponds roughly to the level of the skull base. Venous drainage lies within the connective tissue septa of the orbital fat, making extensive fat manipulation at surgery a risk factor for hemorrhage.

The anterior ethmoid artery is considered the posterior boundary of the frontal recess, and is often encountered in complete ethmoid and frontal dissections. Cadaveric study has shown that 91% of anterior ethmoid arteries are located within the skull base or 1 to 2 mm below, whereas 9% are suspended in a mesentery artery. The precise location of the anterior ethmoid artery can be found on coronal CT scan as a pinch or "nipple" between the medial rectus and superior oblique muscles (**Fig. 3**). The posterior ethmoid artery travels in a less accessible bony canal just anterior to the sphenoid face.

PREVENTION

Meticulous perioperative planning is crucial to avoid complication, and prevention of orbital hemorrhage is no different. Optimization of hemostasis and visualization will help avoid entrance into the orbit or injury to the anterior and posterior ethmoid

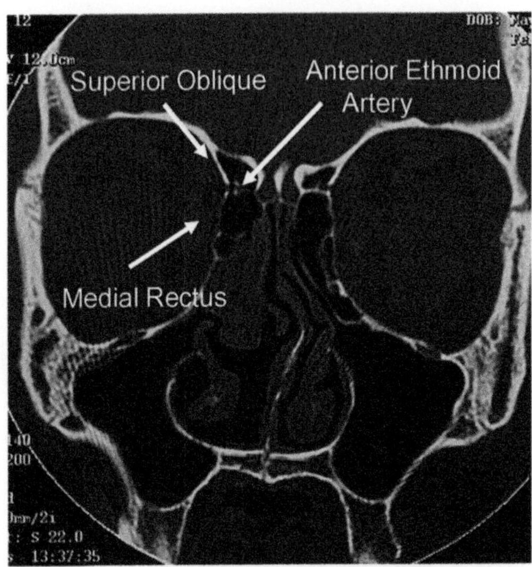

Fig. 3. Coronal CT showing the anterior ethmoid artery exiting the orbit and crossing the ethmoid sinus at the point where the medial rectus and superior oblique muscles converge.

arteries. Preoperative review of patient-specific anatomy should identify the location or presence of (1) the anterior ethmoid artery, (2) the posterior ethmoid artery, (3) medial orbital slope and dehiscence, and (4) atelectasis of the uncinate process (**Fig. 4**). Image guidance may assist certain cases, but is primarily a tool to verify anatomy. The operating surgeon should never rely solely on the image guidance for dissection.[3] At the onset of the case, the registration accuracy should be checked by comparing it with fixed intranasal anatomy, such as the floor of the nasal cavity, the posterior wall of the maxillary sinus, or the anterior face of the sphenoid.

Certain preferences of surgical technique may also minimize the risk for orbital hemorrhage. For instance, the uncinate process may be safely removed in an anterograde fashion with a sickle knife.[4] However, the blind insertion of the knife into the infundibulum is associated with an inherent risk to the orbit. The authors prefer to remove the uncinate process in a retrograde fashion with backbiting forceps. As the infundibulum is opened and the medial orbit is visualized, the remainder of the uncinate can be removed with a through-cutting forceps. During the subsequent ethmoid dissection, identifying the medial orbital wall early is preferable, rather than avoiding it altogether. In this fashion, the orbit can be followed and protected. This philosophy is similar to that for parotid surgery: better to identify the facial nerve and protect it than to blindly try to avoid the nerve, or in this case the lamina papyracea and the medial orbital wall.

After the skull base is identified in the sphenoid or posterior ethmoid sinus, retrograde dissection along the skull base must be performed with care to identify and preserve the anterior and posterior ethmoid arteries. The posterior ethmoid artery is rarely encountered, but the anterior ethmoid artery is reliably encountered posterior to the frontal recess, and can often be on a pedicle that is easily damaged. Use of through-cutting forceps or a curette along the skull base in these regions can directly injure these arteries. In this setting, bipolar electrocautery is preferred over monopolar cautery for hemostasis to prevent current running through the orbit.

Early detection of violation of the lamina papyracea and possible fat exposure is key to avoiding a more serious complication. In the setting of medial orbital wall

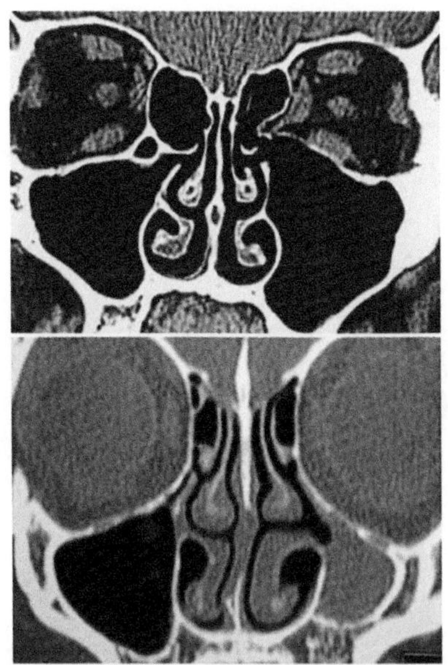

Fig. 4. Coronal CT scans of dehiscent left medial orbital wall (superior) and atelectactic left uncinate process (inferior CT scan).

dehiscence or fat exposure, the microdebrider should not be used, because rapid debridement of soft tissue (fat, muscle, nerve) can occur (**Fig. 5**). The suction portion of the microdebrider can pull not only fat but also the medial rectus muscle into the cutting blade. When the lamina is intact, the microdebrider is used with extreme caution along the medial orbit, and the opening of the debrider tip is never turned toward the orbit. Free mucosa, polyps, and thin bony partitions along the orbit are removed with through-cutting forceps or a microdebrider turned perpendicular to the orbit.

If the lamina papyracea is violated with no other damage, avoidance of nose blowing and strenuous activity is recommended in the postoperative setting. In the recovery room, the head of bed is elevated, ice packs are placed over the midface, and serial visual acuity checks are performed. Orbital hemorrhage may occur in a delayed fashion, and patients should be made aware of worrisome symptoms, although fortunately these are rare. On discharge, patients are counseled to notify the physician immediately or return to the emergency room if they experience eye pain, swelling or bruising around the eye, or decreased vision.

EVALUATION

Two types of orbital hemorrhage have been hypothesized.[1] A slow hemorrhage may occur from venous or capillary bleeding, whereas a sudden hemorrhage is usually attributed to arterial injury. Spontaneous orbital hematoma is usually a slow venous hemorrhage, iatrogenic hematoma is usually arterial, and traumatic hematoma may be either. Evaluation and management of both types of hemorrhage are similar, although arterial causes may result in higher intraorbital pressures. Typical signs include proptosis, resistance to retropulsion, lid edema and ecchymosis, chemosis, subconjunctival hemorrhage, and afferent pupillary defect. Patient who are awake may report pain, diplopia, color vision loss, or loss of acuity.

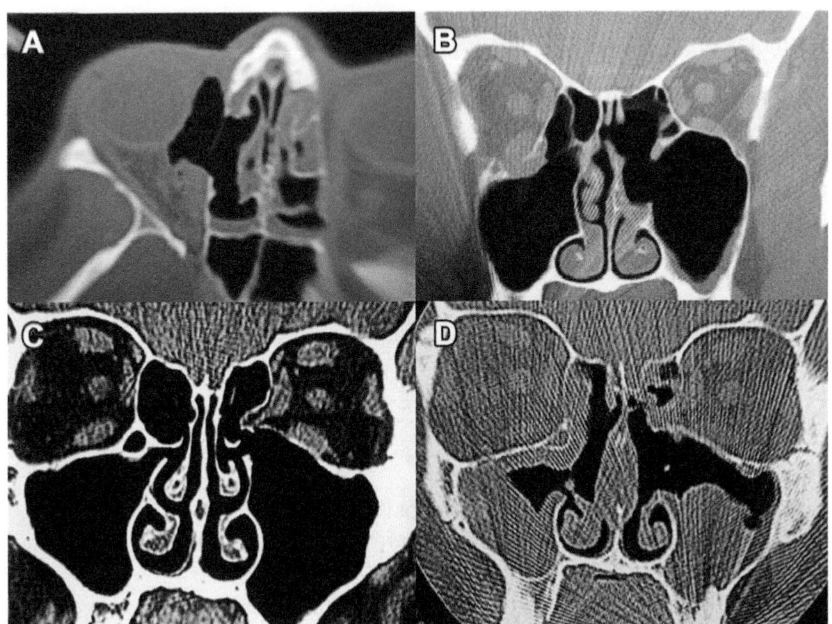

Fig. 5. Multiple images of damage to extraocular muscles during endoscopic sinus surgery. (*A*) Damage to medial rectus muscle and optic nerve. (*B*) Damage to inferior rectus muscle in roof of maxillary sinus. (*C*) Preoperative image of a well-functioning orbit before endoscopic sinus surgery. (*D*) Postoperative image with new-onset medial rectus muscle palsy.

During surgery, the eyes are taped so that they may be frequently examined. A typical sinus surgery case may last a few hours, and if occult orbital hemorrhage occurs without early recognition, irreversible damage may occur before the surgeon is aware of a problem. Intraoperatively, the globes should be periodically balloted as a gross barometer of intraorbital pressure and to endoscopically search for areas of dehiscence.

Intraoperatively, the surgeon's awareness should heighten if the medial orbit is penetrated, orbital fat is visualized, or significant bleeding occurs along the skull base or posterior frontal recess. Postoperatively, if the patient reports pain, diplopia, periorbital ecchymosis or edema, or loss of acuity or color vision, orbital hemorrhage must be suspected. Immediate and serial examination for the above signs must be performed, including resistance to retropulsion, swinging flashlight test, ocular motility, and visual acuity. If hemorrhage is suspected, nasal packing must be removed or minimized and an ophthalmologist should be consulted emergently. The ophthalmologic examination should include tonometric measurement of orbital pressure and retinal examination. Normal intraocular pressure is less than 20 mm Hg. The retina may appear pale if central retinal artery perfusion is restricted. Serial examinations must be performed, because orbital hematoma can be an evolving process.

MANAGEMENT

Management of orbital hematoma and prevention of vision loss require serial examination, and frequently require multiple levels of therapy. Control of epistaxis and hemorrhage is often the first step, and may occur before hematoma development. Bipolar electrocautery is the preferred method of hemostasis along the skull base and orbit. Topical hemostatic agents, such as Avitene (Davol, Cranston, RI, USA) or Flo-seal (Baxter, Fremont, CA, USA), may help with slow-flow bleeding. Nasal packing should be kept to a minimum, because it will force bleeding to stay in the orbital space and further increase intraocular pressure. If bulky nasal packing is present, this should be removed.

Surgeons should remember that in orbital hemorrhage, the actual volume of blood is never life-threatening and would never even require a transfusion; the fact that the hematoma formed is under pressure is what causes blindness. An ophthalmology consult should be called as soon as an orbital hematoma is suspected, and the procedure should be aborted or quickly terminated. Brief orbital massage may stop intraorbital bleeding and redistribute intraocular and extraocular fluids. Orbital massage is contraindicated in patients who have undergone prior ocular surgery.

Several medical therapies exist to decrease intraorbital pressure. Mannitol (20%, 1–2 g/kg over 30 minutes) is administered intravenously and may work quickly. High-dose intravenous steroids Decadron (Merck, Whitehouse Station, NJ, USA), 8–10 mg every 8 hours for 3–4 doses) are also recommended. Acetazolamide (500 mg intravenously) may be administered, but has a slow onset of effect because it functions to decrease aqueous humor production. Timolol drops (0.5%, 1–2 drops topically twice daily) also function to decrease aqueous humor production. Conservative medical therapies may not have a rapid or pronounced effect, and surgeons must work with the ophthalmologists to determine if more intervention is necessary. Consistently elevated pressures, poor or worsening visual acuity, and severe pain may warrant further intervention (**Fig. 6**).

Pressure relief can be achieved rapidly with lateral canthotomy and inferior cantholysis, or orbital decompression. Canthotomy and cantholysis provide the most pressure relief (14–30 mm Hg), and decompression can be expected to relieve an additional 10 mm Hg. Rarely, the anterior or posterior ethmoid artery will need to be identified and ligated. Indications for surgical intervention include intraorbital pressure greater than 40 mm Hg, presence of afferent pupillary defect, poor or worsening visual acuity, severe retro-orbital pain, and visualization of a pale retina with a cherry red macula.

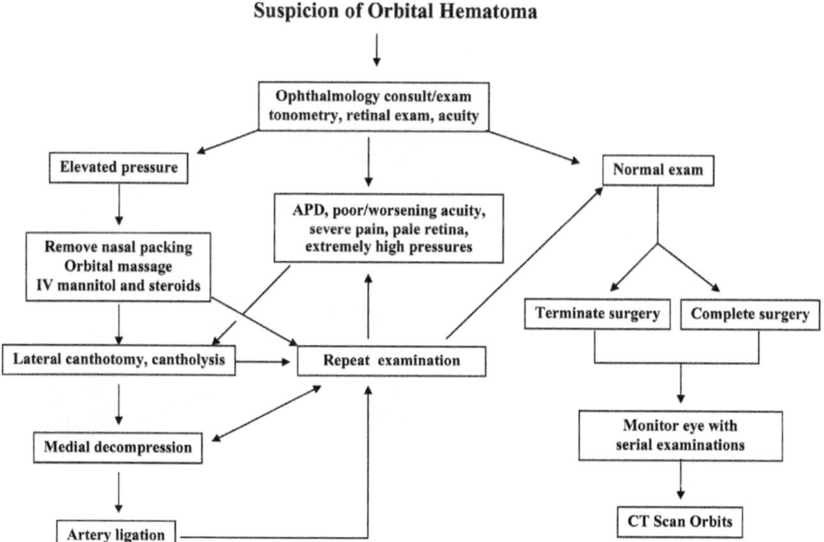

Fig. 6. Algorithm for management orbital hematoma.

Lateral Canthotomy and Cantholysis

All otorhinolaryngologists should understand the principles of lateral canthotomy and cantholysis. Canthotomy and cantholysis allow for pressure release through expansion of the orbital volume anteriorly. The procedure begins with infiltration of the lateral canthal region with 1% lidocaine with 1:100 K epinephrine. A horizontal incision is made from the lateral convergence of the upper and lower lids down to the orbital rim with a #15 scalpel or sharp scissor. The lower lid is then retracted anteriorly and inferiorly, and the inferior portion of the lateral canthal tendon is identified through palpation with the tip of a scissor. Palpation of the taut, retracted tendon is often compared with plucking a guitar string. The inferior crus of the tendon is then cut and the orbital tissues should release anteriorly (**Fig. 7**). The lower lid will freely swing and orbital fat may be visible (**Fig. 8**).

The inferior cantholysis is the most important portion of this procedure. In one study, lateral canthotomy alone decreased intraocular pressure by 14 mm Hg, whereas inferior cantholysis reduced pressure by 30 mm Hg.[5] The wound is left open until the primary disease is adequately controlled, and a delayed repair may be performed with an excellent cosmetic result.

Orbital Decompression

Removal of the middle turbinate may be considered to optimize visualization and instrumentation. Uncinectomy, maxillary antrostomy, total ethmoidectomy, sphenoidotomy, and frontal recess dissection should be complete before decompression. These sinuses are opened widely to provide adequate access to the orbit and prevent postoperative obstruction and sinusitis after orbital fat is ultimately released into the

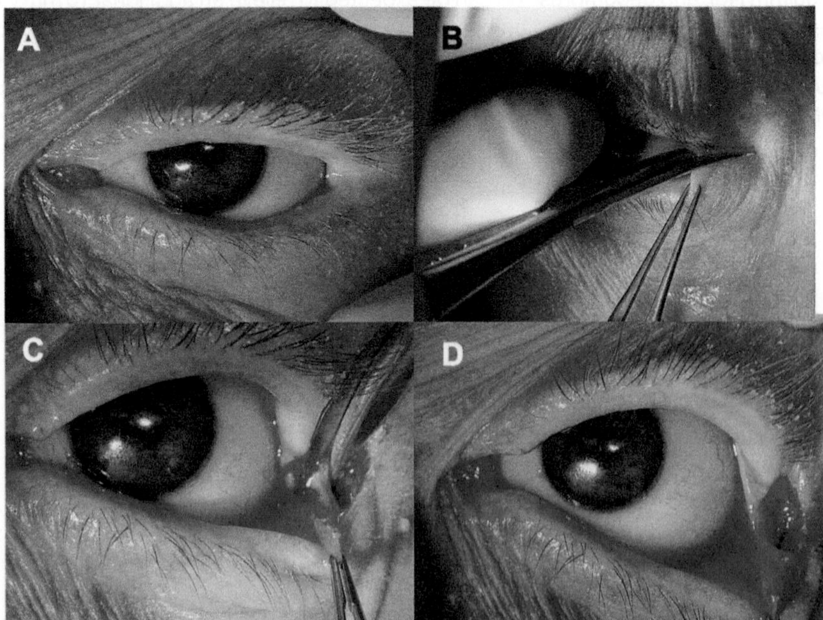

Fig. 7. (*A*) Preoperative view of orbit. (*B*) Incision for lateral canthotomy. (*C*) Identification and incision of inferior canthal tendon, completing cantholysis. (*D*) View after lateral canthotomy and inferior cantholysis, creating maximal immediate decompression by allowing eyeball and orbital contents to move anterior.

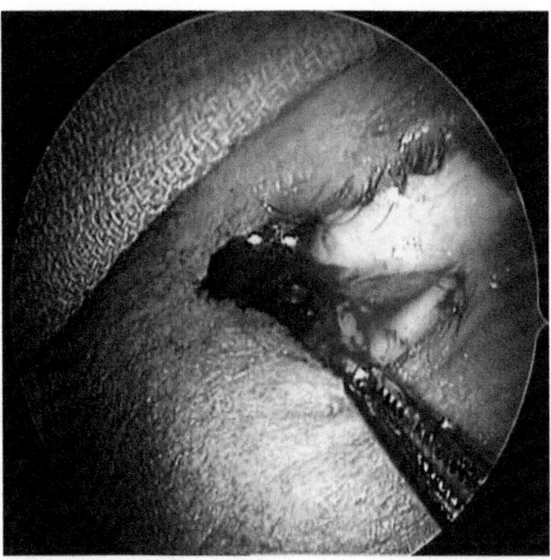

Fig. 8. Lax appearance of inferior lateral canthus after lateral cantholysis and inferior canthotomy.

ethmoid cavity. If the medial orbit is still intact, the lamina papyracea is palpated for its thinnest area, and this site is fractured with an elevator or ball-tipped probe. Surrounding thin bone of the lamina is then flaked away, ideally leaving the periorbita intact. Early entry into the periorbita may spill orbital fat into the operative field and make the ensuing dissection more challenging. Ideally, the entirety of the medial orbital wall is removed, leaving a maxillary orbital strut, and 1 to 1.5 cm around the frontal recess to prevent subsequent frontal sinus obstruction from herniated orbital fat. Thorough removal of the lamina may relieve some orbital pressure, but incision of the periorbita and fat release into the ethmoid cavity will maximize the effect of this procedure. The medial periorbita is incised serially from posterior to anterior, beginning superiorly and finishing inferiorly (**Fig. 9**). The medial portion of the orbital floor may also be decompressed endoscopically; however, this is not routinely performed for treating orbital hematoma.

Approaches to Medial Orbit for Ligation of Ethmoid Arteries

If continued hemorrhage and elevated pressures occur, or suspicion of continued arterial bleeding is high, ligation of the anterior and posterior ethmoid arteries may be of value. The selection of approach is based on the surgeon's experience and comfort. Traditional open approaches are reliable and successful but can be associated with scarring and potential disruption of the medial canthal anatomy and lacrimal system.

The Lynch incision and classic external ethmoidectomy approach can be used to reliably access the medial orbit. A corneal protector or tarsorrhaphy suture is initially placed. A 3-cm incision is created halfway between the medial canthus and nasal dorsum, beginning at the inferior aspect of the medial brow and traveling inferiorly to the level of the medial canthus. The skin and subcutaneous tissues are divided sharply and the angular vessels cauterized.

Subperiosteal dissection with a Freer elevator continues to the point of resistance at the medial canthal ligament. The ligament must be detached from its bony origin, and may be marked with a suture for later reapproximation. The lacrimal sac is elevated from the lacrimal fossa and retracted with the lateral soft tissues. The lamina

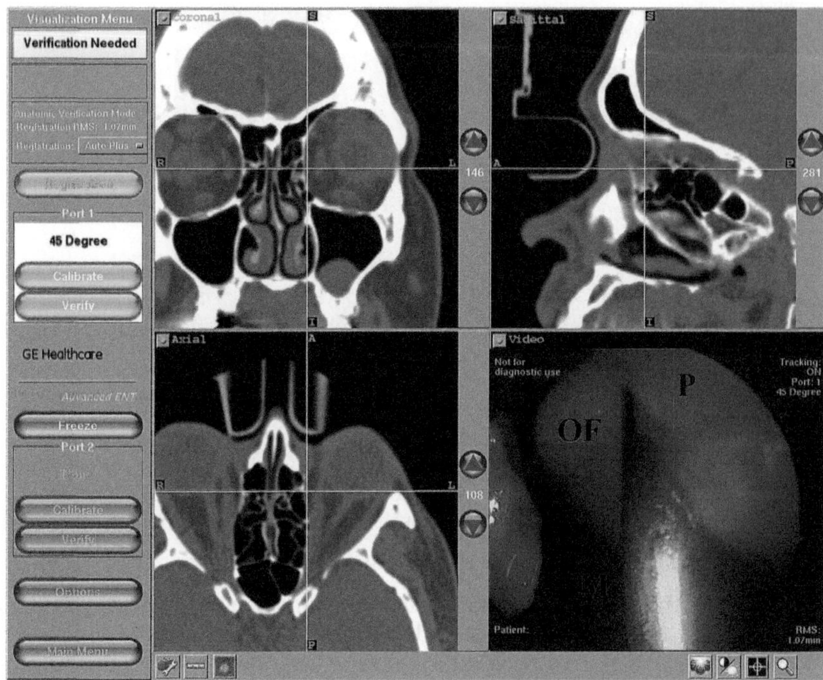

Fig. 9. Endoscopic picture of the lateral nasal wall as the periorbita is pierced by a sickle knife and the fat is allowed to prolapse into the ethmoid sinus as part of a medial orbital wall decompression. M, maxillary sinus; OF, orbital fat; P, periorbita.

papyracea is exposed and the frontoethmoidal suture line identified. The anterior ethmoid artery is usually found within this plane 14 to 18 mm posterior to the lacrimal–maxillary suture, but may range from 9 to 27 mm.[6] The posterior ethmoid artery is found 10 to 11 mm posterior to the anterior ethmoid artery but was found to be absent in 22 of 70 patients in the same anatomic study. Bipolar coagulation and division of the arteries may be performed as they are identified (**Fig. 10**).

Endoscopic transnasal ligation of the anterior ethmoid artery is possible in select cases. With a 30° endoscope, the location of the anterior ethmoid artery is visualized, and may be confirmed with image guidance. A small opening in the medial orbital wall is created with a ball-tipped probe or J-curette, and the lamina papyracea around the artery removed. Here, the periorbita is preserved to prevent herniation of orbital fat into the operative field. A periosteal elevator is used to dissect in the subperiosteal plane anterior and posterior to the artery. An angled clip applier can then be used to clip the isolated vessel.

SUMMARY

Orbital hematoma is an uncommon but serious complication of sinus surgery. Appropriate perioperative attention may minimize risk, but early diagnosis and appropriate management are crucial to preventing vision loss. The surgeon, postoperative care staff, and patient must be aware of the signs and symptoms. Immediate examination must be performed, including pupil size, symmetry, and reactivity, visual acuity, and measurement of intraocular pressure. Immediate consultation from an

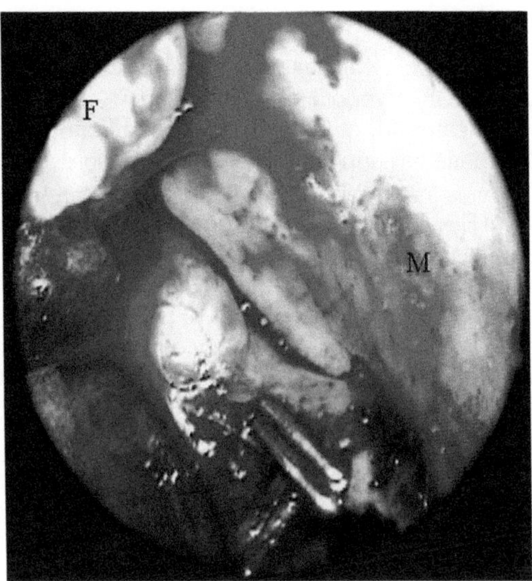

Fig. 10. Clip applied to anterior ethmoid artery. F, orbital fat; M, medial orbital wall.

ophthalmologist or oculoplastic surgeon is mandatory if the diagnosis is suspected. The surgeon and ophthalmologist should follow an algorithm of advancing therapies based on serial examination, ranging from observation only (**Fig. 11**) to immediate surgical intervention.

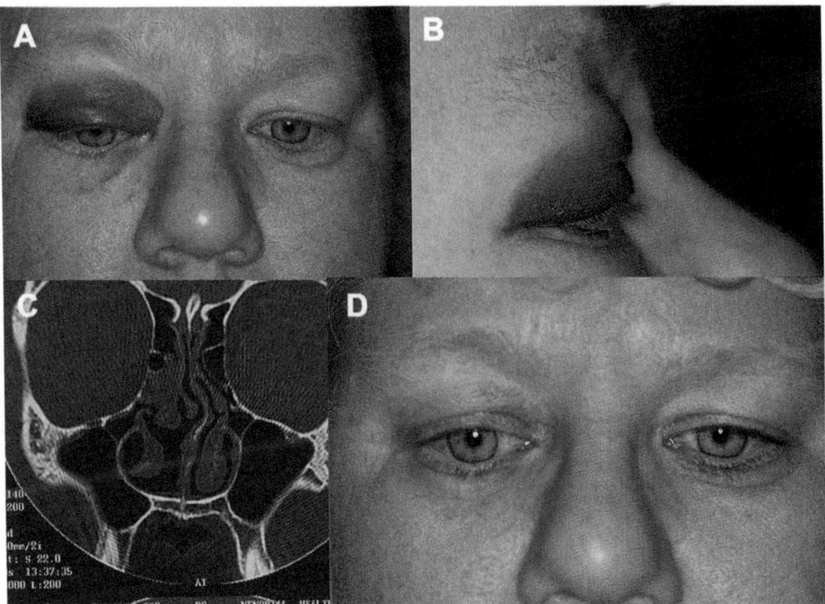

Fig. 11. Inadvertent injury to the anterior ethmoid artery and resultant immediate orbital hematoma. (*A*, *B*) Orbital pressures were not elevated, patient was observed. (*C*) Preoperative CT scan showing exposed anterior ethmoid artery in ethmoid. (*D*) Two weeks postoperative.

REFERENCES

1. Stankiewicz JA, Chow JM. Two faces of orbital hematoma in intranasal (endoscopic) sinus surgery. Otolaryngol Head Neck Surg 1999;120(6):841–7.
2. May M, Levine HL, Mester SJ, et al. Complications of endoscopic sinus surgery: analysis of 2108 patients—incidence and prevention. Laryngoscope 1994; 104(9):1080–3.
3. Kingdom TT, Orlandi RR. Image-guided surgery of the sinuses: current technology and applications. Otolaryngol Clin North Am 2004;37(2):381–400.
4. Wormald PJ, McDonogh M. The “swing-door” technique for uncinectomy in endoscopic sinus surgery. J Laryngol Otol 1998;112:547–51.
5. Yung CW, Moorth RS, Lindley D, et al. Efficacy of lateral canthotomy and cantholysis in orbital hemorrhage. Ophthal Plast Reconstr Surg 1994;10:137–41.
6. Kirchner JA, Yanagisawa E, Crelin ES. Surgical anatomy of the ethmoid arteries. Arch Otolaryngol 1961;74:382–6.

Prevention and Management of Medial Rectus Injury

Benjamin S. Bleier, MD*, Rodney J. Schlosser, MD

KEYWORDS

• Medial rectus injury • Orbital injury • Sinus surgery
• Opthalmology • Complication • Lamina papyracea

Orbital penetration represents a rare but serious complication of functional endoscopic sinus surgery. The proximity of the orbit to the surgical field coupled with the relatively thin bony partition of the lamina papyracea make this region particularly vulnerable to iatrogenic injury. Although violation of the medial orbital wall places the entire orbit at risk, the medial rectus represents the most commonly injured extraocular muscle during sinus surgery. Consequently, early recognition of medial rectus and associated orbital injuries is critical, as immediate diagnosis and intervention may have a dramatic effect on the long-term outcome of these patients.

The lamina papyracea comprises the medial orbital wall and is bounded laterally by orbital periosteum. This layer, which may also be referred to as periorbita, completely surrounds a layer of extraconal periorbital fat that encapsulates the orbit. Medially, this orbital fat is bounded by a fascial layer that ensheaths the extraocular musculature known as Tenon's capsule.[1] The medial rectus muscle originates from the annulus of Zinn and travels along the medial aspect of the globe to insert on the sclera. As the muscle travels anteriorly, it takes a slightly lateral course away from the lamina papyracea (**Fig. 1**). The medial rectus is innervated by the oculomotor nerve that traverses the superior orbital fissure and arborizes, giving off branches to the lateral aspect of the muscle.

PREOPERATIVE PREVENTION

Prevention of medial rectus injury relies on a comprehensive history and physical examination that should include a detailed analysis of the preoperative imaging. A history of prior surgery, maxillofacial trauma, sinonasal neoplasm, expansile inflammatory lesion, or primary orbital pathology should raise the suspicion of a potential

Financial disclosure: None.

Division of Rhinology, Department of Otolaryngology-Head and Neck Surgery, Medical University of South Carolina, 135 Rutledge Avenue, MSC 550, Charleston, SC 29425, USA
* Corresponding author.
E-mail address: bleierb@gmail.com

Otolaryngol Clin N Am 43 (2010) 801–807
doi:10.1016/j.otc.2010.04.007
oto.theclinics.com

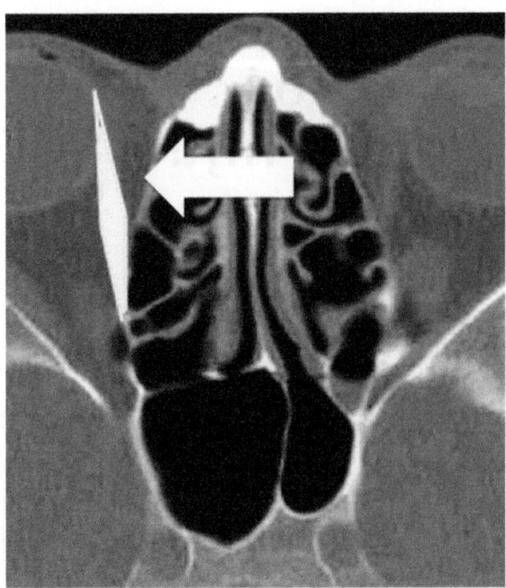

Fig. 1. Axial CT demonstrating increased width (*white arrow*) of the extraconal fat pat between the medial rectus (*white diamond*) and lamina papyracea adjacent to the anterior ethmoid sinuses.

preexisting dehiscence of the lamina (**Fig. 2**). Detailed analysis of the preoperative imaging should include an assessment of the morphology and integrity of the lamina including the position of ethmoid vasculature, complex sinus anatomy, and the presence of any prolapsed orbital contents within the sinonasal cavity. The presence of sinonasal disease may lead to obscuration of the lamina secondary to soft tissue and bleeding, and thus an accurate preoperative knowledge of its position allows the surgeon to safely proceed with the dissection. Image guidance may also be used to aid in the intraoperative identification of the medial orbital wall; however, it should not be used a substitute for rigorous preoperative planning.

INTRAOPERATIVE PREVENTION

Intraoperatively, the lamina should be identified early and skeletonized to provide a consistent anatomic landmark. When dissecting along the lamina, the force should be directed anteriorly, parallel to the face of the lamina, to prevent inadvertent penetration. When using powered instrumentation, the cutting aperture should always be visualized to ensure that tissue aspiration is highly controlled. The head of the debrider should never be pressed against the lamina but rather should remain several millimeters away, allowing the soft tissue to be pulled into the instrument. In regions of particular concern, the instrument should be activated intermittently to prevent the rapid suction and debridement of large volumes of tissue at any given time. During procedures in which the lamina is deliberately violated, such as during an orbital decompression, care should be taken to maintain integrity of the periorbita during the bony dissection (**Fig. 3**). The bone is removed in an anterior to posterior direction, taking advantage of the wider extraconal periorbital fat layer between the medial rectus and lamina in the anterior ethmoid cavity. During incision of the periorbita, the medial

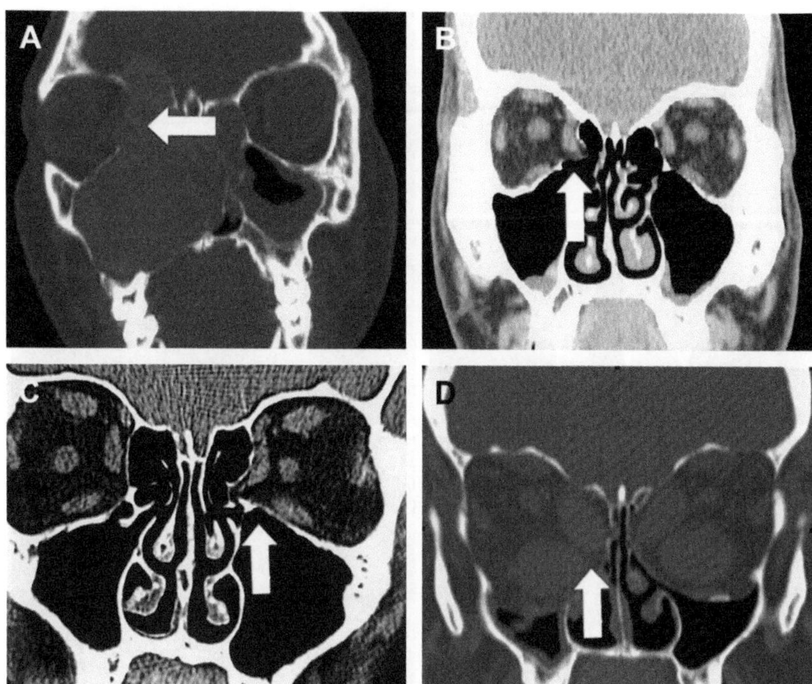

Fig. 2. Examples of preoperative deformities of the medial orbital wall (*denoted by white arrows*): erosion secondary to allergic fungal sinusitis (*A*), congenital dehiscence of the lamina (*B*), medially displaced medial rectus muscle (*C*), and decompressed orbit demonstrating massive extraocular muscle enlargement secondary to Graves' orbitopathy (*D*).

rectus may be visualized and the incision should be made superficially and, if possible, away from the muscle itself.

The overall incidence of medial rectus injury during sinus surgery is difficult to accurately determine because of its low frequency. One of the largest published series gathered a total of 30 cases from 10 large centers and reported an incidence of 1 of 735 over a 5-year period.[2] Although the incidence is low, when orbital injury does occur, the medial rectus is the most common extraocular muscle involved, followed by the inferior rectus.[3]

INTRAOPERATIVE MANAGEMENT

The mechanism of medial rectus injury has evolved over the past decade with the introduction of powered and radiofrequency surgical instrumentation; however, 4 broad patterns of injury are recognized and are associated with distinct symptoms and prognosis. The first pattern represents a complete or near complete transection of the muscle belly. This injury is associated with a large-angle exotropia and marked adduction deficit without an associated abduction deficit. The second pattern results from a contusion or hematoma within the muscle. Patients with this type of injury will exhibit a moderate to large angle exotropia with a combined abduction/adduction deficit. A similar symptom complex will occur with the third injury pattern, which results from damage to the oculomotor nerve as it enters the muscle. The fourth pattern consists of entrapment of the muscle or orbital fat and is associated with relatively mild deviation

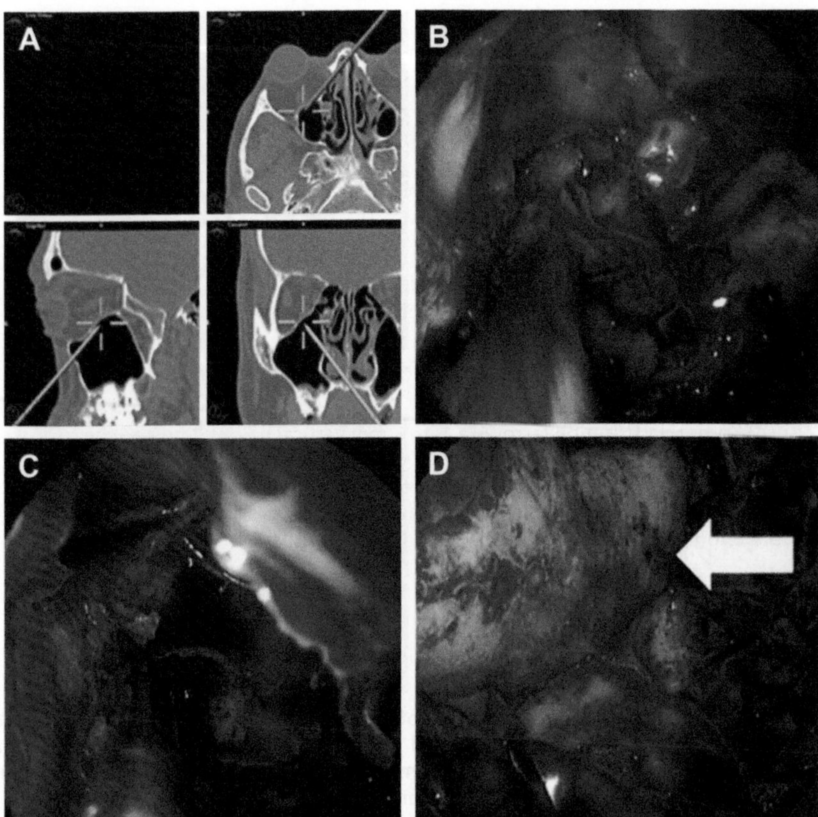

Fig. 3. Right orbital decompression with triplanar imaging of the orbit (*A*), intact lamina papyracea (*B*), anterior to posterior dissection of the lamina with intact periorbita (*C*), and the medial rectus muscle (*white arrow*) visualized through the periorbita at the orbital apex (*D*).

in primary gaze along with a marked abduction deficit.[2,4] This pattern may also result from disruption of Tenon's capsule, which can lead to scarring of the intraconal and extraconal fat with subsequent delayed entrapment symptomatology.[1]

Although there are case reports of temporary medial rectus injury in the setting of sinonasal radiofrequency ablation procedures,[5] it has been the widespread adoption of the powered microdebrider that has had the most dramatic impact on the patterns and severity of medial rectus injury.[1] The combination of suction and rapid tissue debridement allows for tissue to be resected from within the orbit even through very small or trapdoor types of lamina defects. As a result, these types of injuries are often irreparable secondary to the relatively large volumes of tissue loss.[6]

When a medial rectus injury is suspected, rapid assessment of the orbit for associated injuries plays a critical role in determining the need for acute or subacute management. Symptoms of a postoperative adduction deficit, diplopia, or conjunctival hemorrhage should prompt an immediate ophthalmologic consult with an examination including tonometry and fundoscopy to ensure perfusion of the optic nerve and retina.[6] Intraocular pressures (IOP) less than 30 mm Hg can typically be observed, whereas pressures exceeding 40 mm Hg may lead to a poor visual result. Fundoscopically, normal blood flow will result in arterial "flashing" or pulsing when digital pressure on the globe rises above that of diastolic pressure. A pathologically elevated IOP will lead to a loss of this flashing phenomenon when it exceeds systolic pressure. Over the ensuing hours, stagnant blood flow may lead to arterial clot formation or "boxcarring." A "cherry red spot" may also be seen, which results from the contrast of the red macula on the whiter edema of the surrounding ischemic retinal nerve layer. Of note, permanent ischemia has been noted in animal models within approximately 90 minutes.[6]

Pressures exceeding 40 mm Hg with a loss of the flashing phenomenon require immediate surgical decompression of the orbit. Traditionally, this has been done via a lateral canthotomy with upper and lower lid cantholysis, but the orbit can also be decompressed medially via endoscopic approaches. Although these maneuvers will reduce IOP, they may also act to reduce the tamponade effect resulting in continued bleeding. If pressures continue to rise or remain elevated, a formal orbital decompression should be performed. Administration of intravenous (IV) steroids, Diamox, Mannitol, and topical Timoptic eye drops will also help to reduce IOP (**Fig. 4**).[6]

Once the IOP has been addressed and the eye is considered safe, attention can be turned toward the management of the medial rectus injury. Treatment is predicated on an accurate assessment of the site, pattern, and extent of injury. Imaging represents an essential adjunct to the physical examination in determining the nature of the injury.

POSTOPERATIVE MANAGEMENT

Gadolinium-enhanced MRI is considered a superior modality to contrast-enhanced CT, as the normal appearance of muscle on CT does not preclude injury because it will not detect underlying edema in the acute to early subacute stage. Laceration or disruption may even be missed on CT, as the muscle may retract longitudinally and

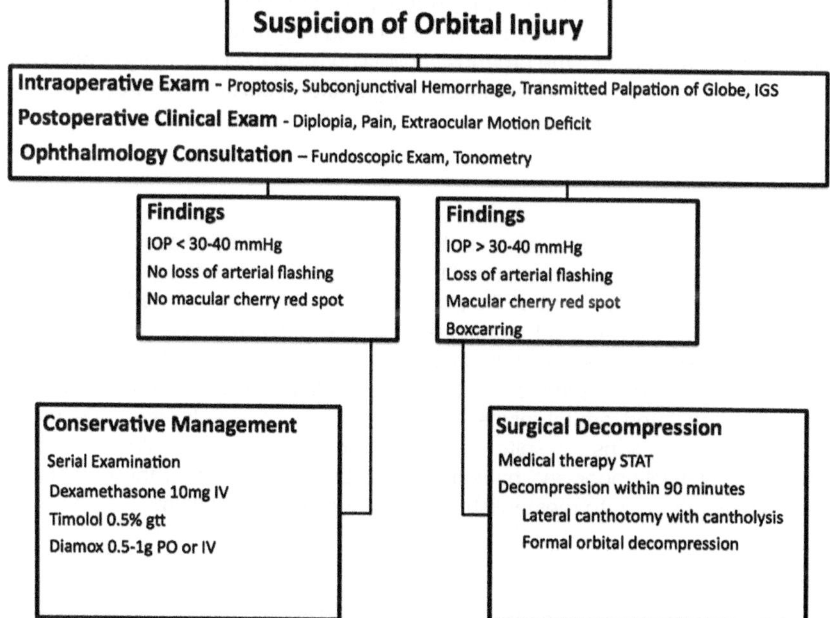

Fig. 4. Treatment algorithm for suspected orbital injury.

thus appear to be artificially enlarged on cross-sectional imaging.[5] MRI using surface coils, gaze-fixation targets, and rapid-sequence contrast techniques is able to generate 312-micron sagittal images, which allows for the visualization of individual muscle fiber bundles as well as motor nerves.[7] MRI is able to delineate different stages of injury as well. Early stages will demonstrate muscle enlargement secondary to edema or intramuscular hemorrhage. In the later stages, muscular atrophy or complete volume loss can be appreciated following partial or complete muscle transection, respectively. Examination of the intraorbital fat should also be performed to look for evidence of the early stages of diffuse edema or hemorrhage, which can lead to long-term scarring and fibrosis.[5]

Surgical management of medial rectus injury seeks to not only restore the adduction function of the muscle itself, but also to limit the fibrosis and contractile forces experienced by the antagonizing extraocular musculature. Although multiple studies have shown that treatment should be initiated within 3 to 4 weeks to prevent permanent scar contracture and fibrosis,[2,4,8] the only indication for immediate reexploration is a suspicion of entrapment.[4] In the setting of a complete transection, orbital exploration with direct reanastomosis is advocated if the posterior 20 mm of the muscle is felt to be present and functional.[3] Unfortunately, the volume loss related to muscle contraction and microdebrider-related injury often precludes a primary reanastomosis.[4] In this scenario, a variety of alternative approaches exist including muscle transposition and muscle-to-muscle anastomosis using an interposition graft or hang-back adjustable sutures. Despite these maneuvers, the involved muscle tends to lose its strength and often leads to restriction of ocular movement even after repair.[9]

Recently, the use of botulinum toxin has emerged as a useful adjunct to the surgical management of medial rectus injury. Botulinum toxin carries multiple potential advantages, as it facilitates single vision more rapidly, prevents secondary contraction of the antagonist muscle during the healing period, and minimizes the force generated against the muscle repair site. Early use of a course of three 5-U injections of botulinum toxin A at a dilution of 50 U/mL to the ipsilateral lateral rectus muscle within the first 3 to 4 weeks is advocated to avoid progressive muscle contracture. Despite these treatment algorithms, the prognosis following medial rectus injury is often quite poor and the reestablishment of a binocular single visual field is considered a successful result in most patients.[4]

SUMMARY

Medial rectus injury is an uncommon but often devastating complication of functional endoscopic sinus surgery. Prevention of these types of injuries is predicated on a thorough preoperative assessment of the position and integrity of the medial orbital wall coupled with excellent surgical technique. The use of powered instrumentation has led to more severe injuries and thus should be used with caution near critical structures such as the lamina papyracea. Early recognition and management of medial rectus and associated orbital injuries is critical to improve outcomes and prevent associated complications. Despite optimal surgical and medical interventions, the prognosis is relatively poor and patients should be counseled that the primary goal of these interventions is to reestablish a binocular single visual field.

KEY POINTS

- Although the overall incidence is low, the medial rectus is the most commonly injured extraocular muscle during functional endoscopic sinus surgery.

- Prevention of medial rectus injury relies on a thorough preoperative assessment including history, physical, and analysis of medial orbital wall on CT or MRI.
- A history of prior surgery, maxillofacial trauma, sinonasal neoplasm, inflammatory expansile lesion, or primary orbital pathology should all raise the suspicion of medial orbital dehiscence.
- Powered instrumentation has increased the severity of medial rectus injury and should be used with caution along the lamina papyracea.
- Orbital or medial rectus injury should be suspected with postoperative adduction deficit, vision changes, or conjunctival hemorrhage and should prompt an immediate ophthalmology consultation including tonometry and fundoscopy.
- Management of a medial rectus injury should be considered only after any associated elevation of intraocular pressure has been addressed.
- Gadolinium-enhanced MRI is useful in determining the site, extent, and pattern of medial rectus injury.
- Medial rectus injury may be managed with a combination of surgical reanastomosis and botulinum toxin injection; however, the primary goal of these interventions is to reestablish a binocular single visual field.

REFERENCES

1. Bhatti MT, Giannoni CM, Raynor E, et al. Ocular motility complications after endoscopic sinus surgery with powered cutting instruments. Otolaryngol Head Neck Surg 2001;125(5):501–9.
2. Huang CM, Meyer DR, Patrinely JR, et al. Medial rectus muscle injuries associated with functional endoscopic sinus surgery: characterization and management. Ophthal Plast Reconstr Surg 2003;19(1):25–37.
3. Thacker NM, Velez FG, Demer JL, et al. Extraocular muscle damage associated with endoscopic sinus surgery: an ophthalmology perspective. Am J Rhinol 2005;19(4):400–5.
4. Hong JE, Goldberg AN, Cockerham KP. Botulinum toxin A therapy for medial rectus injury during endoscopic sinus surgery. Am J Rhinol 2008;22(1):95–7.
5. Bhatti MT, Schmalfuss IM, Mancuso AA. Orbital complications of functional endoscopic sinus surgery: MR and CT findings. Clin Radiol 2005;60(8):894–904.
6. Graham SM, Nerad JA. Orbital complications in endoscopic sinus surgery using powered instrumentation. Laryngoscope 2003;113(5):874–8.
7. Demer JL. Anatomical diagnosis. Br J Ophthalmol 2006;90(6):664.
8. Penne RB, Flanagan JC, Stefanyszyn MA, et al. Ocular motility disorders secondary to sinus surgery. Ophthal Plast Reconstr Surg 1993;9(1):53–61.
9. Hong S, Lee HK, Lee JB, et al. Recession-resection combined with intraoperative botulinum toxin A chemodenervation for exotropia following subtotal ruptured of medial rectus muscle. Graefes Arch Clin Exp Ophthalmol 2007;245(1):167–9.

Prevention and Management of Skull Base Injury

Esther Kim, MD, Paul T. Russell, MD*

KEYWORDS

- Skull base injury • Skull base defect • CSF leak
- Microdebrider • Ethmoid defect

Skull base defects and injuries are rare, but may occur during endoscopic sinus surgery, as a result of facial trauma, or as a result of tumors in the anterior cranial fossa. Iatrogenic injuries resulting in CSF leaks through skull base defects have been noted to have an incidence of 0.46% to 0.85%.[1,2] Injury to the skull base can lead to catastrophic outcomes that include meningitis, brain abscess, neurologic deficits, brain hemorrhage and death. This content discusses ways in which a surgeon may work to prevent or minimize injury to the skull base. We also describe management of these injuries when they do occur, review the current literature, and describe various reconstruction techniques.

PREVENTION

If unrecognized, anatomic variations may contribute to surgical complication along the anterior skull base. One such anatomic variation that may occur along the ethmoid roof is described by the Keros classification, which measures the vertical height between the cribriform plate and the fovea ethmoidalis (**Table 1**).[3] In this classification, the depth of the olfactory fossa is categorized as 1 to 3 mm (Keros I), 3 to 7 mm (Keros II), or 7 to 16 mm (Keros III). As the bone in this region is typically quite thin, increased vertical height lends itself to increased vulnerability. In Keros' original study of 450 cadavers, 12% were found to be Keros I, 70% Keros II, and 18% Keros III. This proportion has been supported by several recent CT studies.[4,5] Also notable in recent studies has been asymmetry of greater than 2 mm in 8% of patients (**Fig. 1**).[5]

Pre-operative CT scans may also be evaluated for the presence of a low-lying skull base. Meyers and Valvassori found that a horizontal line drawn along the roof of the ethmoid passed above the vertical mid-point of the orbit in 88% of the cases studied. Approximately 10% of cases crossed the orbit at the vertical midplane and 2% of

Division of Rhinology, Department of Otolaryngology, Vanderbilt University Medical Center, 7209 Medical Center East-South Tower, 1215 21st Avenue South, Nashville, TN 37232-8605, USA
* Corresponding author.
E-mail address: paul.t.russell@vanderbilt.edu

Otolaryngol Clin N Am 43 (2010) 809–816
doi:10.1016/j.otc.2010.04.018
oto.theclinics.com
0030-6665/10/$ – see front matter

Table 1
Keros classification

Classification	Depth of the Olfactory Fossa
Type I	1–3 mm
Type II	3–7 mm
Type III	8–16 mm
Asymmetric	Asymmetric

cases were below the vertical midplane.[6] Stankiewicz and Chow built on this data from Meyers and Valvassori's study to develop safety zones based on the relationship of the skull base to the level of the orbit. **Fig. 2** depicts this concept with zone 1 being the safest. When the horizontal line drawn from the roof of the ethmoid crosses the upper one-third of the orbit, this is considered the most safe anatomic arrangement.[7] Caution is to be used in cases in which the ethmoid roof crosses below the midplane of the orbit.

Other anatomic considerations when working along the skull base include the extent of sinus disease. Extensive disease can affect visualization during surgery due to increased inflammation and consequent intra-operative bleeding. Intra-operative bleeding has been noted to be significant in several case series that discussed iatrogenic skull base injuries, and this bleeding may be related to the extent of inflammation and sinus disease.[7,8] On the other hand, DelGaudio and colleagues[9,10] found that 74% of skull base injuries occurred in patients with minimal or no mucosal disease. They postulated that injury was a result of less resistance and thinner bone in the less diseased sinuses. Diseased sinuses may have thicker bone as a result of sinus oteoneogenesis.

Use of powered instruments, such as the microdebrider, are commonplace in the surgical management of sinus disease. A microdebrider suctions while a rotating blade cuts through the tissue suctioned into the device. Consequently, a significant amount of tissue can be removed quickly. Due to this aggressive cutting nature, a microdebrider should be used very judiciously along susceptible areas such as

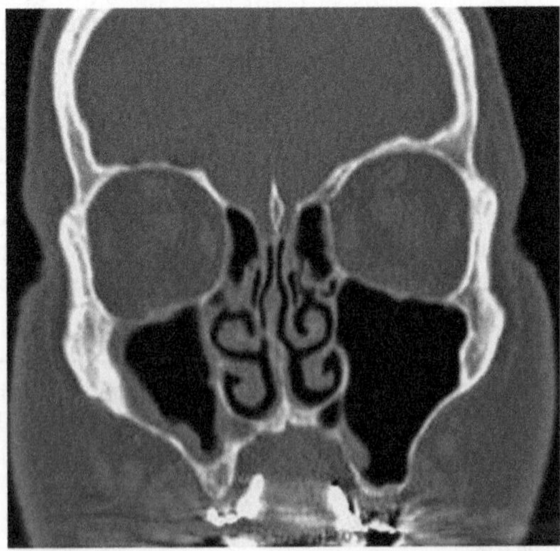

Fig. 1. Asymmetric cribriform plate with Keros Type III.

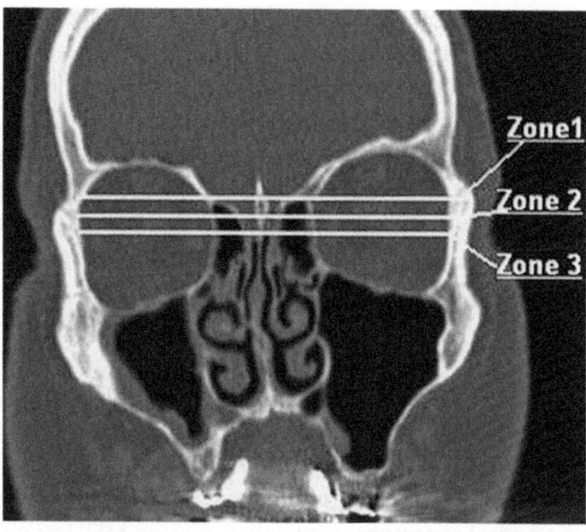

Fig. 2. Zones of safety for skull base. Zone 1: safest skull base position, Zone 3: lowest skull base position.

the skull base. Surgeons may consider using through biting instruments and grasping instruments in these more vulnerable areas.[8] One must always remember that injuries can occur regardless of instrument or technique.

There are two differing approaches when performing sinus surgery. Messerklinger advocated surgery that involved the anterior ethmoid cavities. He did not advocate aggressive surgical dissection beyond the anterior ethmoid for he felt that the larger sinuses improved when the ventilation of these sinuses improved with the ethmoidectomy.[10] As a result, the surgery is often performed in a front to back technique. Alternatively, Wigand describes performing surgery in a back-to-front approach. This technique may allow for easier identification of the skull base earlier in the procedure.[11] We favor this approach in sinus surgery since there is early identification of the skull base, and we believe that the downward angle of the skull base favors a posterior to anterior dissection as a means to avoid inadvertent penetration of the skull base.

Institutions throughout the country train hundreds of residents annually. Close supervision is paramount in sinus surgery. Bumm and colleagues[2] reported the most injuries occurred performed by surgeons in the second half of their residency. These surgeons had performed between 100 and 300 sinus surgeries and typically were unsupervised until the end of the case. The study concluded that this particular group of trainees had enough training to feel falsely safe. This study also noted a difference in location of injury. Early in training, the injuries were noted to be at the anterior ethmoid near the medial concha base (lateral lamella, cribriform plate) whereas, skull base injuries with more experienced surgeons were located in the immediate vicinity of the frontal sinus.[2] Institutions that train residents should consider dissection techniques that allow for the largest margin of safe surgery.

Image guided systems are used regularly in the operating room. When using image guidance, the surgeon should understand the target recognition error (TRE) implicit in this technology. TRE is defined as the location of targets interest compared with the corresponding locations on CT scan. It will vary depending on the position as it relates to the fiducial. Labadie and colleagues[12] concluded that the TRE was approximately 2 mm. Therefore, this technology functions with a built-in margin of error, and is not a substitute for an in-depth understanding of sinus and skull base anatomy.

Meticulous registration and cross checking of the instruments will improve accuracy, however, it is imperative that the surgeon not over rely on the accuracy of the device.

Having a surgical plan with each operation is important. Mapping out a plan of action with a pre-operative CT scan may lessen the likelihood of injury. On a CT scan, the Keros classification, length, height and slope of the skull base, asymmetry of the cribriform plate, and dehiscence of bony structures should be evaluated before surgery. By performing this review with each patient's CT preoperatively, one may develop an increased understanding of which particular anatomic abnormalities to expect during surgery.

MANAGEMENT OF SKULL BASE INJURY

If a skull base injury occurs, the defect should be thoroughly assessed. If evaluated in a post-operative setting, the assessment should include nasal endoscopy. Collection of the rhinorrhea for beta-2 transferrin can confirm a true CSF leak. A preoperative CT scan can help detect the extent of the injury and localization when done in thin slices (1 mm) with coronal and sagittal reconstructions.[13] Often an MRI is performed to assist in diagnosing the contents that have herniated through a defect. Other methods such as radio-nuclide scanning and CT cisternograms may be useful in diagnosis, although we have found their usefulness to be limited.

Intraoperative use of intrathecal fluorescein has been associated with severe complications such as lower extremity weakness, numbness, generalized seizures, opisthotonus, and cranial nerve deficits.[14] Caution must be taken when using intrathecal fluoroscein due to these risks. It may be useful in spontaneous CSF leaks or radiographically non-apparent skull base defects. Several studies have advocated its use with no reported adverse outcome.[15,16] Using the lowest possible concentration is therefore recommended.

Jones and colleagues[17] described a novel use of fluroscein in 1990. They topicalized 10% fluoroscein which is initially yellow and diagnosed the CSF leak with a color change of the fluoroscein that turned green when in contact with CSF. This eliminated the need for intrathecal fluoroscein and eliminated the risks involved with its use. Saafan and colleagues[18] confirmed the efficacy of this technique in diagnosis of CSF leak in their series of 25 patients. The most common site of leakage in this study was the ethmoidal roof (52%). There were five iatrogenic injuries but the study did not specify the location of the iatrogenic injuries. Their conclusion advocated the use of this technique preoperatively, intraoperatively, and postoperatively. Other studies have also categorized the location of the skull base defects. **Tables 1–3** show the distribution of skull base defects by location and etiology, respectively.

Non-operative management is one method to control a skull base injury with CSF leak, and may be necessary in the setting of a sick individual where the risks of undergoing surgery are high. This management includes bed rest and strict precautions against nose-blowing, coughing, and bearing down. A lumbar drain or serial lumbar punctures will divert the drainage of CSF from the site of the injury. The patient is kept as an in-patient for several days until the leak has sealed. Antibiotics are often given intravenously.

The size of the defect can influence the approach for repair. Very large defects resulting from tumors that remove the entire skull base are typically reconstructed using a peri-cranial flap in conjunction with neurosurgery through an open approach. Large lesions of the skull base inflicted by microdebriders have been repaired endoscopically. Church and colleagues[8] described three cases involving skull base defects larger than two centimeters with lasting results. Generally, larger defects may require a layered closure with bone.[19]

Table 2
Skull base injury or defect by location

Study	N	Cribriform	Ant Eth	Post Eth	Frontal	Sphenoid
Banks et al[e]	193	32	64[a]	–[a]	23	64
Harvey et al	106	15	19[a]	–[a]	7	62[d]
Lee et al	39	13	11	5	3	7
Zuckerman et al	42	9	14[a]	–[a]	2	17
Bumm et al	32	14	3	–[b]	6	7[b]
Briggs and Bolger	20	9[c]	–[c]	–[c]	3	8
Zweig et al	53	19	15[a]	–[a]	0	20

[a] Study did not differentiate anterior and posterior ethmoid.
[b] Study grouped posterior ethmoid defects with sphenoid defects.
[c] Study grouped cribriform plate, anterior ethmoid and posterior ethmoid defects.
[d] Study separated CSF leak from sella as a separate location.
[e] Author reports 10 unknown locations.

WE DISCUSS SPECIFIC TECHNIQUES IN TWO CATEGORIES

1. Free tissue grafts
2. Pedicled grafts.

The free graft technique can be further subcategorized into overlay (onlay) and underlay techniques. The overlay technique involves placing free mucosa and mobilized mucosa over an identified defect. The graft is then secured using tissue glue such as fibrin glue. Fibrin glue has been shown in the animal model to reduce failure of CSF leak repairs by improving the graft adherence and strength of repair.[20]

Underlay techniques can be performed using a variety of materials. Typically, the underlay graft is bone, cartilage or fascia. The bone can be harvested from the mastoid bone as described by Bolger K.[19] It can also come from the septum, turbinate, or banked cadavaric bone. The bone must be easily shaped. We found that using banked cadavaric bone provided a shapeable cortical bone that is in regular supply. Cartilage often cracks and turbinate and septal bone is brittle. Using banked cadavaric bone does not cause the patient any additional morbidity that harvesting large graftable bone from the patient could.

Acellular dermal matrix is a readily available product in operating rooms. It can be a useful adjunct to skull base injury repair when a defect requires a pliable material.

Table 3
Skull base defect by etiology

Study	N	Iatrogenic[a]	Traumatic	Spontaneous	Disease/ Congenital
Banks et al	193	89	16	77	11
Harvey et al	106	70	11	18	6
Lee et al	39	20	20	6	0
Zuckerman et al	42	25	5	12	0
Bumm et al	118	52	49	17	26
Briggs and Bolger	52	16	14	11	12
Zweig et al	53	27	11	12	4

[a] Iatrogenic included expected injury from surgery.

Lorenz and colleagues[21] described using Alloderm in two layers for skull base defect less than 3 mm in an underlay technique. In larger lesions, the investigators used bone in between the Alloderm. All of the repairs were then overlaid with free mucosa and fibrin glue. This repair appears redundant with the multiple layers but the authors support a bulky closure for the potential decrease in delayed surgical failures. Snyderman and colleagues[22] described the use of alloderm in repair of a dural defect in which the alloderm was secured to the free edge of the dura. He describes using Duragen as an inlay graft in these repairs. Lee and colleagues,[23] reported no significant difference when comparing the underlay, overlay and fat obliteration techniques for skull base reconstruction.

Fat obliteration is another technique that may be used for repair. This technique can work well in the sphenoid sinus but mucocoeles several years after surgery are well described complications of this technique. It is likely most beneficial when there is a cavity to obliterate such as the sphenoid sinus. It is not a good reconstructive material in which to pack a wound to seal off a CSF leak. This, potentially, can cause fat necrosis and subsequent complications. Hwang reported lipoid meningitis from a fat reconstruction of a skull base defect in neurotologic surgery.[24] Briggs and Wormald describe a "bath plug" technique using fat. It requires a small amount dissection of the intradura which may not be possible near the carotid or optic nerve. The investigators favor this technique because of the intradural seal the fat provides.[15]

Pedicled reconstruction techniques have been described more recently. Hadad and colleagues[25] described a method in which mucoperichondrium and mucoperisoteum are elevated from the nasal septum and rotated over the skull base defect/injury. This flap is based on the nasoseptal artery that branches from the posterior septal artery. It can repair defects that involve the entire anterior cranial base from frontal sinus to the planum sphenoidale. There was a 5% failure using this technique and patients were followed for at least 2 months. Fortes and colleagues[26] described a posterior pedicled inferior turbinate flap as an alternative for patients who have undergone posterior septectomy. This flap is based off the inferior turbinate artery that is a terminal branch of the posterior lateral nasal artery that arises from the sphenopalatine artery. This flap can be applied directly to dura or denuded bone or fat. Crusting was a noted to be a problem over the remnant turbinate bone.

OUR TECHNIQUE IN SKULL BASE INJURY REPAIR

In an operative setting, the first step is to identify the injury. This may mean performing a complete skull base dissection to fully expose the injury. Once identified, the mucosa surrounding the lesion must be cleared away. Encephaloceles or meningoceles must be carefully freed and cauterized using bipolar. Meticulous hemostasis must be achieved. If the defect is large, bone (or cartilage) reconstruction may be considered. If the defect is smaller, overlay versus underlay becomes the next decision. Some defects may be amenable to the overlay technique but our institution leans toward repair using the underlay technique with bone. It is rare for a lumbar drain to be used; however, if one was placed by neurosurgery, it is used. Once the defect is repaired, the nasal cavity is filled with hemostatic foam and splints are placed in the setting of septoplasty. We often use a "finger cot" which is a Merocel pack placed into a surgical glove secured at one end with a silk suture to protect the graft.

We prescribe intraoperative antibiotics and rarely prescribe postoperative antibiotics. Patients are seen 5 days after surgery for splint removal if a septoplasty was performed. Finger cots are removed at this time. Judicious office debridements begin 2 weeks after surgery. Follow up is then dictated by each endoscopic postoperative examination. Patients are followed for 2 to 3 years to assess for any recurrent CSF leakage. This is consistent with the literature that reports recurrent leaks that occur within 2 years.[13] Aside from recurrent CSF leaks, we have seen delayed brain abscesses develop after pneumocephalus related to the original injury. Providers must have a low threshold for patients with late headaches and unexplained fevers. CT scans with contrast easily diagnose these late complications.[27,28]

THE FUTURE OF SKULL BASE INJURY REPAIR

Endoscopic repair of skull base injuries is safe and reliable. Studies have consistently reported repair success rates in excess of 95%.[13,16,19,24] Injury to the skull base is sometimes inevitable and skull base surgeons must be prepared to encounter any type of injury regardless of location and extent. The prevention techniques described above will help reduce the number of injuries but ultimately, injuries may still occur. A surgeon with sound judgement, and safe and effective technique will find a way to repair any defect. We advocate a multidisciplinary approach using otolaryngology, neurosurgery, and endovascular surgeons.

REFERENCES

1. May M, Levine HL, Mester SJ, et al. Complications of endoscopic sinus surgery: analysis of 2108 patients-incidents and prevention. Laryngoscope 1994;104: 1080–3.
2. Bumm K, Heupel J, Bozzato A, et al. Localization in infliction pattern of iatrogenic skull base defects following endoscopic sinus surgery at a teaching hospital. Auris Nasus Larynx 2009;36:671–6.
3. Keros P. On the practical value of difference in the level of the lamina cribrosa of the ethmoid. Z Laryngol Rhinol Otol 1962;41:809–13.
4. Leunig A, Betz CS, Sommer B, et al. Anatomic variations of the sinuses; multiplanar CT-analysis in 641 patients. Laryngorhinootologie 2008;87:482–9.
5. Savvateeva SM, Guldner C, Murthum T, et al. Digital volume tomography measurement of the olfactory cleft and olfactory fossa. Acta Otolaryngol 2009; 0:1–7.
6. Meyers RM, Valvassori G. Interpretation of anatomic variations of computed tomography sans of the sinuses: a surgeon's perspective. Laryngoscope 1998; 108(3):422–5.
7. Stankiewicz JA, Chow JM. The low skull base. The low skull-base: an invitation to disaster. Am J Rhinol 2004;18:35–40.
8. Church CA, Chiu A, Vaughan WC. Endoscopic repair of large skull base defects after powered sinus surgery. Otolaryngol Head Neck Surg 2003;129(3):204–9.
9. Delgaudio JM, Mathison CC, Hudgins PA. Preoperative disease severity at sites of subsequent skull base defects after endoscopic sinus surgery. Am J Rhinol 2008;22:321–4.
10. Messerklinger W. Endoscopy technique of the middle nasal meatus. Arch Otorhinolaryngol 1978;221(4):297–305.
11. Wigand ME. Transnasal, endoscipical sinus surgery for chronic sinusitis. II Endonasal ethmoidectomy. HNO 1981;29:287–93.
12. Labadie RF, Daavis BM, Fitzpatrick JM. Image-guided surgery:what is the accuracy? Curr Opin Otolaryngol Head Neck Surg 2005;13:27–31.
13. Zuckerman JD, DelGaudio JM. Utility of preoperative hight-resolution CT and intraoperative image guidance in identification of cerebrospinal fluid leaks for endoscopic repair. Am J Rhinol 2008;22:151–4.

14. Moseley JI, Carton CA, Stern WE. Spectrum of complications in the use of intrathecal fluorescein. J Neurosurg 1978;48:765–7.
15. Briggs RJ, Wormald PJ. Endoscopic transnasal intradural repair of anterior skull base cerebrospinal fluid fistulae. J Clin Neurosci 2004;11(6):597–9.
16. Banks CA, Palmer JN, Chiu A, et al. Endoscopic closure of CSF rhinorrhea: 193 cases over 21 years. Otolaryngol Head Neck Surg 2009;140:826–33.
17. Jones ME, Reino T, Gnoy A, et al. Identification of intranasal cerebrospinal fluid leaks by topical application with fluorescein dye. Am J Rhinol 2000;14:93–6.
18. Saafan ME, Ragab SM, Albirmawy OA. Topical intranasal flurescein: the missing partner in algorithms of cerebrospinal fluid fistula detection. Laryngoscope 2006;116:1158–61.
19. Bolger WE, Mclaughlin K. Cranial bone grafts in cerebrospinal fluid leak and encephalocele repair: a preliminary report. Am J Rhinol 2003;17:153–8.
20. deAlmeida JR, Ghotme K, Leong I, et al. A new procine skull base model: fibrin glue improves strength of cerebrospinal fluid leak repairs. Otolaryngol Head Neck Surg 2009;141:184–9.
21. Lorenz RR, Dean RL, Hurley DB, et al. Endoscopic reconstruction of anterior and middle cranial fossa defects using acellular dermal allograft. Laryngoscope 2003;113:496–501.
22. Snyderman CH, Kassam AB, Carrau R, et al. Endoscopic reconstruction of cranial base defects following endonasal skull base surgery. Skull Base 2007;17:73–8.
23. Lee TJ, Huang CC, Chuang CC, et al. Transnasal endoscopic repair of cerebrospinal fluid rhinorrhea and skull base defect: Ten-year experience. Laryngoscope 2004;114:1475–81.
24. Hwang PH, Jackler RK. Lipoid meningitis due to aseptic necrosis of a free fat graft placed during neurotologic surgery. Laryngoscope 1996;106:1482–6.
25. Hadad G, Bassagasteguy L, Carrau RL, et al. A Novel reconstructive technique after endoscopic expanded endonasal approaches: vascular pedicle nasoseptal flap. Laryngoscope 2006;116:1882–6.
26. Fortes FS, Carrau RL, Snyderman CH, et al. The posterior pedicle inferior turbinate flap: a new vascularized flap for skull base reconstruction. Laryngoscope 2007;117:1329–32.
27. Becker SS, Russell PT. Intracranial abscess after anterior skull base defect: does pneumocehphalus play a role? Rhinology 2009;47(3):287–92.
28. Harvey RJ, Smith JE, Wise SK, et al. Intracranial complications before and after endoscopic skull base reconstruction. Am J Rhinol 2008;22:516–21.

Prevention and Management of Vascular Injuries in Endoscopic Surgery of the Sinonasal Tract and Skull Base

C. Arturo Solares, MD[a], Yew Kwang Ong, MD[b], Ricardo L. Carrau, MD[c,d,*], Juan Fernandez-Miranda, MD[e], Daniel M. Prevedello, MD[c,d], Carl H. Snyderman, MD[b], Amin B. Kassam, MD[c,d]

KEYWORDS

- Sinus surgery • Endoscopic skull base surgery
- Vascular injury • Carotid artery injury

In the past 2 decades, endoscopic sinus surgery has been widely used as a safe and effective treatment for disorders of the paranasal sinuses that are refractory to medical therapy. Advances in surgical technique, including powered instrumentation and stereotactic image-guided surgery, have improved the efficiency and safety of this procedure. These techniques have been further expanded to manage skull base pathologies. This expansion has been facilitated by a better understanding of the endonasal skull base anatomy. Despite these advances, complications are still encountered. Vascular injuries are particularly troublesome. In a recent issue of this journal, Welch and Palmer[1] extensively discussed interior ethmoid artery injuries during sinus surgery that led to orbital hematoma. Therefore, this article focuses mainly on inadvertent carotid artery injuries during routine sinus surgery and vascular injuries during endoscopic skull base surgery.

[a] Department of Otolaryngology, Medical College of Georgia, Augusta, GA 30907, USA
[b] Department of Otolaryngology, University of Pittsburgh Medical Center, Pittsburgh, PA 15213, USA
[c] John Wayne Cancer Institute, 2200 Santa Monica Boulevard, Santa Monica, CA 92404, USA
[d] Neuroscience Institute, Saint John's Health Center, Santa Monica, CA 92404, USA
[e] Department of Neurosurgery, University of Pittsburgh Medical Center, Pittsburgh, PA 15213, USA
* Corresponding author. John Wayne Cancer Institute, 2200 Santa Monica Boulevard, Santa Monica, CA 92404.
E-mail address: carraur@gmail.com

Otolaryngol Clin N Am 43 (2010) 817–825
doi:10.1016/j.otc.2010.04.008
0030-6665/10/$ – see front matter

OVERVIEW

Avoidance of unintentional injury and complications is an important cornerstone of surgery. The introduction of minimally invasive techniques in any surgical subspecialty has been universally associated with a higher frequency of surgical complications. This increase in complications during the implementation of new techniques, commonly known as the learning curve, can be reduced through proper training and mentorship that promotes and facilitates sequential and progressive learning. Despite its minimally invasive connotation, endoscopic endonasal surgery presents many of the risks and potential for major complications associated with open approaches. Inexperience and lack of proper training with new instruments or techniques, and disorientation with the endoscopic anatomic perspective, are important factors leading to catastrophic vascular injuries.

Although endoscopic sinus surgery has become the standard of care and is taught in residency training programs, endoscopic endonasal skull base surgery is a relatively new concept. In the authors' experience, including more than 1400 endoscopic endonasal skull base surgeries, the incidence and morbidity of catastrophic vascular complications compares favorably with those of traditional approaches. However, otolaryngologists must recognize that endoscopic and traditional approaches are often complementary, and therefore their indications and limitations preclude a direct comparison.

INCIDENCE OF COMPLICATIONS

The literature contains sparse case reports of carotid injuries during endonasal endoscopic surgery;[2–8] however, the true incidence of all vascular injuries during endonasal endoscopic surgery is unknown. In one literature review, Koitschev and colleagues[4] identified 26 cases of carotid artery injuries during sinus surgery, with only 8 occurring during endoscopic sinus surgery. Two additional reports, totaling 3 cases, have since been published.[2,3]

The advent of endoscopic skull base surgery added another level of complexity to endoscopic endonasal procedures, begging the question of whether this operation is associated with an increased incidence of vascular complications. Kassam and colleagues[9] reviewed the early experience at the University of Pittsburgh Medical Center to determine the incidence and nature of complications during endoscopic skull base surgery. Intraoperative vascular injuries were rare and included seven major vascular complications (0.9%). The vascular complications encountered during the first 800 cases performed by the authors' group are listed in **Table 1**. One patient experienced an avulsion of a P1 perforator during the resection of a craniopharyngioma. Two patients experienced an internal carotid artery (ICA) injury, and one an avulsion of the ophthalmic artery. All injuries were controlled intraoperatively before the patients were transferred to the endovascular suite for additional control or sacrifice of the vessel. None of these four patients sustained a new permanent deficit, although the patient with the PCA branch injury had a stroke with a severe aphasia that eventually recovered completely.

The remaining three patients sustained permanent neurologic deficits (0.4%). One patient experienced an avulsion of a frontopolar artery (A2) during the resection of an olfactory groove meningioma. Approximately 2 weeks later, the patient experienced a frontal lobe hemorrhage from a pseudoaneurysm, which required sacrifice of the A2 and the recurrent artery of Huebner, leading to a permanent right hemiparesis and cognitive deficit. Another patient who underwent resection of a clival chordoma with brainstem involvement experienced a delayed postoperative pontine

Table 1
Vascular complications encountered during the first 800 cases at the University of Pittsburgh Medical Center

Patient	Injury	New Deficit
1	Avulsion of P1 perforator	Transient aphasia
2	Laceration of the ICA	None
3	Laceration of the ICA	None
4	Avulsion of the ophthalmic artery	None
5	Avulsion of frontopolar artery (A2)	Permanent right hemiparesis and cognitive deficit after a delayed hemorrhage from pseudoaneurysm formation
6	Delayed pontine bleed	Quadriplegia
7	Avulsion of internal maxillary artery	Subdural hematoma with resulting 4/5 weakness of the left upper limb

Abbreviation: ICA, internal carotid artery.

hemorrhage after an episode of hypertension, resulting in a permanent quadriplegia. The third patient sustained an injury of the internal maxillary artery during the dissection of an infratemporal fossa encephalocele, resulting in an acute subdural hematoma that required transcranial exploration and evacuation. This patient developed a permanent, mild weakness (4/5) of the left upper limb.

This case log represents a 10-year experience, including a wide variety of diagnoses and endonasal surgical approaches. Vascular injuries were not encounter during the authors' early experience, who believe this may be because of the progressive evolution in the technique and indications. Stated differently, the complexity of cases managed by the authors' team progressively increased as the members matured, and thus they did not attempt to operate on complex or high-risk cases until they developed or mastered hemostatic and reconstructive techniques.

PREVENTION OF COMPLICATIONS

Anatomic knowledge with a clear understanding of the paranasal sinus and skull base anatomy from the endoscopic perspective is the first step toward preventing complications. This concept applies to functional endoscopic sinus and skull base surgery. Paranasal sinus anatomy has been reviewed elsewhere.[10]

To progress from sinus surgery to endoscopic skull base surgery requires a thorough understanding of the skull base anatomy. The skull base is a relay station where all the cranial nerves and vessels are distributed to their corresponding areas. With this notion, the authors' group described a modular classification of endoscopic approaches to the skull base based on the identification and control of critical neurovascular structures, particularly the ICA.[11–13] This system aims at minimizing neurovascular complications.

From the ventral perspective, the ICAs are brackets that define the lateral limits of the coronal plane. They define the surgical field, which narrows as the ICAs move from proximal to distal. From the endoscopic view, the ICA can be divided into five segments marked by distinct anatomic points: parapharyngeal or extracranial segment; petrous or horizontal segment; paraclival or vertical segment; parasellar or cavernous segment; and supraclinoid segment (**Fig. 1**). Anatomic variations, space-occupying lesions, prior surgery, and varying degrees of pneumatization of the sinonasal tract also influence the position of each segment of the ICA, and thus the

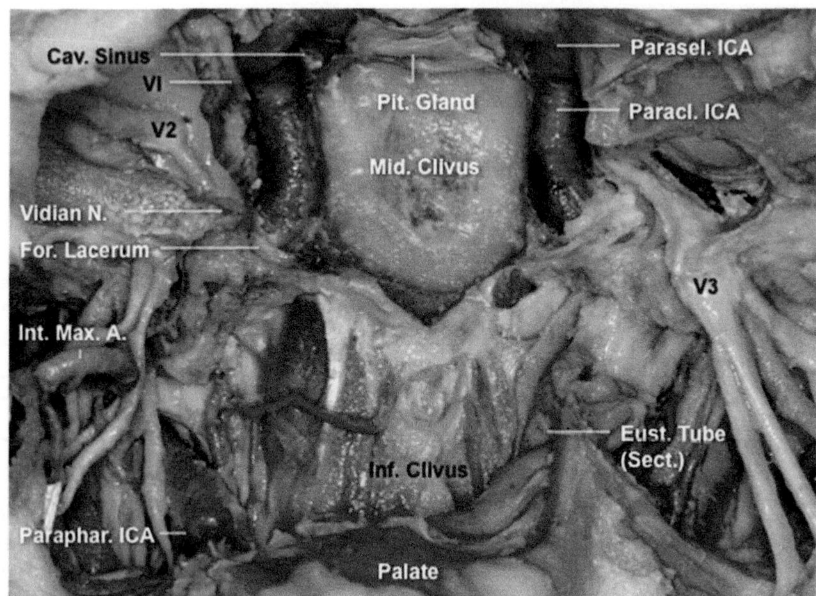

Fig. 1. Segments of the internal carotid artery (ICA). The ICA is divided into five segments marked by distinct anatomic points: parapharyngeal or extracranial segment, petrous or horizontal segment, paraclival or vertical segment, parasellar or cavernous segment, and supraclinoid segment. The transitional segment between paraclival and petrosal is also called the *lacerum segment* because it occupies the upper portion of the foramen lacerum. A, artery; Cav, cavernous; Eust, eustachian; For, foramen; ICA, internal carotid artery; Int, internal; Max, maxillary; Mid, Middle, N, nerve; Paracl, Paraclival; Parasel, Parasellar; Pit, Pituitary; Sect, sectioned.

approach to each segment. The vidian nerve is a useful landmark during surgery for identifying the second genu of the carotid.[14,15] Other anatomic landmarks for the carotid artery are outlined in **Table 2**.

Proper training is also critical for the prevention and management of surgical complications.[16] Although routine endoscopic sinus surgery training is part of the otolaryngology residency, endoscopic skull base surgery is fairly new, with only a handful of fellowships available worldwide. The authors' group proposed guidelines to train endoscopic skull base surgeons. Levels of training are defined by the complexity of the involved anatomy, technical difficulty associated with the surgery, potential risk for neurovascular complications, extent of intradural dissection, and type of pathology. Proficiency in one level must be acquired before the surgeon

Table 2
Anatomic landmarks for various segments of the internal carotid artery

Segment	Anatomic Landmark
Paraclinoid	Medial clinoid
Anterior genu	Medial pterygoid
Horizontal segment	Vidian nerve
Ascending carotid	Eustachian tube

advances to the next. Thus, the surgeon progresses sequentially through the different levels of complexity. In addition to clinical training, animal models and cadaver dissection are essential for the acquisition of technical skills and anatomic knowledge.

INTRAOPERATIVE CONSIDERATIONS

Routine Sinus Surgery

If a vascular injury occurs during routine sinus surgery, specific management strategies are somewhat different from those for a similar injury during skull base surgery. Thorough review of the preoperative CT scans is the first step in preventing carotid injuries.[17] In reviewing the imaging, one must pay special attention to the presence of vascular anomalies of the ICA. Carotid lacerations in the presence of a vascular anomaly are uniformly catastrophic.[4] From a technical aspect, sinus surgery is most often performed one-handed, with the other hand used to hold the endoscope. Thus, in the face of massive bleeding from a carotid artery bleed, maintaining adequate visualization is impossible, and therefore the most important management step is aggressive packing of the nasal cavity to prevent further bleeding. Other sources of bleeding that can be easily cauterized have been excluded. Simultaneously, hemodynamic stabilization is accomplished by the anesthesia team. After these measures, urgent transfer to an endovascular suite is necessary for definitive management. Often, vessel sacrifice with deployable balloons or coils is necessary, although ICA stenting has been reported in the literature. During endovascular exploration, the otolaryngologist should be available to remove nasal packing if it is too tight to prevent adequate localization of the injury.

Endoscopic Skull Base Surgery

Interdisciplinary cooperation is one of the most remarkable advances in skull base surgery. Endoscopic skull base surgery requires a higher level of cooperation, because two surgeons share surgical field rather than work in tandem. A co-surgeon provides visualization of the surgical field and surveillance of its periphery, increases efficiency, assists with problem-solving, provides a continuous second opinion, and balances individual biases.

Neurophysiologic monitoring of cortical and brainstem function is routinely performed. Electromyographic monitoring of cranial nerves is also performed according to the position of the lesion and the required dissection. The authors advocate using CT angiography (CTA) for image guidance, because it highlights the vascular anatomy (except for sellar lesions, for which the authors advocate MRI).[18] Intraoperative CT can be used to provide updated information for image guidance and to detect vascular complications such as brain hemorrhage.

Proper surgical technique helps to avoid complications, especially vascular injuries. The authors strongly advocate bimanual dissection and minimal traction on intracranial tumors to avoid inadvertent avulsion of the surrounding vessels. Following microsurgical principles, the tumor is debulked in a centrifugal direction to allow extracapsular dissection of adjacent neurovascular structures. Hemostasis is achieved using a combination of strategies that include clipping or cauterization of feeding vessels, use of a diamond drill bit for bone removal, application of hemostatic materials, and warm water irrigation.[19] Bipolar electrocautery should be used for any intracranial cauterization and whenever a critical nerve or vessel is adjacent to the bleeding site.

Catastrophic bleeding is better prevented than treated. Its potential increases exponentially in the presence of prior surgery, prior radiation therapy, and tumor encasement. Every team should have a plan following place if this occurs; formulating and executing a plan of action in the middle of a crisis is difficult. Significant bleeding from the cavernous sinus and basilar plexus should be anticipated and its management effected by direct application of hemostatic materials and gentle pressure. Staging a procedure is occasionally warranted for lesions requiring a transclival approach, in which the surgeon encounters significant bleeding from the basilar plexus. During the first stage, the bone is removed to expose the dura of the posterior fossa, which is then cauterized (bipolar electrocautery), and the basilar plexus is thrombosed with any commercially available paste-like hemostatic agents. If deemed appropriate, the surgery can be aborted at this point to stabilize the patient, and a second stage performed 1 to 2 days later.

Injury to small and large arteries produces bleeding proportional to the size of the vessel and injury. Nonetheless, the results of this injury may lead to consequences that are not necessarily proportional to the size of the vessel. Small perforating vessels to the brainstem and optic chiasm provide important blood supply, and their sacrifice or injury often lead to ischemic neurologic deficits. Control of small arteries, however, is best achieved using bipolar electrocauterization or by irrigating warm water (40°C) for several minutes. Alternatively, a hemostatic material can be gently applied using cottonoids, which is repeated as needed until the bleeding stops.

Injury to the ICA is usually accompanied by catastrophic bleeding that must be controlled while maintaining cerebral perfusion. During the crisis, neurophysiologic monitoring is critical because it reflects cerebral perfusion. Digital compression of the cervical carotid may diminish its flow. Hypotensive anesthesia as an attempt to control bleeding is contraindicated because it results in cerebral hypoperfusion. A measure that may seem counterintuitive is the administration of heparin to avoid embolic phenomena.

A two-surgeons-four-hands technique with dynamic handling of the endoscope to preserve an adequate view of the surgical field and the use of two suctions offers the best opportunity to identify and control the site of bleeding. Options at that point include bipolar electrocauterization of the vessel to weld the tear shut or induce thrombosis of the vessel; direct compression; compressive packing; suture repair; reconstruction using aneurysm clips; and circumferential ligation or clipping of the vessel (**Fig. 2**).

Compressive packing is not an option if the dura is opened, because the blood will track into the subdural space. Initially, the bleeding is directed into the suction tips to maintain visualization while focal pressure is applied with a cottonoid. If the hemostasis and resuscitation are successful and vital signs and neurophysiologic monitoring are stable, additional packing can be placed and the patient may be transported to an angiography suite for definitive management. If packing is inadequate or not feasible, the ICA is further exposed to obtain control of the vessel proximal and distal to the injury. Suture repair is possible, albeit technically difficult and in most instances impractical. Preservation of the vessel may be better achieved through reconstructing the vessel with aneurysm clips or using Sundt-Keyes clips. Sacrifice of the ICA is the most commonly used alternative. Although the patency of the ICA could be preserved through use of a covered stent,[3] this may not be available for intracranial use in all institutions. Insertion of a covered stent into the cavernous sinus segment of the ICA is technically challenging; therefore, permanent occlusion is most common. Assessment of collateral blood flow with a balloon occlusion test assesses the risk for ischemic stroke or the need for bypass.

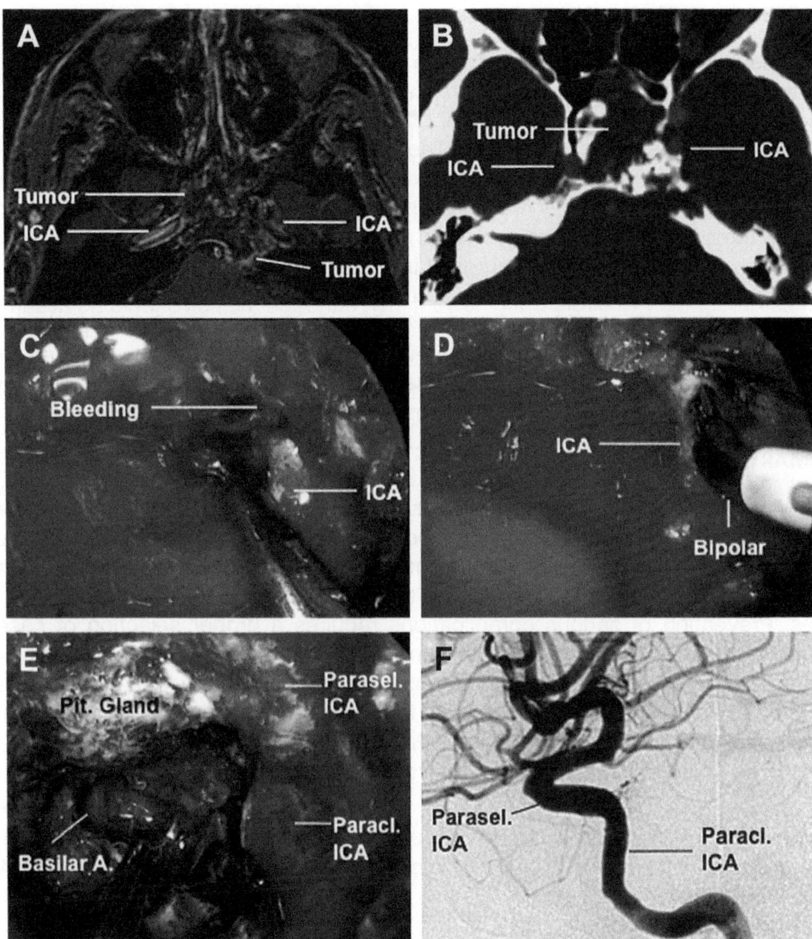

Fig. 2. Case example of a vascular injury. (*A*) Axial T1-weighted MRI of a skull base chondrosarcoma with invasion of the clival and petrous bones especially on the left side with encasement and anterolateral displacement of the left internal carotid artery (ICA) at the petrous segment. (*B*) CT angiogram for same patient. Displacement of the left paraclival ICA is noted again. The intraluminal diameter of the vessel is reduced and irregular, suggesting invasion of the periosteum of the vessel. (*C*) Brisk arterial bleeding was encountered during tumor removal around the left paraclival ICA. The bleeding was easily controlled by gentle compression with a small cottonoid, but when the pressure was relieved the bleeding was copious. (*D*) Digital pressure to the cervical segment of the ICA helped diminish its flow and allowed for accurate identification of the pinhole in the carotid wall. Selective bipolar electrocauterization of the tear was successfully accomplished, with immediate cessation of bleeding. Vital signs and neurophysiologic monitoring were stable throughout. (*E*) The carotid wall was reinforced with fibrin glue and the remaining tumor was subtotally resected. The tumor eroded the clival dura, allowing for identification of the basilar artery. (*F*) Immediate postoperative angiogram showed a patent and completely normal ICA. Follow-up angiogram performed 1 month after the injury to rule out the development of a carotid pseudoaneurysm was unremarkable. A, artery; Paracl, paraclival.

POSTOPERATIVE COMPLICATIONS

A postoperative CT scan, performed in the first 24 hours after surgery, provides early detection of complications, such as cerebral hemorrhage or intracranial hematoma. A CT scanner, built in the operating room, offers the opportunity for intraoperative and immediate postoperative evaluation. The authors encountered two unexpected complications during endoscopic skull base surgery: a subdural hematoma from cerebrospinal fluid loss in an elderly man, and an epidural hematoma from improper placement of a three-pin head fixation system in a pediatric patient. Early identification with intraoperative CT and immediate surgical treatment resulted in the best outcome.

Any significant postoperative epistaxis mandates endoscopic examination of the nasal cavity. Similarly, an immediate angiography is recommended for patients at risk for a carotid blowout or bleed. A follow-up angiography is also recommended after any intraoperative vascular injury, because these patients are at risk for a delayed pseudoaneurysm and rupture that can present weeks to years after the event.[20]

SUMMARY

Despite the fact that endoscopic endonasal surgery is considered minimally invasive, the risk for vascular injury is real. The added complexity of endoscopic skull base surgery requires special skills to manage neurovascular structures, but the incidence of vascular complications is comparable to that for open skull base surgery techniques. Prevention of serious complications requires a proper selection of cases, and a surgeon who has mastered the anatomy from an endoscopic perspective, has completed training in endoscopic techniques, is capable of a meticulous dissection, and provides perioperative care with the utmost attention to detail. Progressive acquisition of skills and experience leads to an acceptable safety profile.

REFERENCES

1. Welch KC, Palmer JN. Intraoperative emergencies during endoscopic sinus surgery: CSF leak and orbital hematoma. Otolaryngol Clin North Am 2008;41: 581–96, ix–x.
2. Reich O, Ringel K, Stoeter P, et al. [Injury of ICA during endonasal sinus surgery and management by endovascular stent application]. Laryngorhinootologie 2009;88:322–6 [in German].
3. Lippert BM, Ringel K, Stoeter P, et al. Stentgraft-implantation for treatment of internal carotid artery injury during endonasal sinus surgery. Am J Rhinol 2007; 21:520–4.
4. Koitschev A, Simon C, Lowenheim H, et al. Management and outcome after internal carotid artery laceration during surgery of the paranasal sinuses. Acta Otolaryngol 2006;126:730–8.
5. Weidenbecher M, Huk WJ, Iro H. Internal carotid artery injury during functional endoscopic sinus surgery and its management. Eur Arch Otorhinolaryngol 2005;262:640–5.
6. Park AH, Stankiewicz JA, Chow J, et al. A protocol for management of a catastrophic complication of functional endoscopic sinus surgery: internal carotid artery injury. Am J Rhinol 1998;12:153–8.
7. Isenberg SF, Scott JA. Management of massive hemorrhage during endoscopic sinus surgery. Otolaryngol Head Neck Surg 1994;111:134–6.
8. Hudgins PA, Browning DG, Gallups J, et al. Endoscopic paranasal sinus surgery: radiographic evaluation of severe complications. AJNR Am J Neuroradiol 1992; 13:1161–7.

9. Kassam AB, Prevedello DM, Carrau RL, et al. Endoscopic endonasal skull base surgery: analysis of complications in our initial 800 patients and literature review. J Neurosurg, in press.
10. Van Cauwenberge P, Sys L, De Belder T, et al. Anatomy and physiology of the nose and the paranasal sinuses. Immunol Allergy Clin North Am 2004;24:1–17.
11. Kassam A, Snyderman CH, Mintz A, et al. Expanded endonasal approach: the rostrocaudal axis. Part II. Posterior clinoids to the foramen magnum. Neurosurg Focus 2005;19:E4.
12. Kassam A, Snyderman CH, Mintz A, et al. Expanded endonasal approach: the rostrocaudal axis. Part I. Crista galli to the sella turcica. Neurosurg Focus 2005; 19:E3.
13. Kassam AB, Gardner P, Snyderman C, et al. Expanded endonasal approach: fully endoscopic, completely transnasal approach to the middle third of the clivus, petrous bone, middle cranial fossa, and infratemporal fossa. Neurosurg Focus 2005;19:E6.
14. Vescan AD, Snyderman CH, Carrau RL, et al. Vidian canal: analysis and relationship to the internal carotid artery. Laryngoscope 2007;117:1338–42.
15. Kassam AB, Vescan AD, Carrau RL, et al. Expanded endonasal approach: vidian canal as a landmark to the petrous internal carotid artery. J Neurosurg 2008;108: 177–83.
16. Snyderman C, Kassam A, Carrau R, et al. Acquisition of surgical skills for endonasal skull base surgery: a training program. Laryngoscope 2007;117:699–705.
17. Lehmann P, Bouaziz R, Page C, et al. [Sinonasal cavities: CT imaging features of anatomical variants and surgical risk]. J Radiol 2009;90:21–9 [in French].
18. Gardner PA, Kassam AB, Rothfus WE, et al. Preoperative and intraoperative imaging for endoscopic endonasal approaches to the skull base. Otolaryngol Clin North Am 2008;41:215–30, vii.
19. Kassam A, Snyderman CH, Carrau RL, et al. Endoneurosurgical hemostasis techniques: lessons learned from 400 cases. Neurosurg Focus 2005;19:E7.
20. Biswas D, Daudia A, Jones NS, et al. Profuse epistaxis following sphenoid surgery: a ruptured carotid artery pseudoaneurysm and its management. J Laryngol Otol 2009;123:692–4.

Prevention and Management of Complications in Frontal Sinus Surgery

Amin R. Javer, MD, FRCSC*, Talal Alandejani, MD, FRCSC

KEYWORDS

• Sinus surgery • Surgical complications • Anatomic variations

PREVENTION OF COMPLICATIONS IN FRONTAL SINUS SURGERY

The frontal sinus remains one of the most complex regions to operate on, with a wide array of anatomic variations between patients and even between 2 sides in the same patient. The frontal sinus surgeon needs to be extremely learned in the different anatomic challenges that may present during surgery in this area. There is no substitute for knowing the anatomy of this region in detail. Performing an adequate functional frontal sinusotomy while minimizing the risk of a complication requires proper planning that starts before the patient enters the operating room.

Preoperative Planning

Computed tomography scan review

A critical preoperative review of the computed tomography (CT) scan is vital and must be performed by the operating surgeon once a decision for surgery has been made. The frontal sinus anatomy should be reviewed on a triplanar imaging system if possible, so that sagittal, coronal, and axial cuts are visualized simultaneously. The presence or absence of cells that may potentially obstruct the frontal recess (frontal cells, intersinusseptal cells, supraorbital ethmoid cells, and so forth), upper attachment of the uncinate process, and the various possible variations of the anatomy need to be identified. It is important that the operating surgeon can mentally create a three-dimensional image of the drainage pathway. Some investigators have recommended creating square line and cube like patterns to imitate the drainage pathway.[1,2] Such an exercise can be helpful for the novice frontal sinus surgeon so that they can be prepared for what might happen during the surgical dissection.

St Paul's Sinus Centre, St Paul's Hospital, University of British Columbia, 1081 Burrard Street, Vancouver, BC V6Z1Y6, Canada
* Corresponding author.
E-mail address: sinussurgeon@drjaver.com

Otolaryngol Clin N Am 43 (2010) 827–838
doi:10.1016/j.otc.2010.04.021
oto.theclinics.com

Preoperative medications

It is important to prime the mucus membrane so that it is in the best possible condition during the operation as it is difficult to operate on an inflamed frontal recess. The presence of inflammation results in increased intraoperative bleeding which, in turn, makes endoscopic exposure difficult. Any medication that may reduce the inflammation in the frontal recess results in a decreased amount of bleeding.

Antibiotics Most sinus cavities are being operated on because they are chronically infected and inflamed. A preoperative antibiotic decreases the amount of inflammation and likely results in a cleaner field with a decreased amount of blood loss. Most of our patients being taken to the operating room for an endoscopic frontal sinusotomy are placed on a 7-day course of antibiotics preoperatively and a 7-day course of antibiotic postoperatively while any spacers or splints are in place.

Prednisone Prednisone is a strong antiinflammatory medication and is also used to reduce the inflammation in a chronically infected and inflamed sinus cavity preoperatively. Patients who do not have a contraindication to oral steroids are started on 0.2 mg/kg of prednisone daily starting 7 days before surgery reducing to 0.1 mg/kg of prednisone daily for 7 days after surgery during the initial healing phase. This has been found to reduce bleeding intraoperatively likely secondary to the reduction in the inflammation of the tissues being operated on.[3] The secondary gain for a significant number of patients is an improvement in their lung function preoperatively, which makes administration of their anesthesia easier and better tolerated.

Topical decongestant Further preoperative preparation of the nasal cavity and mucus membrane is performed by instructing the patient to spray their nose with a topical decongestant (xylometazoline) starting 2 hours before surgery and every 30 minutes thereafter until the patient is wheeled into the operating room. This has a very effective decongestant effect on the mucus membrane of the nose before the operation allowing for an optimal surgical field. This is further enhanced by gently packing the nasal cavity with neuropatties lightly soaked with a topical decongestant (xylometazoline) as soon as the patient has been intubated and before the patient is draped. This results in a wide-open, well-decongested nasal cavity as the operation begins.

Intraoperative Planning

Blood pressure monitoring

We have found that keeping the systolic blood pressure less than 100 mm Hg reduces the amount of blood loss and improves visualization during surgery. We do not inject the lateral nasal wall or the nasal cavity with local anesthetic/epinephrine before beginning the operation. A recently published study from our center showed that injecting the lateral nasal wall with a xylocaine/epinephrine combination at the start of the operation actually increased the amount of blood loss during the operation.[4] We recommend that the nasal cavity not be injected with local anesthetic/epinephrine combination at the start of the operation as long as the patient has been properly prepared for surgery as described earlier. We also recommend against using topical cocaine or topical epinephrine in the nasal or sinus cavity before or during the operation because of concerns regarding the potential for increased cardiovascular complications.[5]

Extent of surgery

It is important to determine the extent of surgery that is necessary before beginning the operation. If the disease is confined strictly to the frontal sinus, then the surgeon may carry out an ethmoid bulla-intact frontal sinusotomy [6] and not disturb the ethmoid cells. On the other hand, if the anterior (and posterior) ethmoid cells are involved, then it is important to complete the ethmoidectomy before focusing on the frontal recess. In such a situation, the surgeon should not start working on the frontal recess before the ethmoidectomy has been completed. Leaving behind shelves at the skull base and starting the frontal sinusotomy with an incomplete ethmoidectomy compromises visualization and access to the frontal recess as well as promoting future scarring.

Approaching the frontal recess

Once the ethmoidectomy is completed, the frontal recess should be approached from a posterior to anterior direction along the skull base. It is important to use through-cutting instrumentation when removing the ethmoid bulla lamellae and other vertical shelves during the approach to the frontal recess. Meticulous preservation of the mucus membrane is important to avoid creating areas of bare bone and therefore the future potential of osteoneogenesis and subsequent iatrogenic scarring that can occur in the frontal recess. If a large, pneumatized agger nasi cell is encountered, it is important to try and identify the posterior or medial edge of the shelf. This allows the surgeon to carefully remove the agger nasi cap in a systematic manner while preserving the mucus membrane within the frontal recess. It is important that the surgeon, with the help of a tridimensional CT scan, creates an imaginary three-dimensional picture of the frontal recess and associated cells in their head. If an image guidance system is being used during the operation, it should simply be used as a guide and not as a final acceptance of the anatomy. The surgeon's own knowledge and instinct should be the most important guide in working on the frontal recess.

It is important to move the instruments from posterior to anterior or from medial to lateral. This reduces the likelihood of mistakenly entering the intracranial cavity. The lateral cribriform plate lamellae can be very thin in the region of the frontal recess where the anterior ethmoid artery crosses the skull base. Using sharp instruments in a rough manner at the level of the anterior ethmoid artery can result in a cerebrospinal fluid (CSF) leak or bleeding from the anterior ethmoid artery. It is also important to identify the anterior ethmoid artery on the CT scan and recognize how low it sits in the skull base so that it is not transected or traumatized during the dissection. Entry into the orbit is difficult because the orbital bone or laminae papyracea is not as thin in the region of the frontal recess as it is in the region of the lacrimal sac or ethmoid region. In rare cases the bone over the orbit can be dehiscent.[7] In such cases it is extremely important to be aware of the dehiscence and to avoid using a powered instrument or microdebrider near the dehiscent area.

At the completion of the endoscopic frontal sinusotomy, the endoscopic surgeon should be able to see a nicely opened internal frontal sinus ostium with well-preserved circumferential mucus membrane. This allows for a well-healed successfully functioning frontal sinus (**Fig. 1**).

Use of powered instrumentation in the frontal recess

At the St Paul's Sinus Center, use of powered instrumentation in the frontal recess is generally avoided. All dissection is performed with 30° or 70° endoscopes complemented with 45° and 90° giraffe forceps and through-cut instruments with meticulous mucus membrane preservation.[8] Advances in angled instrumentation have allowed the frontal sinus surgeons to reach into the frontal recess and sinus at angles previously believed to be unreachable (**Fig. 2**). This has allowed for greater endoscopic success for frontal sinus surgery that previously would have seemed unoperable via an endoscopic-only route.

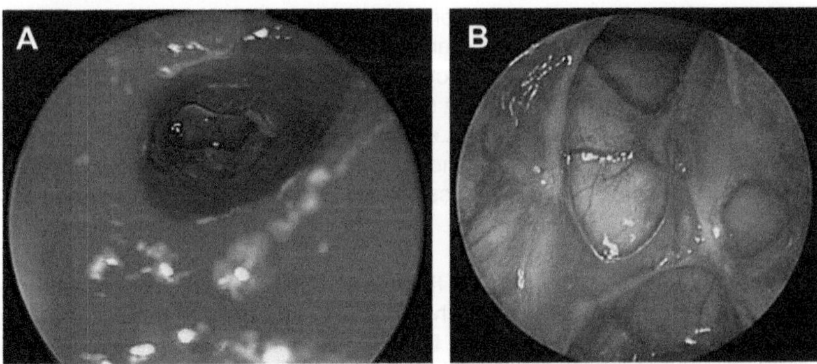

Fig. 1. Intraoperative view of (*A*) a fully opened frontal recess with mucus membrane preservation and (*B*) a completely healed frontal recess at 12 weeks postoperatively.

Powered instrumentation and drilling in the frontal recess can result in bare bone within the frontal recess and ostium. This can lead to scarring and osteoneogenesis with subsequent failure of the frontal sinus from staying open. Use of powered instrumentation in the frontal recess should therefore be avoided as much as possible. A recent, yet unpublished, study of 200 patients at our institution who had undergone endoscopic frontal sinusotomy showed the success rate of endoscopic sinus surgery in a previously unoperated patient was in the 90% plus range. Only 8% of patients in the primary group required a return to the operating room compared with 21% in the group undergoing a revision frontal dissection.[9] Revision surgery, as one would expect, results in a higher failure rate simply from an increased risk of scarring. A modified Lothrop procedure is therefore never indicated for a primary operation in the frontal sinus regardless of how bad the inflammatory disease is in the frontal recess/sinus.

Sinus packing

A middle meatal spacer made out of a downsized merocel sponge placed inside a glove finger is placed within the middle meatus.[10] The objective of the spacer is to allow the middle meatus to stay patent and free of clots. It also allows the middle turbinate to stay medialized during the early healing process. The spacer is removed

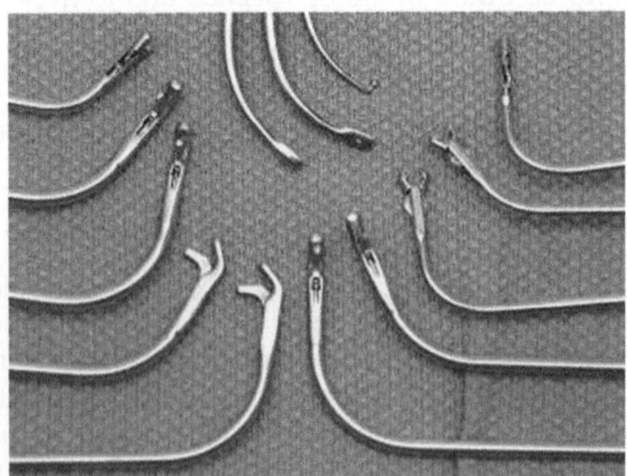

Fig. 2. A sample of the large number of single and double curved instrumentation available for frontal sinus surgery.

at the first postoperative visit between 5 and 7 days after surgery. We are currently investigating medicated merocel sponges as spacers in the early postoperative period, but it is too early to make any conclusive comments.

Postoperative Planning

Postoperative irrigation

Patients are instructed to start irrigating their nasal/sinus cavities 3 times a day with saline starting on the first postoperative day. This allows for autodebridement of the nasal cavity washing out all clots and fibrin debris. After the first visit at 6 days postoperatively, irrigation is reduced to once a day for the next 6 to 12 weeks. We have found that heavy irrigation (more than once a day) after the first 2 weeks can actually result in significant discomfort for the patient.

Postoperative medication

All patients are started on a 7-day course of prednisone at 0.1 mg /kg and antibiotics. This keeps the early postoperative inflammation under control while the sinuses are actively draining mucus and blood clots. If the patient has met the criteria for a diagnosis of allergic fungal sinusitis, then the patient is instructed to place 2 mL of budesonide (0.5 mg/2 mL) into 240 mL of isotonic saline for irrigation of the sinonasal cavity twice a day.

Postoperative visits

Patients are seen at 6 days postoperatively (5 to 7 days) at which time the middle meatal spacers are removed and the sinus cavities are very gently suctioned free of clots and mucus. It is important to avoid creating new bleeding in the frontal recess at this visit because this will obscure the surgeons view and create further clotting. Leaving clots behind in the frontal recess risks the formation of fibrin and therefore scarring, and increases the risk of infection. The frontal recess and sinus are visualized with a pediatric 45° or 70° scope to ensure patency and absence of infection. Any evidence of purulence results in cultures being taken and the sinuses being lavaged with saline using double curved suctions or Van Alyea cannulas, followed by placement of a topical steroid and antibiotic mixture within the affected sinus cavity.[11]

The second and third visits are planned depending on what the cavity looks like at the first visit. In most cases, if all looks well, the second visit is at 4 weeks postoperatively and the third visit at 12 weeks postoperatively at which point the sinuses are usually well healed and patent as shown in **Fig. 1**B. The frontal recess and ostium are visualized at each visit and if needed the frontal sinus is lavaged with saline. If edema is identified within the recess or sinus, a mixture of gentamycin and a topical nasal steroid is placed within the sinus with the patient in a dependent position. If scar bands or remnant slivers of bone are seen within the frontal recess during the first few visits, they are removed in the clinic under local anesthesia.

COMPLICATIONS IN FRONTAL SINUS SURGERY

Several major intraoperative complications can occur during frontal sinus surgery depending on the approach used (endoscopic vs external). Although, these different types of approaches may share some of the general complications (eg, bleeding and CSF leak), each technique can also have specific complications related to it. These can be broadly divided into 2 categories

(1) Transnasal endoscopic procedures:
   - Endoscopic frontal sinusotomy
   - Modified endoscopic Lothrop procedure (MEL).

(2) External procedures:
- Frontal sinus trephine
- Osteoplastic flap with/without obliteration
- Frontal sinus cranialization
- Combined above and below approaches (external plus endoscopic).

The complications from each type of surgical technique can be further subdivided into intraoperative complications and early and late postoperative complications.

Endoscopic Frontal Sinusotomy Complications

(1) Entry into the orbit
(2) Excessive bleeding from transection of the anterior ethmoid artery
(3) Intracranial entry
(4) Excessive denudation of the mucosal membrane.

Managing Complications

Orbital entry

Orbital entry can range from simple orbital fat exposure to intraorbital hemorrhage to actual damage to the intraorbital muscles with powered instrumentation. Analysis of the preoperative CT scan to identify any areas of dehiscence of the lamina papyracea should be performed before surgery. Exposure of the periorbita can usually be identified endoscopically and confirmed by palpation of the orbit with associated movement of the periorbita. If the periorbita has been violated and fat exposed, it should be immediately recognized and the use of any suction and/or powered instrumentation in the area should be strictly avoided. The area of orbital fat exposure should be covered with a small piece of silastic or epifilm (Medtronic Xomed) and, if there is adequate space around it, the operation can be carefully completed. Once surgery is complete, the exposed area should be covered with a small piece of epifilm. On the other hand, if there is a major orbital complication (ie, intraorbital hemorrhage from a retracted and resected anterior ethmoid artery), then the surgeon should be prepared to carry out a lateral canthotomy and cantholysis and follow the protocol outlined in the next section.

A medial rectus muscle injury caused by suction-assisted powered instruments (debriders) is considered the most devastating complication from sinus surgery. The resulting diplopia is permanent and devastating to the patient's quality of life and its treatment is seldom successful.[12] When it does occur, immediate ophthalmology consultation should be obtained (**Fig. 3**).

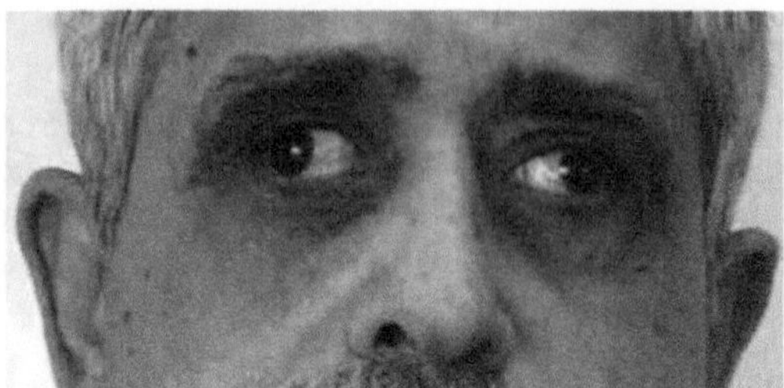

Fig. 3. A right medial rectus injury secondary to use of a powered debrider in an area of boney dehiscence.

Hemorrhage from anterior ethmoid artery

If the anterior ethmoid artery is low lying in the skull base, it can easily be damaged with through-cut instruments or the debrider during approach to the frontal sinus. It is therefore extremely important for the operating surgeon to have critically analyzed the preoperative CT scan to determine the position of the anterior ethmoid artery, the presence or absence of bone over the artery, the possible presence of more than 1 branch, and any other oddities in the anatomy of the artery before attempting surgery in the frontal recess.[13] A partial transection of the artery can result in a significant amount of bleeding but as long as the artery does not retract into the orbital cavity there is no significant danger posed to the patient's vision. A bipolar or unipolar suction cautery can be used to cauterize and control the bleeding vessel.

Complete transection of the anterior ethmoid artery may result in retraction of the artery. Retraction into the orbit may produce the rapid onset of an orbital hematoma. Orbital hematomas may be either arterial or venous in origin. Arterial bleeds are of rapid onset and usually present with intraoperative proptosis.[14] The globe usually becomes rock hard within seconds to minutes. The most important factor in managing these patients is maintaining or restoring blood flow to the optic nerve, thereby preventing visual compromise. Because vision cannot be assessed while the patient is under a general anesthetic, decisions on hematoma management must be made as if the least favorable outcome is likely. Ophthalmology assistance should be sought immediately. In reality, immediate ophthalmologic assistance may not always be available or the ophthalmologist may have limited expertise in orbital surgery. In such situations, the patient relies on the judgment and skills of the otolaryngologist. Surgical and medical management should commence immediately because ischemia time to the optic nerve is an essential factor. A lateral canthotomy with upper and/or lower cantholysis is indicated and should be performed immediately. This immediately increases orbital volume and decreases orbital pressure thereby allowing blood flow to the optic nerve once again. Simultaneous medical management includes intravenous mannitol (1 g/kg intravenously), which also decreases intraorbital pressure. The use of intravenous steroids in such a situation remains unproven and controversial. If the intraorbital pressure does not decrease despite these measures, endoscopic orbital decompression with removal of lamina papyracea should be considered.

Orbital hematomas as a result of a venous bleed usually occur in the postoperative period and present as a slowly progressive proptosis and visual loss. The patient's vision should be closely assessed, especially the color vision, because it is first to deteriorate. If the vision is within normal limits and the proptosis is mild, the patient should be observed very closely. Any nasal/sinus packing on the ipsilateral side should be removed. Orbital massage has been suggested in the literature to redistribute the blood clot within the orbit; we do not recommend this technique at our center. Ophthalmology should be consulted to assess vision, do a fundoscopy, as well as measure intraocular pressure. Medical management, including mannitol, may be started if the situation continues to worsen. If the patient's vision starts deteriorating, then surgical intervention should be performed as discussed earlier.

Intracranial entry/CSF leak

If intracranial entry and a resulting CSF leak occurs, it should be recognized and dealt with immediately.[15] The violated region of the skull base should be cleared of any sinus disease and the site of entry prepared for repair. Site preparation is the most important aspect for successfully repairing a CSF leak. The immediate area around the defect should be denuded of mucus membrane as a first step in the repair.

Depending on the skull base defect and the skill of the surgeon, a variety of underlay and overlay options using autograft and allograft material can be used for the repair.[16] At our institution, a 2- to 3-layer repair using septal bone, temporalis fascia, and a mucosal membrane graft is usually used and has been found to be very successful. A lumbar drain is not required if the repair is performed immediately. The sinus operation can then be continued and completed in the usual manner. Support to the repair site is essential. A merocel sponge in a finger glove cot is placed against the repair site for the first 7 days. Another sponge may be placed under the first one to create snug support for the repair site. During this time the patient is given oral antibiotics and advised on the importance of minimal activity and reduced physical stressors.

The only exception to not repairing the defect intraoperatively is if the surgeon remains anatomically disoriented. In such a case, any attempt at surgical repair could result in further complications, such as brain parenchymal injury or orbital injury. It is recommended that the patient be transferred to the nearest tertiary sinus center where a properly trained team can complete the repair.

If the CSF leak is not diagnosed until the postoperative period, the patient usually presents with unilateral rhinorrhea. If not identified early, the patient may suffer from serious sequelae, including meningitis, pneumocephalus, and possibly coma or death. All patients suspicious of having a CSF leak should have the secretions tested for β2-transferrin. Once a CSF leak is confirmed, investigation to seek the exact site of the leak should be sought. High-resolution, fine-cut coronal CT scan of the sinuses is performed. A search for bony defects in the area of previous surgery is attempted. The most common location for an iatrogenic CSF leak is the lateral lamella of the cribiform plate where the anterior ethmoid artery enters the intracranial cavity. Special attention should be given to opacification or air fluid levels within sinuses that may give a clue to a leak in the area.

If the site of the leak is not apparent on CT, then a magnetic resonance cisternogram should be performed.[17] It is a highly sensitive and specific test if done when the patient is actively leaking and will identify any CSF that has pooled within the sinuses. All patients with suspected meningoceles or meningoencephaloceles should undergo magnetic resonance imaging to confirm the diagnosis and for proper management.

We usually use pre- or intraoperative placement of a lumbar drain and intrathecal fluorescein for patients undergoing a CSF leak repair. Because intravenous fluorescein is not approved for intrathecal use, a separate consent designed specifically for this purpose is obtained. A lumbar puncture and placement of drain is performed while the patient is awake. Ten milliliters of CSF are removed and mixed with 0.1 mL of 10% intravenous fluorescein using a tuberculin syringe. The mixture is then re-injected into the intrathecal space at a rate of 1 mL per minute (ie, 10 minutes). Potential risks of intrathecal fluorescein injection include parasthesias and convulsions. These side effects have been reported in the past but with much higher doses of fluorescein than used currently. The fluorescein stains the CSF a fluorescent yellow-green color allowing precise confirmation of the leak site. A blue light filter placed on the light source helps to identify the presence of fluorescein even in very small quantities. If the leak is not visible, the patient may be placed in a head down position and the anesthesiologist may perform a valsalva maneuver. Once the site of the leak is identified, the repair process is similar to that described earlier for CSF leaks diagnosed intraoperatively.

Bone denudation of mucus membrane

If the mucus membrane is inadvertently damaged/removed during the dissection in the frontal recess, the risk of osteoneogenesis and scarring of the frontal recess increases significantly. This requires that the surgeon be very careful when dissecting in the frontal recess/sinus region. If an area of denudation does occur and it is in the region of the frontal sinus ostium, a free mucosal membrane graft can be considered to cover the area and thereby avoid osteoneogenesis and scar formation. If it is not possible to cover the denuded area then the denuded area should be washed out with an antibiotic/steroid gel at the end of the operation and watched carefully during the postoperative period.

MEL Procedure Complications

The MEL procedure is a more extensive form of endoscopic frontal sinusotomy with loss of mucus membrane in a critical area with the possibility of significant potential complications. Re-stenosis of the frontal recess secondary to denudation of the bone from this procedure continues to remain high. Long-term patency and re-stenosis is the most concerning complication and has received a good deal of attention.[18] The drilling in the agger and anterior buttress region destroys the lateral frontal recess mucous membrane. This particular mucous membrane carries the ciliary mucous transport mechanism for exit out of the frontal sinus. Destruction of this important mucus membrane puts the frontal sinus at risk for mucociliary clearance failure, neoosteogenesis, and re-stenosis (**Fig. 4**). Denuded bone results in the formation of crusting, chronic infections, and persistent symptoms. Wormald[19] showed that 21 out of the 83 patients who had MEL procedures continued to have symptoms. Their group also demonstrated in another study that all patients undergoing MEL procedures had a 33% narrowing of the neoostium at 1 year after surgery. Twenty-two of 77 patients had significant stenosis (>60%) and 9 patients (12%) required revision surgery.[20] The accompanying endoscopic picture (see **Fig. 4**) shows extensive scarring from a MEL procedure after 2 years.

Frontal Sinus Trephine

Misdirected attempts to enter the frontal sinus may result in intracranial entry. The consequences depend on the depth of intracranial entry and structures injured. In all circumstances, the worst should be suspected as major complications may occur

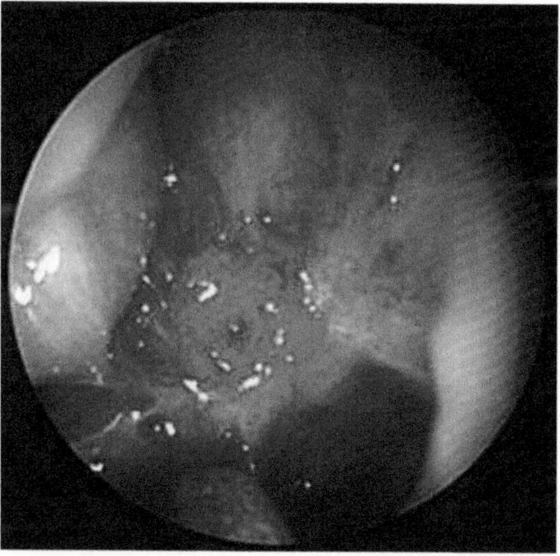

Fig. 4. Endoscopic view of a scarred MEL procedure 2 years after surgery.

ranging from CSF leaks to intracranial bleeds to postoperative brain abscess formation. Neurosurgical assistance should be sought if needed, and further management may be performed either endoscopically or through external approaches depending on the type of injury and experience of the surgeon. The surgeon should be aware of the potential of damage to the supraorbital and/or supratrochlear nerves resulting in numbness or parasthesias in the forehead region.

Osteoplastic Frontal Sinus Procedures Complications

Complications from osteoplastic frontal sinus procedures can vary widely depending on the type of incisions used, extent of frontal sinus pneumatization, type of disease being treated, and the need of obliteration.

An unfavorable or visible scar may result if the incision is not positioned properly. Multiple types of incisions have been discussed in the literature. If the disease is unilateral and the procedure limited, we prefer to use a brow or half gull-wing incision. In case of bilateral but limited disease, a gull-wing incision may be used. The incision is beveled and hidden in the eyebrow to preserve hair follicles and provide a more cosmetically acceptable scar. The supratrochlear and supraorbital nerves are identified and preserved by working around them in most instances.

If the amount of work required in the sinus is extensive, eyebrow incisions may not be appropriate, in which case a bicoronal incision and osteoplastic flap may be used. The incision may be placed behind the hairline. Great care should be taken so that branches of the facial nerve are not injured when elevating the flap. Numbness does occur over the scalp, posterior to the area of incision.

Dural lacerations and inadvertent intracranial entry may occur during the initial raising of the bony flap and entry into the frontal sinus. Several methods have been described to mark the boundaries of the frontal sinus ranging from the use of a 1.8-m (6-ft) Caldwell film to transilluminate the frontal sinus to using image-guided navigation devices.[21] We have been using the image guidance system to enter the frontal sinus in almost all our cases for the last decade and have found it to be very accurate. In the event of a dural tear and intracranial entry, neurosurgical help should be sought to avoid further damaging consequences.

Mucoceles have been considered the most common long-term complication of the frontal sinus obliteration procedure. They can occur from 1 to 42 years after surgery with an average of 7.5 years.[22] The most common site of a late mucocele is the frontal recess. This occurs because of persistent mucosa trapped between the fat and unresected mucus-producing cells trapped within the frontal recess. Great care must be taken to meticulously remove and drill all the mucosa from the frontal sinus and recess if an obliteration procedure is being performed. This can be difficult and in some situations impossible to achieve. If there is any question about the complete removal of all frontal sinus mucosa, obliteration should be avoided.

Infection of the adipose graft may occur in the postoperative period. This may occur with or without evidence of mucocele formation. When this occurs, the frontal sinus unobliteration procedure is recommended.[23] When unobliterating the frontal sinus, the primary task is to remove the diseased tissue within the frontal sinus and connect the mucosalized areas to a functional internal frontal ostium. Some practitioners prefer to use the MEL procedure to attempt this. At our center, every effort is undertaken to preserve the remaining mucus membrane by performing an endoscopic revision frontal sinusotomy and using silastic or biliary t-tube stents to keep the drainage pathway patent and functional. A T-shaped 0.25-mm (0.01-inch) thick silastic template is placed onto the posterior sinus table with the upper flanges sitting within the neo-frontal sinus. The inferior flap is rolled and passed down through the frontal ostium to act as a stent. In this manner, every part of the sinus outflow tract is protected from synechiae formation. The stent is left in place for a minimum of 6 months but usually longer if tolerated by the patient.

SUMMARY

Successful endoscopic frontal sinus surgery is reliant on a good working knowledge of frontal recess anatomy, mucosal-sparing techniques, and meticulous postoperative care. Good practice of these principles aid in avoiding complications and insuring good surgical outcomes.

REFERENCES

1. Kew J, Rees GL, Close D, et al. Multiplanar reconstructed computed tomography images improves depiction and understanding of the anatomy of the frontal sinus and recess. Am J Rhinol 2002;16(2):119–23.
2. Wormald PJ. Surgery of the frontal recess and frontal sinus. Rhinology 2005; 43(2):82–5.
3. Wright ED, Agrawal S. Impact of perioperative systemic steroids on surgical outcomes in patients with chronic rhinosinusitis with polyposis: evaluation with the novel Perioperative Sinus Endoscopy (POSE) scoring system. Laryngoscope 2007;117(11 Pt 2 Suppl 115):1–28.
4. Javer AR, Gheriani H, Mechor B, et al. Effect of intraoperative injection of 0.25% bupivacaine with 1:200,000 epinephrine on intraoperative blood loss in FESS. Am J Rhinol Allergy 2009;23(4):437–41.
5. Thevasagayam M, Jindal M, et al. Does epinephrine infiltration in septoplasty make any difference? A double blind randomized controlled trial. Eur Arch Otorhinolaryngol 2007;264:1175–8.
6. Landsberg R, Friedman M. A minimally invasive endoscopic approach to chronic isolated frontal sinusitis. Operat Tech Otolaryngol Head Neck Surg 2006;17(3): 184–8.
7. Moulin G, Dessi P, Chagnaud C, et al. Dehiscence of the lamina papyracea of the ethmoid bone: CT findings. AJNR Am J Neuroradiol 1994;15(1):151–3.
8. Kuhn FA, Javer AR. Primary endoscopic management of the frontal sinus. Otolaryngol Clin North Am 2001;34(1):59–75.
9. Philpott CM, McKiernan DC, Javer AR. Selecting the best approach to the frontal sinus. Submitted for publication.
10. Shoman N, Gheriani H, Flamer D, et al. Prospective, double-blind, randomized trial evaluating patient satisfaction, bleeding, and wound healing using biodegradable synthetic polyurethane foam (NasoPore) as a middle meatal spacer in functional endoscopic sinus surgery. J Otolaryngol Head Neck Surg 2009; 38(1):112–8.
11. Kuhn FA, Wong KK, Mechor B, et al. Creating the "double curved" suctions for sinus endoscopy and surgery. Laryngoscope 2007;117(8):1450–1.
12. Raham SM, Nerad JA. Orbital complications in endoscopic sinus surgery using powered instrumentation. Laryngoscope 2003;113(5):874–8.
13. Simmen D, Raghavan U, Briner HR, et al. The surgeon's view of the anterior ethmoid artery. Clin Otolaryngol 2006;31(3):187–91.
14. Welch KC, Palmer JN. Intraoperative emergencies during endoscopic sinus surgery: CSF leak and orbital hematoma [review]. Otolaryngol Clin North Am 2008;41(3):581–96, ix–x.

15. Platt MP, Parnes SM. Management of unexpected cerebrospinal fluid leak during endoscopic sinus surgery [review]. Curr Opin Otolaryngol Head Neck Surg 2009; 17(1):28–32.
16. Artin TJ, Loehrl TA. Endoscopic CSF leak repair [review]. Curr Opin Otolaryngol Head Neck Surg 2007;15(1):35–9.
17. Sillers MJ, Morgan CE, el Gammal T. Magnetic resonance cisternography and thin coronal computerized tomography in the evaluation of cerebrospinal fluid rhinorrhea. Am J Rhinol 1997;11(5):387–92.
18. Anderson P, Sindwani R. Safety and efficacy of the endoscopic modified Lothrop procedure: a systematic review and meta-analysis [review]. Laryngoscope 2009; 119(9):1828–33.
19. Wormald PJ. Salvage frontal sinus surgery: the endoscopic modified Lothrop procedure. Laryngoscope 2003;113(2):276–83.
20. Tran KN, Beule AG, Singal D, et al. Frontal ostium restenosis after the endoscopic modified Lothrop procedure. Laryngoscope 2007;117(8):1457–62.
21. Melroy CT, Dubin MG, Hardy SM, et al. Analysis of methods to assess frontal sinus extent in osteoplastic flap surgery: transillumination versus 6-ft Caldwell versus image guidance. Am J Rhinol 2006;20(1):77–83.
22. Bockmühl U, Kratzsch B, Benda K, et al. [Paranasal sinus mucoceles: surgical management and long term results]. Laryngorhinootologie 2005;84(12):892–8 [in German].
23. Javer AR, Sillers MJ, Kuhn FA. The frontal sinus unobliteration procedure. Otolaryngol Clin North Am 2001;34(1):193–210.

Prevention and Management of Complications in Sphenoidotomy

Carl W. Moeller, MD, Kevin C. Welch, MD*

KEYWORDS

- Sphenoid sinus • Sinus surgery • Endoscopic sphenoidotomy
- Surgical complications

Chronic rhinosinusitis is a common disorder accounting for an estimated 20 million visits to physician offices in the United States each year. The aggregated cost of sinusitis is approximately $1.8 billion annually, affecting an estimated 16% of the population in the United States. Despite multiple attempted treatments, including an estimated 500,000 surgeries per year, the disease continues to be a major health problem, both in expenditures and poor quality of life.[1,2] Functional endoscopic sinus surgery is reserved for patients for whom medical therapy including intranasal steroids, systemic steroids, oral antibiotics, oral and intranasal antihistamines, leukotriene inhibitors, and saline irrigation has failed.

When medical therapy fails to treat patients with chronic rhinosinusitis, surgery is indicated. This article discusses surgery of the sphenoid sinus and its complications. The completion of a safe sphenoidotomy depends on familiarity with its anatomy and its related structures and their variations. A careful review of preoperative CT scans and identification of intraoperative landmarks is paramount to a safe and successful operation. Despite detailed analysis of preoperative CT images and meticulous surgical technique, complications can occur.

Complications of sphenoid sinus surgery can be divided into two categories: intraoperative complications and postoperative complications. Intraoperative complications can be devastating and include vascular and neurologic injury, including those that lead to cerebrospinal fluid (CSF) leaks. Postoperative complications are typically less severe and can be considered functional complications leading to poor long-term surgical outcomes. Examples of these complications include epistaxis, ostial stenosis, and delayed mucocele formation.

Disclosures: None.
Department of Otolaryngology–Head and Neck Surgery, Loyola University School of Medicine, 2160 South First Avenue, Maguire Building, Maywood, IL 60153, USA
* Corresponding author.
E-mail address: kwelch1@lumc.edu

Otolaryngol Clin N Am 43 (2010) 839–854
doi:10.1016/j.otc.2010.04.009 **oto.theclinics.com**

ANATOMY

The paired sphenoid sinuses result from progressive pneumatization of the body of the sphenoid bone, which is situated centrally at the base of the skull. Aeration begins at approximately 3 months gestational age with the invagination of the cartilaginous cupolar recess and progresses through the teenage years.

The sphenoid sinus itself is bounded anterosuperiorly by the sphenoid crest, which articulates with the ethmoid plate and anteroinferiorly by the rostrum, which articulates with the vomer. Lateral to the sphenoid crest are the sphenoid ostia, which measure approximately 2 mm in dimension, are located 10 to 22 mm from the floor of the sphenoid and approximately 7 cm from the anterior nasal spine.[3–6] Lateral to the rostrum lie the vaginal processes and the pterygopalatine (vidian) foramina. The lateral limit of the sphenoid sinus is variable depending on the extent of pneumatization into the greater wings of the sphenoid bone and pterygoid processes. Typically, the lateral limit of the sphenoid sinus is flush with the cavernous sinus. Pneumatization may extend laterally between the maxillary and vidian nerves, superior to the infratemporal fossa and inferior to the middle cranial fossa. The floor of the sphenoid sinus forms the roof of the nasopharynx and is contiguous with the anterior aspect of the clivus posteroinferiorly.

The roof and posterior boundaries of the sphenoid sinus depend largely on a well-described sphenoid bone pneumatization pattern. As originally described by Hamberger,[7] pneumatization of the sphenoid bone is classified as conchal, presellar, or sellar. The conchal pattern is uncommon and defined by absent (or rudimentary) pneumatization of the sphenoid bone. In the presellar pattern, pneumatization extends to the anterior face of the sella turcica, whereas pneumatization extending to the posterior face of the sella turcica is defined as sellar pneumatization (**Fig. 1**). The sellar configuration is the most common pattern and is found in 86% of the population, whereas presellar and conchal pneumatization patterns account for only 11% and 3% of the population, respectively.[7] Other surgeons[4,8–10] use a modified version of the Hamberger classification by defining a presellar configuration (anterior to the sella turcica), a sellar configuration (flush with the face of the sella turcica), and a postsellar configuration (pneumatization inferior to the sella turcica). As with Hamberger, pneumatization beyond the limits of the sella turcica is found most frequently. In patients with postsellar pneumatization, the sella forms part of the sphenoid roof, and the remainder is formed by the planum sphenoidale.

Sphenoid sinus dimensions vary but typically measure approximately 2 cm × 2 cm × 3 cm,[4,5] with a volume ranging from 5.8 to 7.5 mL.[4,5,11,12] Although paired in nature, the

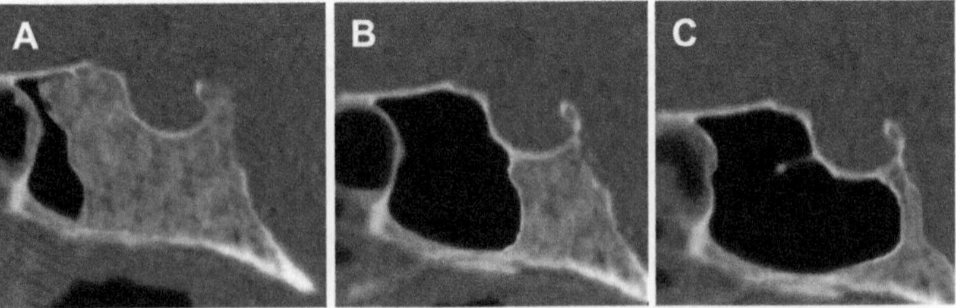

Fig. 1. Sagittal CT demonstrations of pneumatization patterns of the sphenoid sinus. The conchal pattern (*A*) represents underpneumatization of the sphenoid bone. The presellar pattern (*B*) is defined by pneumatization of the sphenoid bone to the sella turcica. The sellar pattern (*C*) is demonstrated by pneumatization inferior to the sella turcica.

bilateral sphenoid sinuses are infrequently symmetric. The degree of septation within the sphenoid sinus creates this lack of symmetry. A single septum is identified in 20% to 95% of specimens,[5,9,10] with accessory septations in 11% to 41%.[5,9,13] More importantly, when a single septum is identified, this septation commonly is located off of the midline,[13] indicating that the septum inserts off the midline in most cases (and may mislead the surgeon when identifying the midline). When more septations are present, these septations frequently insert on one or both carotid prominences[13] (**Fig. 2**) and are oriented in the sagittal plane. Septations that are transverse or horizontal may indicate the presence of a sphenoethmoidal cell (discussed later).

Several neurovascular structures are intimately related to the sphenoid sinus. The largest most important vascular structure is the carotid artery, located medially within the cavernous sinus. The carotid artery indents the lateral wall of the sphenoid sinus in 71% to 98% of cases[8,14,15] and may be dehiscent in 4% to 22%.[4,8,14,16,17] In the superolateral wall of the sphenoid sinus, the optic nerve is identified, typically by a bulge in 8% to 100% of patients,[5,14,15,18] and is dehiscent in 4% to 8%.[16,18] Together, the optic nerve and the carotid artery form the opticocarotid recess (**Fig. 3**). Autonomic fibers contained within the pterygopalatine (ie, vidian) nerve run along the lateral floor of the sphenoid sinus within the pterygopalatine canal, inferior and medial to the maxillary nerve (V_2), which can be exposed when significant lateral pneumatization of the sphenoid bone is present.

The sphenoid sinus may be related to a sphenoethmoidal[19] (ie, Onodi[20]) cell, which may be present in 3% to 42% of patients.[21–24] A sphenoethmoid cell pneumatizes superolaterally to the sphenoid sinus, and can be recognized radiographically by the presence of a horizontal septation within the sphenoid sinus on coronal imaging (**Fig. 4**). When a sphenoethmoidal cell is present, the optic nerve travels immediately lateral to this ethmoid sinus rather than the sphenoid sinus itself. This anatomic variation places the optic nerve at risk if a sphenoidotomy is performed in a haphazard fashion.

Given the complex anatomy and vital structures surrounding the sphenoid sinuses, great care must be taken when operating within or around the sphenoid sinuses. An in-depth understanding of the regional anatomy lessens the risk for operative complications during sphenoidotomy.

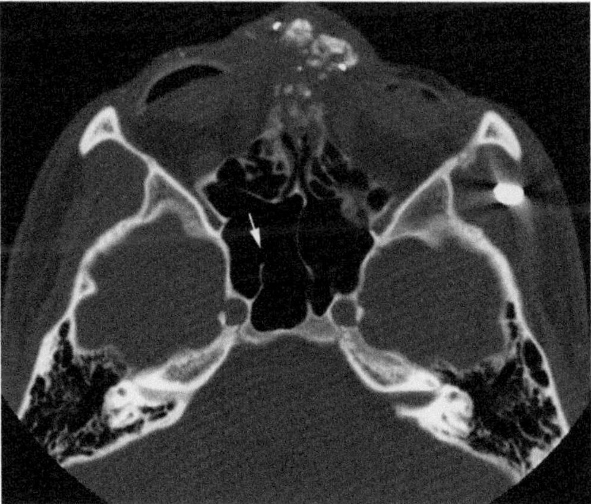

Fig. 2. Septations within the sphenoid sinus are best identified with a CT scan viewed in the axial plane. In this figure, a septation can be seen inserting on the right carotid canal (*arrow*). A larger septation arises and inserts essentially in the midline; however, it inserts posteriorly near the left carotid canal.

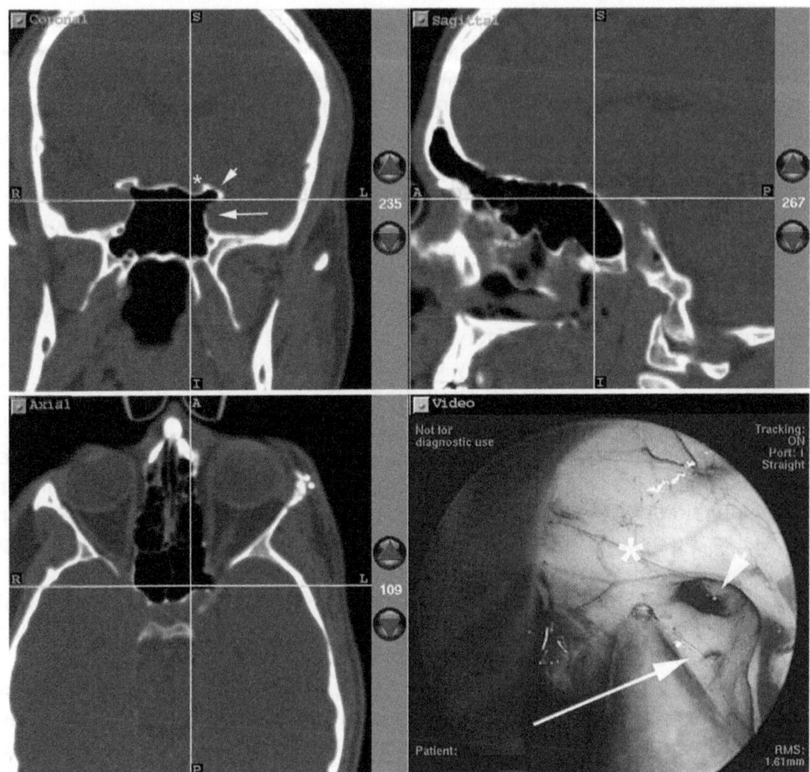

Fig. 3. These triplanar images show the relationship between the optic nerve (*asterisk*) and the carotid artery (*arrow*). Together, they form the opticocarotid recess (*arrowhead*). In this patient, the anterior clinoid process is aerated, making the recess easy to identify (and placing these structures at increased risk for injury).

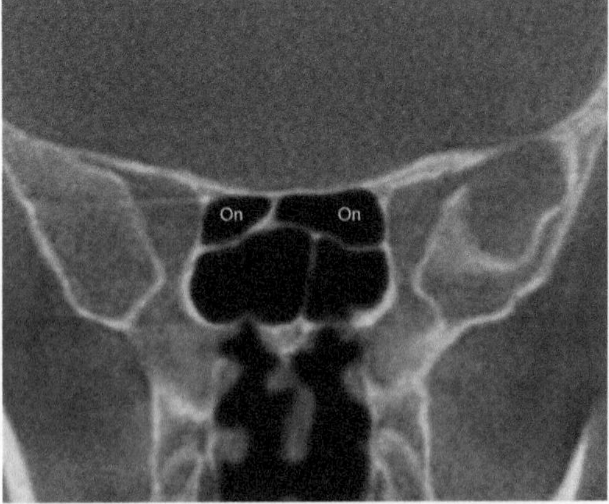

Fig. 4. Horizontal septations within the sphenoid sinus signify the presence of possible sphenoethmoidal (Onodi) cells (On). These cells are best viewed with CT images viewed in the coronal plane. If sagittal reformations are available, the sphenoethmoidal cell can be seen pneumatizing superior to the sphenoid sinus.

OPERATIVE TECHNIQUE

The sphenoid sinus can be safely entered through the posterior ethmoid or the nasal cavity, medial to the superior turbinate.[25–28] When the sphenoidotomy is performed through the ethmoid route, the superior turbinate is identified after perforating the basal lamella (**Fig. 5**). Once the superior turbinate is identified, the surgeon is directed toward the sphenoid os, which lies medial to the superior turbinate. A parallelogram is then envisioned, with its boundaries being the skull base superiorly, the lamina papyracea laterally, the septum and superior turbinate medially, and the horizontal portion of the basal lamella inferiorly. The parallelogram is divided superomedially to inferolaterally (**Fig. 6**).

Surgeons generally may safely enter the sphenoid sinus in the inferomedial portion of this "box"[28] without significant risk to the carotid artery or the optic nerve. Entry into a sphenoethmoidal cell may be avoided when using this technique. If difficulty identifying the superior turbinate is encountered, lateralizing the middle turbinate with an elevator and introducing a 0° camera medial to the middle turbinate to locate the sphenoid ostium medial to the superior turbinate is often helpful.

When entering the sphenoid sinus through the transnasal route, the os is usually located 7 cm from the limen nasi and approximately 30° from the nasal floor.[3,6] A measured beaded probe or stereotactic probes may be used to confirm these distances.[26,29] If entering the sphenoid from this route, the superior turbinate need not be manipulated further; however, when entering the sphenoid through the ethmoid route, removing the lower third or half using a through-cutting punch typically helps visualize the sphenoid ostium.

Using a curette or suction, the os can usually be cannulated without much difficulty. Bleeding in the region of the os can obstruct visualization. If not performed already, a transoral pterygopalatine fossa injection with 1% lidocaine and 1:100,000 epinephrine may help constrict the sphenopalatine artery and its branches, and additional injection around the septal branch of the sphenopalatine artery may further induce vasoconstriction. Pledgets moistened with 0.05% oxymetazoline or a mixture of

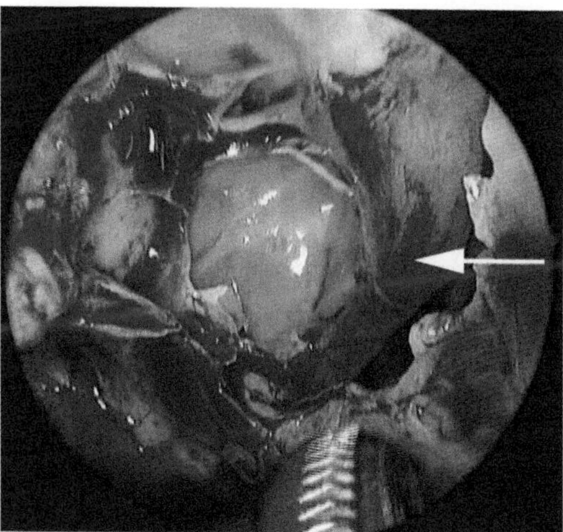

Fig. 5. Endoscopic view of the right sinonasal cavity. The superior turbinate (*arrow*) is the gateway to the sphenoid sinus. After the basal lamella is perforated, the superior turbinate is easily identified as it arises from the posterior aspect of the middle turbinate. The sphenoid os is located medial to the superior turbinate.

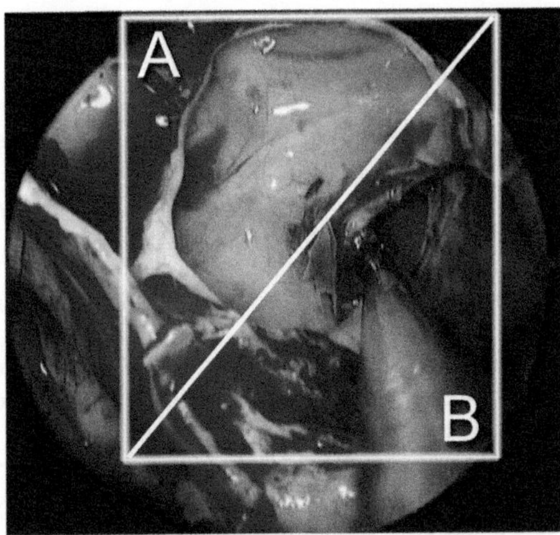

Fig. 6. Endoscopic view of the right sinonasal cavity. After the superior turbinate is partially resected, an imaginary parallelogram is drawn with the boundaries being the lamina papyracea laterally, skull base superiorly, and superior turbinate lamella both inferiorly and medially. Entering the sphenoid sinus in the superolateral half is unsafe (*A*), whereas entering the sphenoid through the inferomedial half is usually safe (*B*).

1:1000 epinephrine and 10,000 units of thrombin are also useful to help control bleeding. If bleeding near or on the skull base cannot be controlled with pledgets, cautery may be necessary. Electrocautery should be used with discretion around the sphenoid sinus and, when necessary, bipolar electrocautery should be used, because monopolar cautery can cause inadvertent CSF leak when used close to the skull base.

After the sphenoid sinus is entered through the ostium, it is enlarged superiorly and laterally using a circular sphenoid punch. When opened maximally, the superior limit of the sphenoidotomy is the roof of the sinus, which is an invaluable landmark and particularly useful when clearing posterior ethmoid cells from the skull base. Laterally, the sphenoidotomy can be widened to the lateral wall of the sinus, taking care to note the position of the optic nerve, the presence or absence of a sphenoethmoidal[19] (Onodi[20]) cell, and the position of the pterygopalatine neurovascular bundle. Aggressive enlargement inferiorly is discouraged to avoid the septal branch of the sphenopalatine artery. Furthermore, the vidian nerve runs along the inferolateral floor of the sinus and could be damaged if the sphenoidotomy is extended too far inferiorly and laterally.

When performing surgery for mild to moderate chronic sinusitis, opening and widening the natural os is typically all that is required. When polyps are present or if inspissated secretions or fungal material may need to be extracted, a larger sphenoidotomy is performed. Instrumentation within the sphenoid sinus, however, is fraught with potential complications and should be avoided.

INTRAOPERATIVE COMPLICATIONS

Local Hemorrhage

Several vascular structures can be injured during sphenoidotomy: the posterior ethmoidal artery (PEA), the artery of the pterygoid canal, the artery of the palatovaginal canal, and the septal branch of the sphenopalatine artery. When these vascular structures are injured, they typically cause local hemorrhage, which jeopardizes the surgical field and may require termination of the case if not adequately controlled. In rare circumstances, injury can constitute a surgical emergency.

The PEA is a branch of the ophthalmic artery that usually passes through the posterior ethmoidal canal to give branches to the posterior ethmoid cells before it enters into the cranium to supply the dura through its meningeal branches. Additionally, it emanates branches that anastomose with the branches of the sphenopalatine artery to supply the superior portion of the posterior septum. The relationship of the PEA has been characterized by CT[30] and endoscopic dissection.[31] Typically, the artery is embedded within the skull base; however, it may be suspended within a bony mesentery if significant supraorbital ethmoid cells are present (**Fig. 7**).

Using CT images, Gotwald and colleagues[30] identified indentations in the medial orbital wall and the relationship between the medial rectus muscle and the superior oblique muscle as reliable radiologic landmarks for the PEA. Han and colleagues[31] performed dissections on 24 cadaver heads and used an image guidance system to record the location of the PEA in reference to the anterior wall of the sphenoid sinus. The mean distance from the PEA to the anterior face of the sphenoid sinus was 8.1 mm and the artery was located anterior to the sphenoid face in 98% of specimens, and on average 14.9 mm posterior to the anterior ethmoidal artery.

Avoidance of this artery involves correlating preoperative and intraoperative (stereotactic, when used) imaging with endoscopic visualization (**Fig. 8**). It is best to avoid overly aggressive removal of the anterior face of the sphenoid sinus or high posterior ethmoid partitions to avoid the PEA. When the artery is injured, it is best controlled with bipolar electrocautery. If not controlled, it not only can cause local hemorrhage but also may retract within the orbit and lead to devastating orbital complications.[32] In this circumstance, an external incision may need to be performed to ligate the ethmoidal arteries.

The artery of the pterygoid (vidian) canal has dual origins: the external carotid artery (by way of the internal maxillary artery [IMA]) and the C2 segment of the internal carotid artery,[33,34] although it more commonly arises from the IMA. It gives rise to an anastomotic network supplied also by the ascending pharyngeal artery and the accessory meningeal artery. This vessel is uncommonly encountered in routine sinus surgery unless the surgeon has performed a wide sphenoidotomy that includes removal of the sphenoid bone laterally and inferiorly near the pterygoid plate. Brisk bleeding

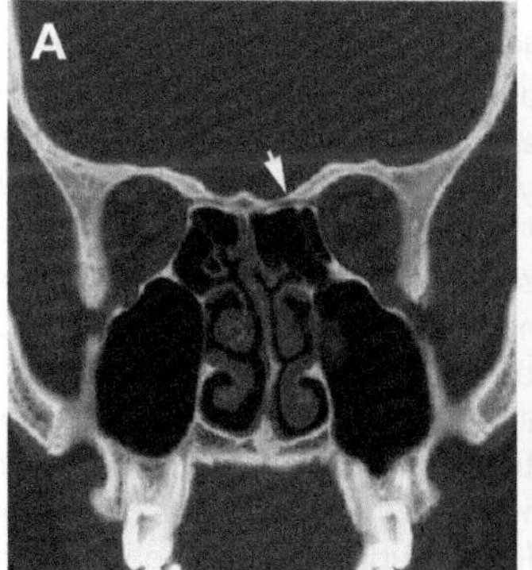

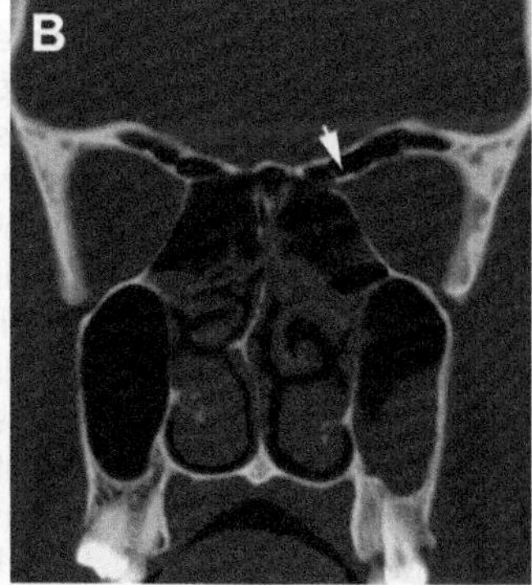

Fig. 7. The posterior ethmoidal artery (*arrowhead*) commonly traverses within the skull base (*A*); however, it may be seen suspended from the skull base within a bony mesentery (*B*) in patients with extensively pneumatized ethmoid sinuses or supraorbital ethmoid cells.

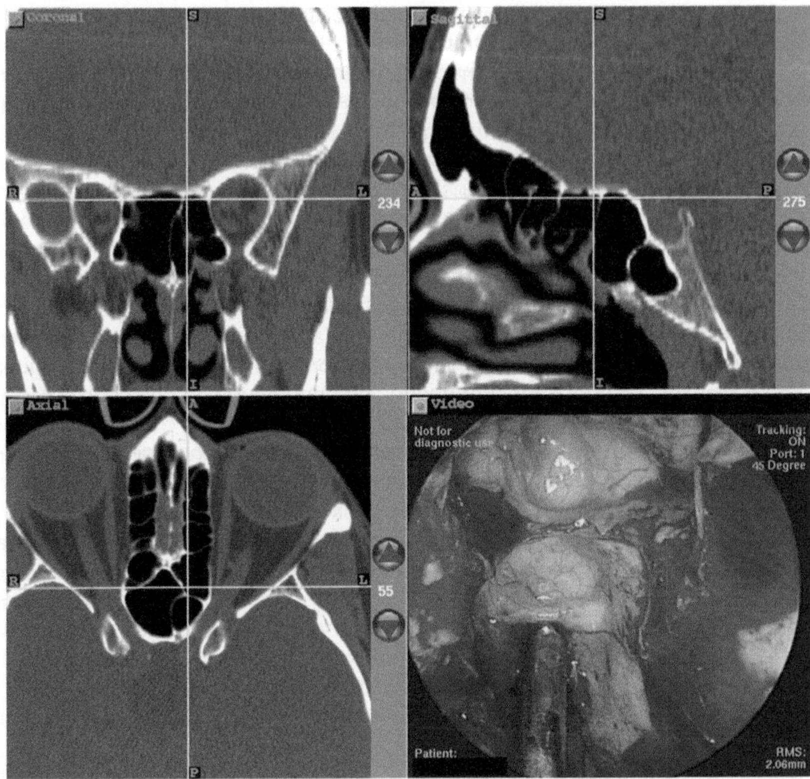

Fig. 8. These triplanar images show the location of the posterior ethmoidal artery as it courses across the skull base near the sphenoid sinus. Overly aggressive removal of the anterior face of the sphenoid sinus can lead to injury to this artery.

and injury to the vidian nerve may be encountered, requiring subsequent control of hemorrhage. This neurovascular structure, however, presents a legitimate issue when addressing lateral sphenoid sinus defects (eg, meningoencephaloceles), but further discussion is beyond the scope of this article.

The pharyngeal branch of the IMA passes through the palatovaginal canal, located on the undersurface of the body of the sphenoid bone. The canal is formed by the articulation of the vaginal process of the sphenoid bone and sphenoidal process of the palatine bone. It is flanked laterally by the medial pterygoid plate and medially by the sphenoid rostrum and vomer. The vessel may be injured when opening the sphenoid sinus inferiorly and laterally, but is easily controlled with monopolar cautery.

The most prominent vascular structure encountered when performing a sphenoidotomy is the septal branch of the sphenopalatine artery, which is a distal branch of the IMA. The septal branch of the sphenopalatine typically is one of two main branches directly arising from the sphenopalatine artery within the sphenopalatine foramina,[35–37] and traverses across the anterior face of the sphenoid sinus near the insertion of the superior turbinate posteriorly and superior to the posterior lateral nasal arterial branch, which supplies the middle turbinate.[36] After crossing the anteroinferior face of the sphenoid sinus (**Fig. 9**), the artery typically branches to supply the septum and anastomose in Little's area anteriorly.[38] This vessel is typically encountered when

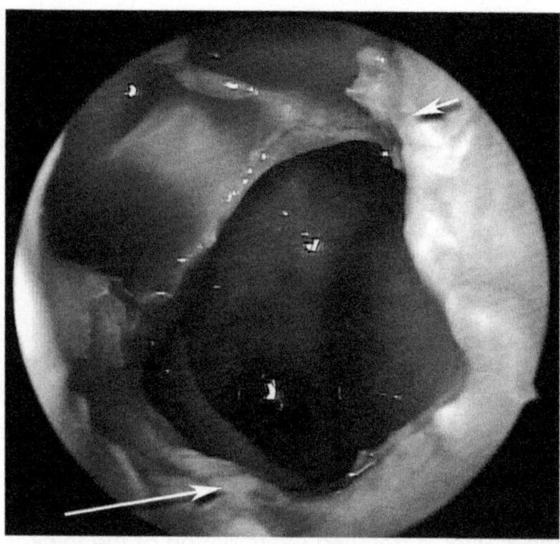

Fig. 9. In this latex-injected cadaveric specimen, the septal branch of the sphenopalatine artery (*arrow*) can be seen traversing the inferior aspect of the sphenoid sinus face. The septum and superior turbinate remnant (*arrowhead*) are seen on the medial aspect of the sinus.

opening the sphenoid sinus too inferiorly near the horizontal portion of the superior turbinate. When the vessel is encountered, it is easily controlled with monopolar cautery; however, this action can typically lead to postoperative crust formation, scarring, and stenosis of the ostium. When necessary, the sphenopalatine artery itself may be ligated near the sphenopalatine foramen or crista ethmoidalis if bleeding persists.

Local hemorrhage can typically be controlled with epinephrine-soaked pledgets and patience. Communication with the anesthesiologist is vital when encountering localized hemorrhage, because managing the mean arterial pressure and the heart rate are helpful in decreasing local hemorrhage. If packing and control of hemodynamics are unsuccessful, judicious monopolar cautery is highly effective at controlling local bleeding. However, indiscriminate cautery should be avoided, because it may contribute to postoperative scarring and stenosis. Biosynthetic topical powders and sponges are also useful adjuncts for achieving and maintaining hemostasis in these circumstances.

Catastrophic Hemorrhage

The internal carotid artery (ICA) consists of seven segments;[39] however, only the cavernous portion (C4) is relevant during routine sinus surgery because it is intimately associated with the lateral wall of the sphenoid sinus. The ICA indents the lateral wall of the sphenoid sinus in 71% to 98% of cases[8,14,15] and may be dehiscent in 4% to 22% (**Fig. 10**).[4,8,14,16,17] Fujii and colleagues[16] noted a 98% incidence of the ICA bulging into the sphenoid sinus, an 8% incidence of bony dehiscence, and an 88% incidence of bone less than 0.5 mm covering the artery. Kennedy and colleagues[17] assessed ICA dehiscence clinically as opposed to pathologically or radiographically, defining dehiscence as an area over the artery that was soft to palpation. The study reports a 22% incidence of clinical dehiscence in 147 sphenoid sinuses studied, which is significantly higher than frequently cited in the literature. Others have reported the more extreme: a grossly dehiscent carotid artery presenting as a sphenoid sinus mass.[40] Therefore, although preoperative identification of the carotid artery's course

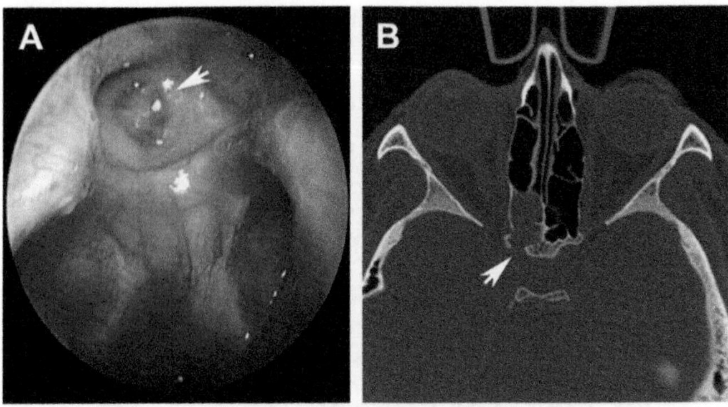

Fig. 10. Endoscopic (*A*) and radiographic (*B*) views of a dehiscent carotid artery (*arrowhead*).

and presence of bone is vital, a detailed examination of the thickness of bone is also necessary to help avoid injury to the carotid artery, especially when bone can be as thin as 0.5 mm.

Entering and enlarging the natural os minimizes the risk for ICA injury during routine sphenoidotomy. However, significant anatomic variability exists, and therefore the potential for catastrophic carotid injury. Delayed carotid injures (namely development of a carotid artery pseudoaneurysm and carotid-cavernous fistula) are rare and have been successfully treated with endovascular intervention.[41–43] Typically, however, the sequelae of ICA injury will be dramatic and immediate, characterized by massive hemorrhage. Management of carotid artery injury during endoscopic sinus surgery was proposed by Sofferman[44] and has become to be known as the *carotid drill* (**Fig. 11**). If available, balloon occlusion with EEG monitoring, followed by endovascular embolization, offers the least invasive method that minimizes the chances for permanent neurologic sequelae. If angiography is unavailable, the neck is opened immediately and the carotid is ligated. Ligature in the neck is followed by clipping the carotid artery below the anterior cerebral artery through craniotomy, successfully trapping the injured segment between the two sites of ligature.

Optic Nerve Injury

The opticocarotid recess is identified within the lateral posterosuperior corner of the sphenoid sinus and represents the confluence of the ICA and the optic nerve, and serves as a landmark for the anterior clinoid process. The optic nerve courses along the superolateral aspect of the sphenoid sinus and a lateral bulge or prominence can often be appreciated intraoperatively and radiographically. In a prospective review of 150 CT scans, Dessi and colleagues[18] noted an 8% incidence of optic nerve protrusion into the sphenoid sinus. In these circumstances, the nerve is covered by a thin layer of mucosa. Fujii and colleagues[16] reported a 4% incidence of bony dehiscence, with only sinonasal mucosa covering the nerve; 78% of specimens were covered by bone less than 0.5 mm thick. Furthermore, in the presence of a laterally pneumatized sphenoid sinus (especially when a sphenoethmoidal cell is present), the nerve can actually be suspended within the sinus (**Fig. 12**), placing it at significant risk for injury.

Avoidance of the optic nerve requires diligent preoperative assessment of all CT images to ascertain the course of the optic nerve, the absence of bone covering the optic nerve, and whether any sphenoethmoidal cells are present. As Onodi warned,[20]

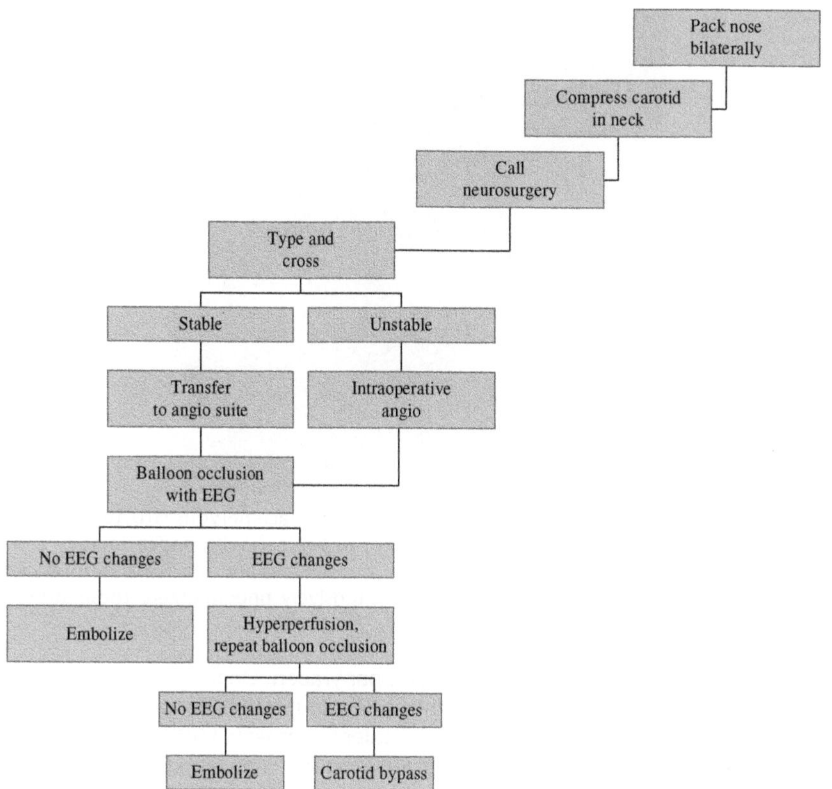

Fig. 11. The Sofferman protocol.

it is a mistake to assume that the sphenoid sinus can be entered directly posteriorly to the ethmoids or by following the lamina papyracea posteriorly. Following the lamina papyracea into the sphenoid is a recipe for optic nerve injury. When injured, management of the optic nerve depends on the extent of injury. It the nerve is visibly transected, the damage is irreparable. In this circumstance, it is prudent to examine the orbital apex and the optic canal to ensure that a CSF leak has not occurred, and to repair any leak that has. Hemostasis should be achieved, and patients should be emerged from anesthesia for evaluation by an ophthalmologist.

A paucity of data relates to lesser injury of the optic nerve during endoscopic sinus surgery. Intravenous corticosteroid administration and optic nerve decompression are common treatments for traumatic optic neuropathy; however, their usefulness in endoscopic sinus surgery has not been adequately studied. If a direct injury to the nerve has occurred, decompression of the nerve is recommended with removal of bone fragments. Further management should be addressed on a case-by-case basis with the help of an ophthalmologist.

Cerebrospinal Fluid Leak

During routine sinus surgery, the regions most at risk for CSF leak within the posterior ethmoid region are the fovea ethmoidalis, lateral cribiform lamella, and cribiform plate. Posteriorly, these structures abut the planum sphenoidale, which comprises the roof the sphenoid sinus. Skull base injury is best avoided by entering sphenoid through

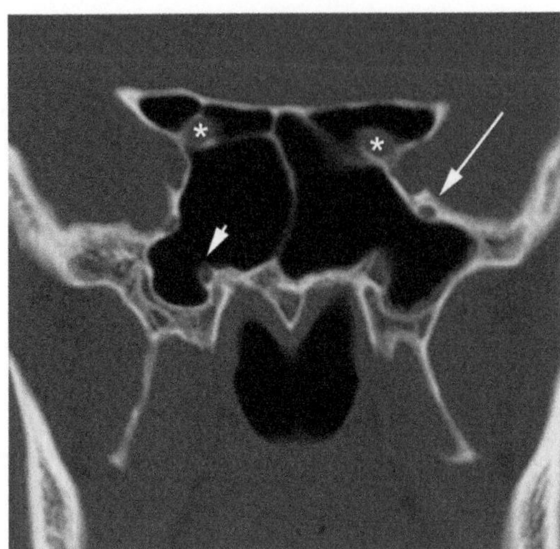

Fig. 12. Extensive pneumatization in some patients can place nervous structures at risk. In this coronal CT figure, the optic nerves (*asterisk*) can be seen with approximately 270° of exposure within the sphenoid sinus. The vidian (*arrowhead*) and maxillary (*arrow*) nerves also can be seen. When the sphenoid bone is extensively pneumatized, these structures are at increased risk for injury.

the natural ostium and away from the lamina papyracea. Once the sphenoid sinus is entered, carefully identifying the roof of the sphenoid through incrementally removing the anterior wall with a sphenoid punch is the safest approach. More aggressive instruments, such as the Hajek-Kofler punch or Kerrison punches, can be used for thicker bone but also have the potential to fracture bone in an unpredictable pattern. Therefore, they must be used with caution near the skull base. Manipulation of structures within the sphenoid sinus is fraught with complications and is generally unnecessary in routine (or revision) sinus surgery. Given the number of possible areas of dehiscence (eg, carotid, optic nerve, sella turcica), sphenoidotomy should be performed with caution.

If a CSF leak occurs, the most important step is identification. When the location is identified, repair is generally straightforward but requires patience. Hemostasis should be achieved rapidly and, although no conclusive evidence exists for their use, intravenous antibiotics administered (typically a third-generation cephalosporin). If the defect is less than 2 mm, the site may be repaired with a mucosal or fascial overlay graft and fibrin glue. The graft is placed after denuding the mucosa surrounding the defect. If the defect is 2 to 6 mm, a composite graft composed of mucosa, periosteum, and bone is useful. For defects greater than 6 mm, a multilayered closure should be undertaken with the use of a bone underlay, followed by a mucosal or fascial overlay graft.[45] A fat graft may also be used to "plug" the sphenoid sinus. Elevated head of bed, strict bed rest, and straining precautions are mandatory in the immediate postoperative period. Placement of a lumbar drain is typically not advised unless signs of intracranial hypertension are present (high flow leak, empty sella, or arachnoid pits). In experienced hands, the success rate of endoscopic CSF leak repair is greater than 90%.[46,47]

POSTOPERATIVE COMPLICATIONS

Complications of sphenoidotomy that occur after surgery result from a combination of overly aggressive surgery and local or systemic host factors. The most prominent complications arising in the postoperative setting are stenosis of the sphenoidotomy and mucocele formation.

Stenosis and Mucocele Formation

Late complications of sphenoidotomy are namely stenosis and synechiae, both of which dictate the long-term success or failure of sphenoid surgery. Stenosis of the surgical ostium typically occurs when the ostium is not widened enough or if the ostium is enlarged circumferentially. Mucosal defects contract as they heal through secondary intention, and therefore circumferential defects tend to form cicatricial stenosis (**Fig. 13**). Avoiding instrumentation of the medial and inferior aspect of the sphenoid sinus os decreases the risk for postoperative cicatricial stenosis by leaving an intact mucosal margin.

If identified early in the postoperative period, stenosis may be addressed without much difficulty in the clinic setting. In patients who tolerate instrumentation under local anesthesia, early scarring can be removed with a Stammberger punch or a balloon catheter. If the os stenosis is complete, the patient will likely develop symptomatic sphenoid disease. Targeted revision surgery of the sphenoid ostium should be straightforward; however, given the vital structures surrounding the sinus, and the loss of operative landmarks, image guidance should be considered.

The formation of sphenoid sinus mucoceles can result from long-standing postoperative obstruction of the sphenoid sinus, usually caused by postoperative scarring and stenosis of the neo-ostium. Sphenoid sinus mucoceles are uncommon and should be treated in symptomatic patients to prevent long-term sequelae related to expansion. Endoscopic decompression of sphenoid sinus mucoceles has been described previously[48] and is straightforward. Principles guiding primary sphenoid sinus surgery should be used, and the mucocele entered in a low and medial position. A wide sphenoidotomy should be performed to achieve marsupialization.

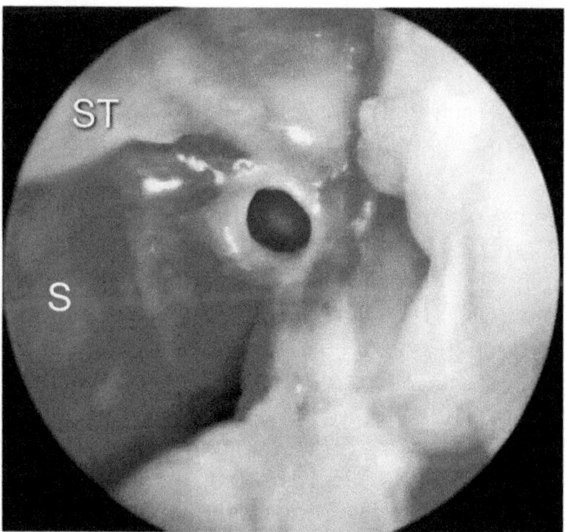

Fig. 13. Circumferential scar formation around the sphenoidotomy is apparent in this figure. The left septum (S) and superior turbinate (ST) are seen in relation to the os. The stenosis may result in loss of function if the ostomy becomes occluded. Revision sphenoidotomy may be performed in the office with topical or local anesthesia and a sickle knife and circular sphenoid punch.

SUMMARY

Endoscopic sphenoidotomy is a common surgical procedure that often accompanies routine sinus surgery. Safe completion of a sphenoidotomy depends on a thorough understanding of the surrounding anatomy, reviewing preoperative imaging, and maintaining intraoperative orientation. Intraoperative complications include local hemorrhage, catastrophic hemorrhage caused by internal carotid injury, optic nerve injury, and CSF leak. Postoperative complications tend to be less severe and include postoperative stenosis and mucocele formation. Regarding surgery of the sphenoid sinuses, the best management of complications truly is prevention, making pre- and intraoperative vigilance vital to a successful outcome.

REFERENCES

1. Benson V, Marano M. Current estimates from the National Health Interview Survey, 1995. Hyattsville (MD): National Center for Health Sciences. Vital Health Stat 1998;10:76.
2. Bhattacharyya N. The economic burden and symptom manifestations of chronic rhinosinusitis. Am J Rhinol 2003;17:27–32.
3. Kim HU, Kim SS, Kang SS, et al. Surgical anatomy of the natural ostium of the sphenoid sinus. Laryngoscope 2001;111(9):1599–602.
4. Elwany S, Yacout YM, Talaat M, et al. Surgical anatomy of the sphenoid sinus. J Laryngol Otol 1983;97(3):227–41.
5. Sareen D, Agarwal AK, Kaul JM, et al. Study of sphenoid sinus anatomy in relation to endoscopic surgery. Int J Morphol 2005;23(3):261–6.
6. Turgut S, Gumusalan Y, Arifoglu Y, et al. Endoscopic anatomic distances on the lateral nasal wall. J Otolaryngol 1996;25(6):371–4.
7. Hamberger CA, Hammer G, Norlen G, et al. Transantrosphenoidal hypophysectomy. Arch Otolaryngol 1961;74:2–8.
8. Renn WH, Rhoton AL Jr. Microsurgical anatomy of the sellar region. J Neurosurg 1975;43(3):288–98.
9. Hamid O, El Fiky L, Hassan O, et al. Anatomic variations of the sphenoid sinus and their impact on trans-sphenoid pituitary surgery. Skull Base 2008;18(1):9–15.
10. Idowu OE, Balogun BO, Okoli CA. Dimensions, septation, and pattern of pneumatization of the sphenoidal sinus. Folia Morphol (Warsz) 2009;68(4):228–32.
11. Ridpath FR. Disease of the nose, throat and ear. 3rd edition. Philadelphia (PA): W.B. Saunders Company; 1947.
12. Simpson JF, Robin IG, Ballantyne JC, et al, editors. Synopsis of otolaryngology. 2nd edition. Bristol (UK): John Wright and Sons Ltd; 1967. p. 148.
13. Fernandez-Miranda JC, Prevedello DM, Madhok R, et al. Sphenoid septations and their relationship with internal carotid arteries: anatomical and radiological study. Laryngoscope 2009;119(10):1893–6.
14. Sethi DS, Stanley RE, Pillay PK. Endoscopic anatomy of the sphenoid sinus and sella turcica. J Laryngol Otol 1995;109(10):951–5.
15. Elwany S, Elsaeid I, Thabet H. Endoscopic anatomy of the sphenoid sinus. J Laryngol Otol 1999;113(2):122–6.
16. Fujii K, Chambers SM, Rhoton AL Jr. Neurovascular relationships of the sphenoid sinus. A Microsurgical Study. J Neurosurg 1979;50(1):31–9.
17. Kennedy DW, Zinrich H, Hassab M. The internal carotid artery as it relates to endoscopic spheno-ethmoidectomy. Am J Rhinol 1990;4:7–12.

18. Dessi P, Moulin G, Castro F, et al. Protrusion of the optic nerve into the ethmoid and sphenoid sinus: prospective study of 150 CT studies. Neuroradiology 1994;36(7):515–6.
19. Stammberger HR, Kennedy DW. Paranasal sinuses:anatomic terminology and nomenclature. The Anatomic Terminology Group. Ann Otol Rhinol Laryngol Suppl 1995;167:7–16.
20. Onodi A. The optic nerve and the accessory sinuses of the nose. New York: William Wood & Co; 1910.
21. Driben JS, Bolger WE, Robles HA, et al. The reliability of computerized tomographic detection of the Onodi (sphenoethmoid) cell. Am J Rhinol 1998;12(2): 105–11.
22. Habal MB, Maniscalco JE, Lineaweaver WC, et al. Microsurgical anatomy of the optic canal: anatomical relations and exposure of the optic nerve. Surg Forum 1976;27(62):542–4.
23. Kainz J, Stammberger H. Danger areas of the posterior rhinobasis. An endoscopic and anatomical-surgical study. Acta Otolaryngol 1992;112(5):852–61.
24. Maniscalco JE, Habal MB. Microanatomy of the optic canal. J Neurosurg 1978; 48(3):402–6.
25. Kennedy DW. Functional endoscopic sinus surgery. Technique. Arch Otolaryngol 1985;111(10):643–9.
26. Stankiewicz JA. The endoscopic approach to the sphenoid sinus. Laryngoscope 1989;99(2):218–21.
27. Stammberger H, Kopp W. Functional endoscopic sinus surgery: the Messerklinger technique. Philadelphia (PA): BC Decker; 1991.
28. Bolger WE, Keyes AS, Lanza DC. Use of the superior meatus and superior turbinate in the endoscopic approach to the sphenoid sinus. Otolaryngol Head Neck Surg 1999;120(3):308–13.
29. Welch KC, Stankiewicz JA. A contemporary review of endoscopic sinus surgery: techniques, tools, and outcomes. Laryngoscope 2009;119(11):2258–68.
30. Gotwald TF, Menzler A, Beauchamp NJ, et al. Paranasal and orbital anatomy revisited: identification of the ethmoid arteries on coronal CT scans. Crit Rev Comput Tomogr 2003;44(5):263–78.
31. Han JK, Becker SS, Bomeli SR, et al. Endoscopic localization of the anterior and posterior ethmoid arteries. Ann Otol Rhinol Laryngol 2008;117(12):931–5.
32. Stankiewicz JA, Chow JM. Two faces of orbital hematoma in intranasal (endoscopic) sinus surgery. Otolaryngol Head Neck Surg 1999;120(6):841–7.
33. Kassam AB, Vescan AD, Carrau RL, et al. Expanded endonasal approach: vidian canal as a landmark to the petrous internal carotid artery. J Neurosurg 2008; 108(1):177–83.
34. Osborn AG. The vidian artery: normal and pathologic anatomy. Radiology 1980; 136(2):373–8.
35. Lee HY, Kim HU, Kim SS, et al. Surgical anatomy of the sphenopalatine artery in lateral nasal wall. Laryngoscope 2002;112(10):1813–8.
36. Midilli R, Orhan M, Saylam CY, et al. Anatomic variations of sphenopalatine artery and minimally invasive surgical cauterization procedure. Am J Rhinol Allergy 2009;23(6):e38–41.
37. Simmen DB, Raghavan U, Briner HR, et al. The anatomy of the sphenopalatine artery for the endoscopic sinus surgeon. Am J Rhinol 2006;20(5):502–5.
38. Fujii M, Goto N, Shimada K, et al. Demonstration of the nasal septal branches of the sphenopalatine artery by use of a new intravascular injection method. Ann Otol Rhinol Laryngol 1996;105(4):309–11.

39. Bouthillier A, van Loveren HR, Keller JT. Segments of the internal carotid artery: a new classification. Neurosurgery 1996;38(3):425–32 [discussion: 432–3].
40. Christmas DA, Mirante JP, Yanagisawa E. Endoscopic view of the carotid artery appearing as a sphenoid sinus mass. Ear Nose Throat J 2009;88(8):1028–9.
41. Biswas D, Daudia A, Jones NS, et al. Profuse epistaxis following sphenoid surgery: a ruptured carotid artery pseudoaneurysm and its management. J Laryngol Otol 2009;123(6):692–4.
42. Feuerman TF, Hieshima GB, Bentson JR, et al. Carotid-cavernous fistula following nasopharyngeal biopsy. Arch Otolaryngol 1984;110(6):412–4.
43. Pedersen RA, Troost BT, Schramm VL. Carotid-cavernous sinus fistula after external ethmoid-sphenoid surgery. Clinical course and management. Arch Otolaryngol 1981;107(5):307–9.
44. Sofferman R. Complications: prevention and management – carotid artery and optic nerve injury. In 1st International Symposium on Contemporary Sinus Surgery. Pittsburgh (PA), November 4–6, 1990.
45. Welch KC, Palmer JN. Intraoperative emergencies during endoscopic sinus surgery: CSF leak and orbital hematoma. Otolaryngol Clin North Am 2008; 41(3):581–96, ix–x.
46. Hegazy HM, Carrau RL, Snyderman CH, et al. Transnasal endoscopic repair of cerebrospinal fluid rhinorrhea: a meta-analysis. Laryngoscope 2000;110(7): 1166–72.
47. Lanza DC, O'Brien DA, Kennedy DW. Endoscopic repair of cerebrospinal fluid fistulae and encephaloceles. Laryngoscope 1996;106(9 Pt 1):1119–25.
48. Stankiewicz JA. Sphenoid sinus mucocele. Arch Otolaryngol Head Neck Surg 1989;115(6):735–40.

The Prevention and Management of Complications in Ethmoid Sinus Surgery

Zara M. Patel, MD, Satish Govindaraj, MD*

KEYWORDS

- Ethmoid sinus surgery • Endoscopic ethmoidectomy
- Anterior ethmoid artery

Prevention of complications during ethmoid sinus surgery begins with sound knowledge of the relevant anatomy, preoperative planning with use of radiologic imaging, and careful, thoughtful dissection intraoperatively. In spite of these measures surgeons are bound to have complications. This article will highlight potential complications and treatment techniques to salvage good outcomes following endoscopic ethmoidectomy.

ANATOMY

The ethmoid sinuses arise from a series of evaginations of the nasal mucosa into a lateral ethmoid mass during the sixth fetal month. Pneumatization will continue until 7 years, and these cells will reach their adult size at 12 years of age.[1]

Superomedially, the ethmoid sinus is bordered by the thinner bone of the lateral lamella of the cribriform plate, and superolaterally by the thicker bone of the fovea ethmoidalis. The sphenoid sinus or skull base forms its posterior border. Superolaterally, the ethmoid sinus is bordered by the thinner bone of the lateral lamella of the cribriform plate, and superomedially by the thicker bone of the fovea ethmoidalis. The length of the lateral lamella has been categorized into three types, as defined by Keros. In Keros type 1, the fovea ethmoidalis lies 1 mm to 3 mm above the level of the cribriform plate; thus the lateral lamella is shortened. In type 2, the difference in height is 4 mm to 7 mm, and in type 3, the difference in height is 8 mm to 16 mm. The longer the lateral lamella, the greater chance there is for inadvertent entry through the skull base.[2]

Additional important anatomic structures of the skull base include the anterior and posterior ethmoidal arteries. The anterior ethmoid artery (AEA) originates from the

Department of Otolaryngology/Head and Neck Surgery, Mount Sinai Medical Center, One Gustave L. Levy Place, PO Box 1191, New York, NY 10029, USA
* Corresponding author.
E-mail address: satish.govindaraj@mountsinai.org

Otolaryngol Clin N Am 43 (2010) 855–864
doi:10.1016/j.otc.2010.04.010

ophthalmic artery in the orbit, enters the ethmoids through the frontoethmoidal suture, traverses the skull base, and ends in the nasal cavity. By following the face of the ethmoid bulla superiorly to the ethmoid roof and examining the region a few millimeters posterior to this point, the artery often can be found.[3] The canal runs anywhere between 1 mm inferior to the height of the cribriform plate to 4 mm superior, and it often can be dehiscent.[4] It is because of this variability that special care must be taken when dissecting bony septae projecting down from the ethmoid roof. Damage to the artery can cause bleeding, and if it retracts into the orbit, a retrobulbar hematoma can develop, which left untreated, can lead to blindness. This danger also exists in regards to the posterior ethmoid artery (PEA). But with its more posterosuperior location, entering the bony roof of the posterior ethmoid cells at the junction between the lamina papyracea and the frontal bone 2 to 8 mm anterior to the optic nerve, there is less risk for intraoperative injury.

The ethmoid sinuses are divided into anterior and posterior cells by the basal lamella of the middle turbinate. The anterior cells drain into the ethmoid infundibulum, and the posterior cells drain into the sphenoethmoidal recess. The ethmoid infundibulum is a three-dimensional space, running anterosuperiorly to posteroinferiorly, bounded by the ethmoid bulla, the lateral nasal wall, and the uncinate process. The uncinate process is a thin semilunar piece of bone that acts as the anteromedial border of the infundibulum. The superior edge of this bone, although most often free, can attach to either the skull base or the lamina papyracea.[4]

The largest of the anterior ethmoid cells is called the ethmoid bulla. This cell sits posterosuperiorly to the infundibulum. The space behind the bulla is referred to as the sinus lateralis. If the bulla does not reach the skull base superiorly, the resulting space above the bulla is called the suprabullar recess. The most anterior of the ethmoid cells is termed the agger nasi cell, a pneumatization of the lacrimal bone. It is found anterosuperior to the attachment of the middle turbinate to the lateral wall. The posterior wall of the agger nasi usually forms the anterior wall of the frontal recess, and it is present in 93% to 98% of cases.

Ethmoid cells that extend into the maxillary sinus above the ostium are called infraorbital ethmoid cells. Infraorbital ethmoid cells often have been found incidentally, with one study finding these cells in 45.9% of patients undergoing CT scan for sinus complaints and in 41.6% of patients scanned for nonsinus reasons.[5] These cells are often not clinically significant; however, they sometimes can cause obstruction of the ostiomeatal complex.

Ethmoid cells that grow posteriorly and superolaterally to the sphenoid sinus have the potential for pneumatizing around the optic nerve or carotid artery. These cells are called Onodi cells, and they occur in approximately 9% to 12% of the general population.[6] Dissection in and around these cells holds the possible danger of injuring the optic nerve or carotid artery.

PREOPERATIVE PLANNING

If a patient fails maximal medical therapy and the decision is made to go ahead with functional endoscopic sinus surgery (FESS), there are important preoperative steps that will make the surgery not only easier for the surgeon, but safer for the patient.

Reviewing the radiology before surgery is the most important of these steps. A patient undergoing sinus surgery should have a computed tomography (CT) scan of the paranasal sinuses to identify any and all anatomic variations. The ethmoid labyrinth is very complex, and without prior knowledge of the individual patient's anatomy the surgery can be fraught with potential complications. Knowing preoperatively the location of ethmoid variants like agger nasi cells, infraorbital ethmoid cells, and Onodi cells allows the surgeon to predict areas where important structures like the lamina papyracea, optic nerve, and carotid artery may be at risk (**Figs. 1** and **2**). The lamina papyracea may be dehiscent or medially deviated, and the lateral lamellae of the cribriform plate can be extremely deep, asymmetric, or even eroded from chronic disease (**Figs. 3** and **4**). It is also important to identify the location of the anterior ethmoid artery as it traverses the ethmoid roof (**Fig. 5**).

The preoperative medical clearance should proceed just as indicated for all surgeries, and for FESS in particular, the cardiovascular status of each patient becomes an important factor in how much controlled hypotension can be used intraoperatively. Proper positioning, the request for controlled hypotension, and total intravenous anesthesia (TIVA) should be a collaborative effort with the anesthetic team and discussed preoperatively.

The patient also should have preoperative placement of pledgets soaked in a vasoconstrictive agent, such as cocaine, phenylephrine, or oxymetazoline, followed by transoral or transnasal injection of 1cc of 1% lidocaine with epinephrine (1:100,000) to region of the greater palatine or sphenopalatine foramen respectively.

All patients at the authors' institution are given a course of antibiotics and steroids to be started 1 week preoperatively. Lastly, all patients are given a long list of medications that have been implicated in increased bleeding during or after surgery, both traditional and naturopathic, to avoid 2 weeks before and 2 weeks after surgery.

The authors have found all these measures work together to allow for more meticulous dissection by controlling mucosal inflammation and subsequent intraoperative bleeding.

INTRAOPERATIVELY

Prevention and Management of Anterior or Posterior Ethmoid Artery Transection

The AEA and PEA are crucial structures to identify when clearing superior ethmoid partitions off of the anterior skull base. As the AEA traverses the skull base, there can be variability in its height, as 8.5% can be suspended in a bony mesentery 2 mm to 3 mm below the skull base.[7] Coronal cuts from the preoperative CT scan may be the most useful in verifying its location by identifying a bony nipple that protrudes from the orbit between the junction of the medial rectus and superior

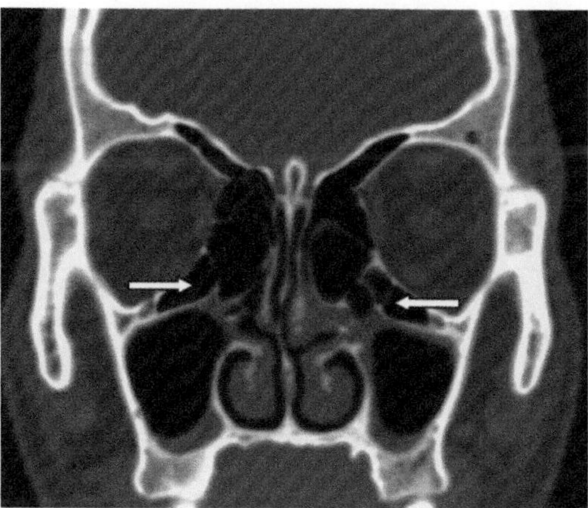

Fig. 1. Bilateral Haller cells (*white arrows*). Note that there are multiple Haller cells on the patient's left side.

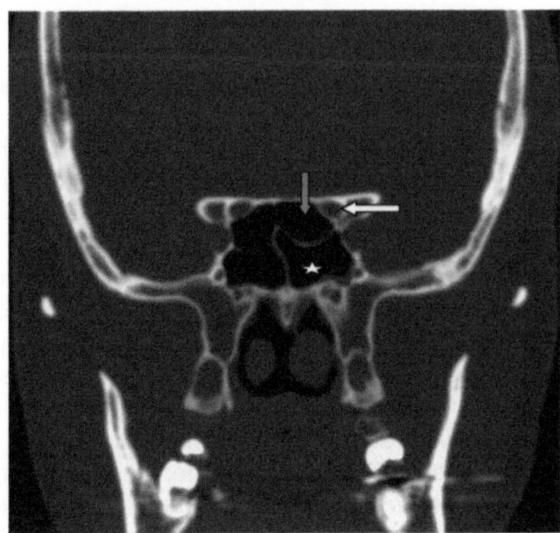

Fig. 2. Left Onodi cell (*light grey arrow*) with optic nerve (*white arrow*) at lateral aspect. The sphenoid sinus lies below (*star*).

oblique muscle. The PEA is smaller, and therefore slightly more difficult to visualize endoscopically, and while it can often be found 10 mm to 13 mm posterior to the AEA, recent studies have demonstrated considerable variability in this relationship. A more constant relationship to look for endoscopically may be to first identify the anterior face of the sphenoid and then look approximately 8 mm anterior to that at the level of the skull base.[8]

If either artery is injured during surgery, pressure and application of hemostatic material within a pledget should be applied to slow the bleeding. If a full transection has occurred, however, bipolar cauterization may be used to control the hemorrhage in these cases. Unipolar suction cautery should be avoided when controlling bleeding at the skull base to avoid the creation of a cerebrospinal fluid (CSF) leak. If bipolar cautery is not sufficient to stop the bleed, and the transected end of the artery is still visible, endoscopic ligation with surgical clips is an option.[9]

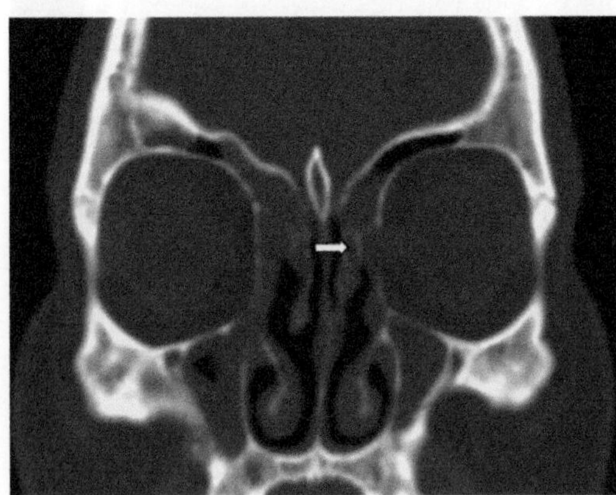

Fig. 3. Left lamina papyracea with dehiscence. Note fragment of bone in ethmoid cavity (*arrow*).

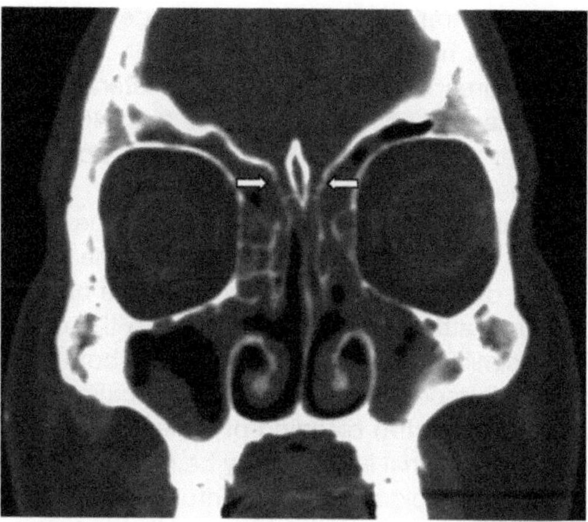

Fig. 4. Bilateral lamina lateralis of the fovea ethmoidalis showing signs of early erosion from polypoid disease (*arrows*).

It is not uncommon for the AEA to retract into the orbit after transection. The retraction of a bleeding artery into the orbit will lead to a rapidly expanding orbital hematoma, a serious and potentially devastating complication. This can quickly lead to orbital compartment syndrome, which can result in vision loss from compression of the optic nerve. If ischemia time is greater than 90 minutes, permanent injury to the optic nerve can be expected. Preseptal edema, ecchymosis, orbital proptosis, and elevated intraocular pressures are all early signs of an orbital hematoma.[10] If the AEA is transected and seen to retract intraoperatively, an emergent ophthalmologic consult should be called for evaluation, and temporizing medical measures such as

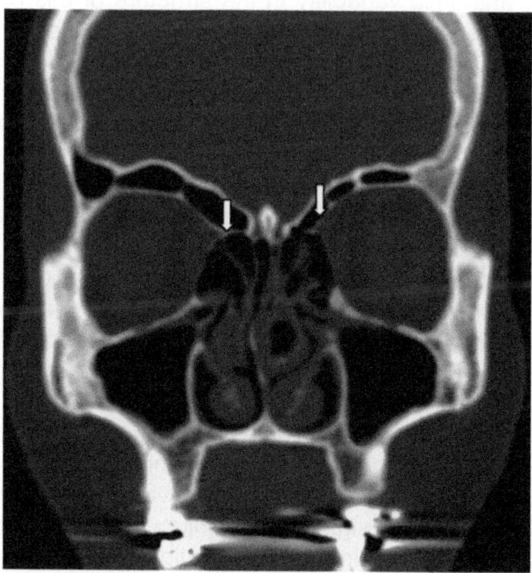

Fig. 5. Bilateral demonstration of bony nipple marking entrance of anterior ethmoid arteries into the nasal cavity (*white arrows*). Note that the vessels course below the skull base.

orbital massage and administration of mannitol and acetazolamide should be instituted. If the bleed is arterial, however, these are unlikely to work rapidly enough to decrease intraocular pressures. Absolute indication for lateral canthotomy in the anesthetized patient is an intraocular pressure greater than 40 mm Hg. In the awake patient, severe retrobulbar pain, Marcus-Gunn pupil, or a cherry red macula are all signs that indicate the need for a lateral canthotomy.[11]

To perform a lateral canthotomy, local anesthetic can be infiltrated at the lateral canthus, and a hemostat can be used to clamp across the soft tissue from skin to bony orbital rim and then divided with a sharp scissor or a blade. The lateral canthal tendon then can be found, attached 4 mm posterior to the orbital rim at Whitnall's tubercle, and should be similarly divided. The division of both soft tissue and tendon has the potential to lower intraocular pressures by approximately 33 mm Hg.[12]

If endoscopic intervention to stop bleeding of either anterior or posterior ethmoid arteries is unsuccessful, an external incision may be necessary to identify the vessels as they traverse the fronto-ethmoidal suture line into the nasal cavity from the orbit. A Lynch incision is used and carried down to the level of the periosteum. The periosteum is elevated anteriorly and posteriorly, with care taken to preserve the lacrimal sac. After the lacrimal crest and fossa with the medial canthal tendon are identified and preserved, the elevation can proceed posteriorly until the fronto-ethmoidal suture is identified. Here the AEA can be identified and ligated. A clue to confirm AEA identification is the presence of periorbita exiting the orbit through the foramen. If the PEA is the culprit, the elevation can proceed even more posteriorly, and this vessel usually is found approximately 12 mm back from the AEA. It is important to keep in mind the proximity of the PEA to the optic nerve, which often runs just 5 mm posterior[13] to the artery.

Prevention and Management of Damage to the Lamina Papyracea and Medial Rectus

The lamina papyracea demonstrates by its very name the fragility of the paper-thin bone dividing the nasal cavity and the orbit. It lies superior and lateral to the natural maxillary sinus ostium. Examining the CT scan preoperatively will allow the surgeon to assess for any dehiscences or anatomic variability in the structure of this bone. Studies have demonstrated an increase in orbital complications on the left side for a right-handed surgeon standing on the right side of the patient, so there should be a heightened awareness when operating on this side.[14] The difference is probably reflective of scope orientation changing from straight to slightly angled when operating across the body, causing the lamina to appear more lateral than it truly is. Intermittent palpation of the eye when dissecting in this region is paramount in being able to identify the lamina without penetrating it. There have been several case reports suggesting the rapidity and severity of orbital injury following powered instrumentation use.[15] Powered instruments never should be angled directly at the lamina, and it may be more judicious to use traditional instruments when skeletonizing the medial wall of the orbit.

If the lamina is disrupted, often the exposure of orbital fat, in and of itself, is not of any consequence. If periorbital veins are disrupted, however, this may cause a slow onset bleed into the orbit. If orbital fat is seen to herniate into the nasal cavity after disruption of the lamina, the surgeon should immediately check the eye for edema, ecchymosis, and proptosis. If the eye remains within normal limits, the dissection can be continued if the orbital fat has not obstructed view of more posterior structures. At the end of the case, even if no sign of orbital injury is evident, nasal packing within the middle meatus should be avoided. Any questions about the status of the orbit necessitate an ophthalmology consult for measurement of intraocular pressures. If there are any clinical signs of an orbital hematoma, the patient should be admitted for monitoring. As mentioned previously, medical measures include orbital massage, administration of mannitol or acetazolamide, and in the awake patient, timolol eye drops to decrease intraocular pressure. Eye massage helps to redistribute intraocular and extraocular fluid, but is absolutely contraindicated in any patient with a history of corneal, retinal, or glaucoma filtering surgery. Acetazolamide is given 500 mg intravenously, and acts to reduce intraocular pressures by decreasing production of aqueous humor, but it is relatively slow in onset. Mannitol is given in a dose of 1 to 2 g/kg over 20 to 30 minutes, acts by osmotically drawing fluid out of the orbital spaces, and has a much quicker onset of action.

As mentioned previously, the advent of powered instrumentation has brought to the literature several reports of serious orbital complications, including severe damage to the medial rectus muscle. When patient information was gathered from 10 ophthalmologic centers over 6 years, a pattern emerged detailing four general types of injury to the medial rectus (MR): complete MR transection, partial MR transection, mild contusion, and entrapment.[16] In cases of entrapment, it is important to look intraorbitally to evaluate if the muscle itself has been damaged or if there is a piece of bone that may be impinging on the muscle. If so, this should be removed immediately, and a resorbable barrier can be placed along the medial orbital wall to prevent re-entrapment. Autogenous tissue such as septal cartilage is a good candidate, and some have used nonadhesive synthetic materials also. In cases of complete or partial muscle transection, an ophthalmologic surgeon can try to reapproximate the cut ends of muscle, but only rarely will this bring back true realignment of the eye.[16]

Prevention and Management of Postoperative Synechiae

Although a seemingly minor concern compared with those complications listed previously, postoperative synechiae can negate a successful surgery and leave a patient with the same or worsened sinus complaints than what they had preoperatively. Prevention of scar band formation begins at the outset of surgery with the use of meticulous atraumatic technique from the moment the intranasal injection is given to the end of the operation. Any bony spicules without mucosal covering should be removed completely, and surgery should be limited to those structures involved with disease. Although some authors have considered a middle turbinectomy to alleviate scar formation, others have found this technique to either worsen the condition by having the middle turbinate remnant scar over the frontal recess, or they have found that removing this structure can lead to further nasal complaints. Many surgeons now opt to leave the middle turbinate intact and place a small stent within the middle meatus to prevent lateralization. Some use a technique known as Bolgerization, which is to cauterize a point on the medial aspect of the middle turbinate and then a correlating point on the septum to facilitate scarring of the middle turbinate to the septum. Others will suture both middle turbinates through and through to fix them medially to the septum bilaterally. Whichever method is used, the goal is the same: to prevent lateralization of the middle turbinate and scarring of the ostiomeatal complex.

Meticulous debridement in the postoperative period will have the greatest impact on prevention of synechiae formation, but if they are noted postoperatively, good topical anesthesia will allow for removal of these bands of scar tissue in the office.

Prevention and Management of Mucocele Formation and Secondary Obstruction of the Frontal Recess

A potential long-term complication of endoscopic ethmoidectomy is mucocele formation. If not all septae are removed from the ethmoid labyrinth, there is the potential for scarring and closing of the drainage pathway of remnant ethmoid air cells. When this occurs, the normal physiologic mechanism of mucus production is met with an outflow obstruction, and the mucosal lining of that cell will begin to expand under the pressure of the mucus trapped inside. If the mucosa expands to the bony limits of the sinus cavity, the patient will begin to experience pressure and pain in that region. Specifically in the case of ethmoid mucoceles, the mucosa can expand to the point where there is erosion of the medial orbital wall and skull base (**Fig. 6**). The underlying periorbita and dura are often intact, providing a protective barrier to underlying structures; however, if the mucocele becomes infected (mucopyocele), more serious complications may ensue such as orbital cellulitis, meningitis, and osteomyelitis. The prevention of this occurrence lies in the precise dissection of the skull base and clearance of all bony partitions in the ethmoid cavity.

The exception to this rule is an ethmoidectomy performed in the absence of frontal sinus disease. In this setting, the frontal recess should be left undissected; however, remnants of the agger nasi, bulla ethmoidalis, or frontal recess cells may form synechiae resulting in secondary frontal sinus obstruction and infection or mucocele formation. Methods to prevent this delayed complication are to avoid creation of adjacent raw surfaces. For example, the cut edges of the residual agger nasi and bulla ethmoidalis should be at different heights to avoid scarring. In addition, any mobile or unstable partitions should be resected to avoid displacement, synechiae, and obstruction. Meticulous debridements after surgery also prevent the development of scar tissue in the frontal recess. The use of either a 45° or 70° scope in the office to examine the frontal recess is advised in the postoperative period.

If a mucocele does occur, it may not be for many years, with some authors noting a median time to presentation for fronto-ethmoidal-orbital mucoceles of 14.8 years.[17] Techniques for managing mucoceles include endoscopic marsupialization, a modified endoscopic Lothrop procedure, and for some mucoceles that have expanded far into the frontal sinus and broken through the bony walls of the sinus cavity, or those cases in which there is extensive scarring of the frontal recess, some authors choose an open approach for drainage, with an osteoplastic flap, preferably without obliteration of the frontal sinus.[18–20]

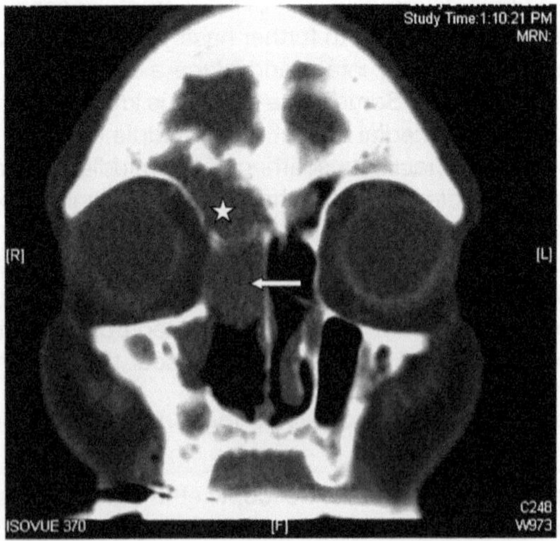

Fig. 6. Right ethmoid mucocele (*white arrow*) obstructing the frontal recess, resulting in frontal sinus (*star*) opacification.

POSTOPERATIVE CARE

All sinus surgeons have their own particular regimen of postoperative medications. Most regimens include antibiotics to prevent infection of the raw surgical surfaces, oral steroids to reduce swelling and immediate polyp formation, pain medicine, and saline spray or irrigation. The senior author generally uses two separate antibiotics for 2 weeks post operatively as well as placing patients on a prednisone taper, starting at 20 to 30 mg. Antibiotic therapy may be refined based on intraoperative culture results. Both saline spray and saline irrigation are given to the patient with specific instructions for the irrigation to be used at least three times daily for the first 2 weeks. It is important to emphasize proper cleaning of the irrigating syringe to prevent the introduction of new bacteria into the sinonasal cavity.

The same medications held preoperatively should be held postoperatively, unless medical necessity dictates immediate reinstitution of those drugs. The patient should be instructed not to lift heavy objects or strain, participate in strenuous activity, blow his or her nose, or hold in coughs or sneezes, all of which raise blood pressure in the head and may cause postoperative bleeding.

The schedule for postoperative debridement also varies between individual surgeons, but general consensus is that patients need debridements for anywhere between 4 and 8 weeks postoperatively. If stents have been placed within the middle meatus, these are removed at the first postoperative visit. The following visits pertain to the aforementioned meticulous debridement to prevent formation of synechiae and the removal of crusting, devitalized bone, and mucosa. The senior author generally will see a patient every week for the first weeks and then increase the length between visits based on how well patients are healing to every 1 to 3 months for the first year. Those patients with signs of ostial stenosis or adverse scarring are followed more frequently.

SUMMARY

Prevention of complications during ethmoid sinus surgery begins with sound knowledge of the relevant anatomy, preoperative planning with use of radiologic imaging, and careful, thoughtful dissection intraoperatively. In spite of these measures, surgeons are bound to have complications. Having the ability to recognize and treat these complications is paramount for good surgical outcomes and patient satisfaction.

REFERENCES

1. Lee KJ. Essential otolaryngology, head and neck surgery. 8th edition. New York (NY): McGraw-Hill; 2003.
2. Keros P. [On the practical value of differences in the level of the lamina crib Rosa of the ethmoid]. Z Laryngol Rhinol Otol 1962;41:808–13 [in German].
3. Becker SP. Applied anatomy of the paranasal sinuses with emphasis on endoscopic surgery. Ann Otol Rhinol Laryngol 1994;103(Suppl 162):1–32.
4. Rice DH, Schaefer SD, editors. Endoscopic paranasal sinus surgery. 2nd edition. New York: Raven Press; 1993. p. 27.
5. Bolger WE, Butzin CA, Parsons DS. Paranasal sinus bony anatomic variations and mucosal abnormalities: CT analysis for endoscopic sinus surgery. Laryngoscope 1991;101:56–64.
6. Van Alyea OE. Ethmoid labyrinth: anatomic study, with consideration of the clinical significance of its structural characteristics. Arch Otolaryngol 1939;29: 881–902.

7. Moon HJ, Kim HU, Lee JG, et al. Surgical anatomy of the anterior ethmoid canal in the ethmoid roof. Laryngoscope 2001;111:900–4.
8. Han JK, Becker SS, Bomeli SR, et al. Endoscopic localization of the anterior and posterior ethmoid arteries. Ann Otol Rhinol Laryngol 2008;117(12):931–5.
9. Pletcher SD, Metson R. Endoscopic ligation of the anterior ethmoid artery. Laryngoscope 2007;117:378–81.
10. Stankiewicz JA, Chow JM. Two faces of orbital hematoma in intranasal (endoscopic) sinus surgery. Otolaryngol Head Neck Surg 1999;120:841–7.
11. Welch KC, Palmer JN. Intraoperative emergencies during endoscopic sinus surgery: CSF leak and orbital hematoma. Otolaryngol Clin North Am 2008;41:581–96.
12. Yung CW, Moorthy RS, Lindley D, et al. Efficacy of lateral canthotomy and cantholysis in orbital hemorrhage. Opthal Plast Reconstr surg 1994;10:137–41.
13. Cooke ET. An evaluation and clinical study of severe epistaxis treated by arterial ligation. J Laryngol Otol 1985;99:745–9.
14. Dessi P, Castro F, Triglia JM, et al. Major complications of sinus surgery: a review of 1192 procedures. J Laryngol Otol 1994;108(3):212–5.
15. Bhatti MT, Giannoni CM, Raynor E, et al. Ocular motility complications after endoscopic sinus surgery with powered cutting instruments. Otolaryngol Head Neck Surg 2001;125:501–9.
16. Huang CM, Meyer DR, Patrinely JR, et al. Medial rectus muscle injuries associated with functional endoscopic sinus surgery: characterization and management. Ophthal Plast Reconstr Surg 2003;19(1):25–37.
17. Meetze K, Palmer JN, Schlosser RJ. Frontal sinus complications after frontal craniotomy. Laryngoscope 2004;114(5):945–8.
18. Chiu AG, Vaughan WC. Management of the lateral frontal sinus lesion and the supraorbital cell mucocele. Am J Rhinol 2004;18(2):83–6.
19. Wormald PJ, Ananda A, Nair S. Modified endoscopic lothrop as a salvage for the failed osteoplastic flap with obliteration. Laryngoscope 2003;113(11):1988–92.
20. Herndon M, McMains K, Kountakis S. Presentation and management of extensive fronto-orbital-ethmoid mucoceles. Am J Otol 2007;28(3):145–7.

Prevention and Management of Complications in Maxillary Sinus Surgery

Esther Kim, MD, James A. Duncavage, MD*

KEYWORDS

- Maxillary antrostomy • Management of complications
- Prevention of complications • Caldwell-Luc
- Maxillary sinoscopy • Balloon dilatation

Maxillary sinus surgery has continued to evolve ever since George Caldwell and Henri Luc described an anterior approach to the maxillary sinus in the late 1800s. Notable changes came in the 1980s with the introduction of endoscopes for use in the paranasal sinuses. The use of angled endoscopes gave the surgeon views of the middle meatus and maxillary ostium that were previously not possible.[1] The development of the coronal bone window for CT scans, introduced in 1987, also gave sinus surgeons a much-needed diagnostic test for the maxillary sinus.

This article is divided into six sections that are related to six commonly used operations for surgery on the maxillary sinus. The authors discuss maxillary sinoscopy, the Caldwell-Luc procedure, extended middle meatus antrostomy, endoscopic maxillary sinus antrostomy, minimally invasive sinus technique, and balloon sinus procedures. In each of these procedures, the authors discuss potential complications (**Table 1**) and address prevention and management strategies.

MAXILLARY SINOSCOPY

Maxillary sinoscopy is a surgical technique that allows the surgeon to look inside the maxillary sinus with a telescope and to treat the diseased anterior half of the maxillary

---

James Duncavage is a stockholder and serves on the scientific advisory board for Entellus Medical, Inc.
Division of Rhinology, Department of Otolaryngology, Vanderbilt University Medical Center, 7209 Medical Center East, South Tower, 1215 21st Avenue South, Nashville, TN 37232-8605, USA
* Corresponding author.
E-mail address: james.duncavage@vanderbilt.edu

Otolaryngol Clin N Am 43 (2010) 865–873
doi:10.1016/j.otc.2010.04.011
oto.theclinics.com

Table 1
Complications by procedure

Procedure	Complication
Maxillary sinoscopy	Pain, facial swelling, dental numbness, facial numbness
Caldwell-Luc	Pain, facial swelling, dental numbness, facial numbness, facial asymmetry, oroantral fistula, gingival-labial wound dehiscence, dacryocystitis, devitalized tooth, bleeding, persistent sinusitis
Extended middle meatus antrostomy	Chronic crusting, empty nose syndrome, circular flow around stump, injury to nasolacrimal duct
Endoscopic middle meatus antrostomy	Missed natural os, scarring, injury to nasolacrimal duct-epiphora, orbital penetration, facial numbness
Balloon dilatation (Acclarent)	Missed natural os, submucosal passage of balloon, orbital penetration
Balloon dilation (Entellus)	Pain, facial swelling, dental numbness, facial numbness, failure to pass balloon catheter
Minimally invasive sinus technique	Missed natural os, scarring, circular flow

sinus. This procedure is often performed in association with an endoscopic endonasal middle meatal approach. For the sinoscopy, the surgeon uses an endoscopic trocar to traverse the canine fossa into the maxillary sinus. During this approach, branches of the infraorbital and anterior superior alveolar nerve (ASAN) may be harmed because of their proximity to the canine fossa.[2] Resultant complications from injury to these nerves include facial pain, dental numbness, and local hypoesthesia. Other notable complications of the sinoscopy procedure include facial swelling and cellulitis.

Robinson and Wormald described an ideal point of anterior entry into the sinus at the intersection of the mid-pupillary line and the horizontal line through the floor of the nasal vestibule.[3] **Fig. 1** depicts this point. Once this landmark is identified, a trocar is twisted to remove bone of the anterior wall of the maxillary sinus. The trocar should not be hammered into the sinus because of the possibility of fracture of the anterior wall through the branches of the infraorbital nerve and ASAN with resultant facial numbness. Careful attention to these guidelines will diminish the risk for dental numbness and facial hypoesthesia. To decrease postoperative facial emphysema, patients should be instructed to not blow their nose for 24 hours after surgery. Pre- and postoperative antibiotics should also be considered to prevent facial cellulitis as a consequence of dragging the trocar through the facial soft tissues. In the authors' experience, placing ice over the cheek area postoperatively has reduced the bruising and swelling often associated with this approach.

CALDWELL-LUC

Until the mid 1980s, the Caldwell-Luc operation was the main operation used to manage maxillary sinus disease. Currently, it is rare for the sinus surgeon to resort to the Caldwell-Luc operation. The Caldwell-Luc operation is, however, the authors' mainstay of surgical treatment for failed middle meatus antrostomy maxillary sinus disease. This procedure is the authors' last-resort operation after exhausting surgical and medical treatments of the diseased sinus, including revision antrostomies, biofilm management, use of culture-directed antibiotics, nasal irrigations, systemic steroids,

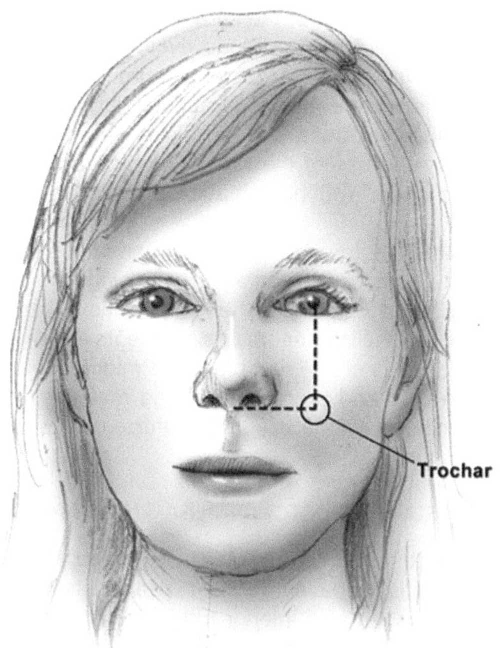

Fig. 1. Location of trocar placement for maxillary sinoscopy, Caldwell-Luc, Entellus balloon procedure adapted from Wormald. (*Courtesy of* Megan Rojas, MA, Nashville, TN; with permission.)

multiple office debridements, and intravenous antibiotics on occasion. When patients state that they are tired of all the treatment, it becomes time to look at other options: the authors offer Caldwell-Luc at this point.

This procedure has been noted to have varying rates of complication and morbidity in the literature. Cutler and Duncavage reviewed 133 Caldwell-Luc procedures with a follow-up of 1 to 6 years. They found a 92% success rate with an average follow-up of 23.5 months. The most common risk for the Caldwell-Luc procedure is the failure of the surgery to cure the infection. Eight percent (n = 3) of subjects in this review did not respond to the surgery. In two of these three cases, failure was caused by trapped mucosa and these cases were successfully salvaged with a repeat Caldwell-Luc procedure. Mild postoperative discomfort was reported in 37% and facial numbness or deformity was identified in 2%.[4,5] Defreitas and Lucente published the largest, single institutional review of 670 cases of the Caldwell-Luc operation in 1988. The immediate postoperative complications in 522 subjects were facial swelling in 89% of subjects, cheek discomfort in 33% of subjects, temperature more than 101°F in 12% of subjects, and significant hemorrhage in 3% of subjects. They reported long-term complications of facial asymmetry in 0.7% of subjects, facial numbness or paresthesia in 9.0% of subjects, oral antral fistula in 1.0% of subjects, gingival-labial wound dehiscence in 1.0% of subjects, dacryocystitis in 2.0% of subjects, devitalized dentition in 0.4% of subjects, recurrent sinusitis in 12.0% of subjects, and recurrent polyposis in 5.0% of subjects.[6]

How do we prevent the previously mentioned complications? The authors recommend using the previously described anatomic landmarks for entry into the maxillary sinus to minimize injury to branches of the infraorbital nerve and ASAN.[3] By twisting the trocar through the canine fossa, one can avoid fracture of surrounding bone. Care must also be taken when elevating the periosteum to avoid injury to the adjacent nerves. The authors do not extend the bone removal lateral to the point of entry to protect the lateral maxillary buttress and to minimize potential facial asymmetry. Bleeding is minimized by the use of the topical clotting agents and, at the end of the procedure, the sinus is filled with hemostatic agents, such as Surgifoam (Ethicon, Inc, Somerville, NJ, USA).

To avoid an oroantral fistula, the authors perform an inferior meatal antrostomy at the time of the Caldwell-Luc procedure to assist with sinus drainage. The placement of this antrostomy is important to not injure the valve of Hasner, and should be directed in the posterior two thirds of the inferior meatus.[7] Patients are seen postoperatively at 1 week to remove and debride crusts that block the middle meatus, which seems to help with postoperative pain and pressure over the maxillary sinus. Wound dehiscence is prevented by closure with absorbable suture using a running, non-locking, horizontal mattress closure.

EXTENDED MIDDLE MEATUS ANTROSTOMY/MEGA-ANTROSTOMY

The extended middle meatus antrostomy[8] was described in 1996 to help manage persistent maxillary sinusitis in patients with a previously placed inferior meatus antrostomy and a surgically reduced inferior turbinate. To correct the postoperative maxillary sinus circular flow that was often present in these patients, the natural maxillary ostium was connected to the inferior meatus antrostomy with removal of the inferior turbinate posterior to the valve of Hasner. Duncavage and Cho reported resolution of sinusitis in all six subjects on whom they first performed this procedure.[8] Cho and Hwang also studied 28 subjects (42 procedures) who underwent a similar procedure for recalcitrant maxillary sinusitis and reported 74% of the subjects with complete or marked resolution of symptoms. They concluded this was a reasonable intermediate salvage procedure for maxillary sinusitis for which radical mucosal exenteration is not desirable.[9]

The authors have identified several possible complications that can be associated with this procedure. The first is exposed bone of the posterior attachment of the inferior turbinate that can lead to crusting. This complication can be easily treated by endoscopic removal of any exposed bone. Another complication is incomplete removal of the posterior inferior turbinate resulting in circular flow around the stump. This complication can be corrected by removing the posterior stump of the remaining inferior turbinate. Bleeding is also a risk, and meticulous hemostasis around the posterior aspect of the inferior turbinate is especially important. Empty nose syndrome or atrophic rhinitis may also occur; it is for this reason that the anterior aspect of the inferior turbinate is meticulously preserved.[10] Injury to the nasolacrimal duct is also a consideration and avoiding the anterior one half of the inferior turbinate will assure the nasolacrimal system from injury.[7]

ENDOSCOPIC MIDDLE MEATAL ANTROSTOMY

Kennedy and colleagues[11] introduced the middle meatal antrostomy as a better surgical approach to the maxillary sinus in the mid 1980s. Proof that the mucociliary clearance through the natural os persisted despite inferior meatal antrostomies led to the development of this procedure. Kennedy argued that careful enlargement of the natural os was the key to treatment of this sinus. The endoscopic middle meatal antrostomy is one of the most common endoscopic sinus procedures sinus surgeons perform today. The maxillary sinus is often misunderstood and a mere surgical opening is not enough; it must include the natural os. The surgery can be performed in various ways but the key steps of the procedure include removal of the uncinate process, identification of the natural os, and enlargement of the ostium. This procedure can be accomplished through a variety of instruments, including biting instruments and powered microdebriders. The patency of the middle meatal antrostomy in the original Kennedy study was reported to be 98%.[11] In a more recent study that involved 90 antrostomies, 84 (93.5%) remained patent after 18 to 30 months.[12] The size of the antrostomy does not appear to affect the outcome of symptoms or chronic maxillary sinusitis.[13]

Scarring in a postoperative setting is commonly seen and can easily be revised in the office. It is often the result of a circular injury to the ostium. Care must be taken when dissecting the natural os to leave the anterior superior aspect of the antrostomy intact. Scarring can also result in circular flow when the scar tissue separates the natural ostium from the surgical antrostomy. A missed natural ostium is also another cause for circular flow. Whether the scar tissue forms or a missed ostium is the cause for the circular flow, Albu discovered that this finding has the strongest correlation in persistent postoperative symptoms.[13] Similarly, the accessory os should be included in the enlargement to prevent circular flow. **Fig. 2** is a pictorial sequence of circular flow in the setting of missed natural ostia. One can follow the air bubble to see the flow pattern.

Several complications can occur intraoperatively. Injury to the nasolacrimal duct can occur with excessive dissection anteriorly, most commonly with a back biter. The nasolacrimal sac lies 8.8 mm above the insertion of the middle turbinate and drops about 11 mm inferiorly where it then becomes the nasolacrimal duct. It is closest to the maxillary os at the midpoint of the maxillary line, which is described as a curvilinear line from the middle turbinate attachment to the roof of the inferior turbinate.[7] The initial management of this complication is by observation. If postoperative epiphora is persistent, ophthalmologic consultation and subsequent operative treatment may be needed, including a dacryocystorhinostomy. Orbital penetration during uncinectomy is a potential complication and is especially important in the setting of hypoplastic maxillary sinus surgery. The uncinate may often be adherent to the medial orbital wall in some situations, and care must be taken to dissect the uncinate away before removal is attempted. Using a sickle knife to perform an uncinectomy would be inappropriate in the example of a severely atelectatic, retracted uncinate. Entering the maxillary sinus inferiorly first and then following the contour of the orbit is the safest technique to avoid orbital penetration. Even less common is injury to the infraorbital nerve. A dehiscent nerve will be evident on coronal CT scan and when this anatomic variation occurs, care must be taken to not injure the nerve by avoiding aggressing dissection within the sinus.

During endoscopic sinus surgery, the middle turbinate is often preserved. In the setting of preservation, it can become destabilized and cause scarring of the middle

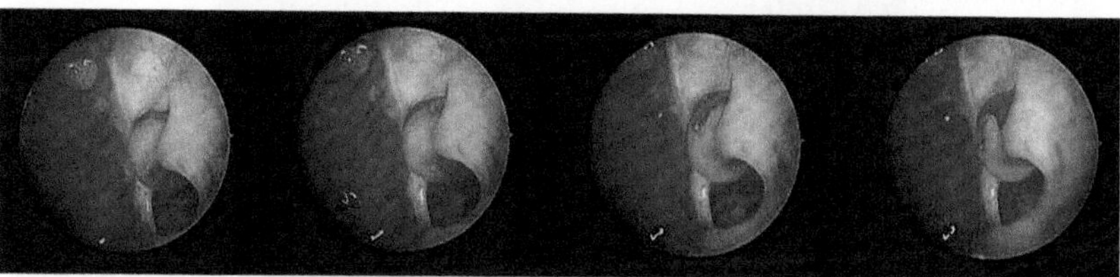

Fig. 2. Circular flow of maxillary sinus as a result of missing natural os, following the bubbles will give the reader the direction of movement.

meatus. To prevent this, a spacer must be placed postoperatively or care must be taken to prevent lateralization with either the Bolger technique, excoriating the medial surface of the turbinate and septum, or suture technique. If scarring results, often simple office revision is all that is necessary, but operative revisions are not uncommon.

BALLOON PROCEDURES

Balloon technology has become a relevant tool in sinus surgery. It has enabled sinus surgeons to address treatment of the maxillary sinus while avoiding some of the surgical pitfalls previously mentioned. There are two products that are able to address the maxillary sinus. Each product has shown efficacy in treatment of chronic rhinosinusitis of the maxillary sinus.

Acclarent Inc uses balloon technology that introduces a balloon catheter over a wire through an angled sheath. The sheaths are specific to each sinus: 70° for frontal, 110° for maxillary, and 0° for sphenoid. The wire is either used under fluoroscopy or a lighted wire can be used. The initial clinical evaluation to confirm safety and efficacy of sinuplasty in the paranasal sinuses (CLEAR) study reported a patency of 113 out of 124 (91%) maxillary ostia. It was non-patent in 1 (1%) and indeterminate in 10 (8%).[14]

The most common complication of this technology is failure to pass the catheter. In the CLEAR study, prior scar tissue was the cause in six subjects, anatomic restrictions in four subjects, and polyps in one subject. The study did not delineate the failure by sinus.[14] The wire can be malpositioned and miss the natural os. As a result, dilatation of the accessory os, submucosal passage of the balloon, and orbital penetration can occur.[15] **Fig. 3** shows the guidewire appropriately coiled into the maxillary sinus. The wire must be fully visualized coiling in the maxillary sinus to be assured correct placement. Rotation of the sheath medially and caudally also improves the correct trajectory of the wire. One way to reduce this malpositioning is to use a lighted guidewire (Luma, Acclarent Inc, Menlo Park, CA, USA). **Fig. 4** shows the maxillary sinus with the Relieva Luma catheter. Device failure has also been described and may be easily addressed with replacement. Non-patency of the balloon-dilated ostia required revision in 7 out of 195 (3.6%) of the sinuses.[16] The CLEAR study at 2 years did not specify which sinuses required revision. The PatiENT Registry reported a 2.4% revision rate.[17]

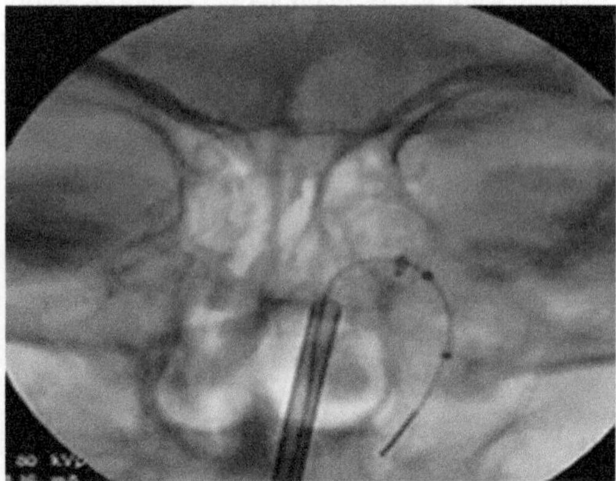

Fig. 3. Fluoroscopy view of the left maxillary sinus with the guidewire appropriately coiled in the maxillary sinus. (*Courtesy of* Acclarent, Inc, Menlo Park, CA; with permission.)

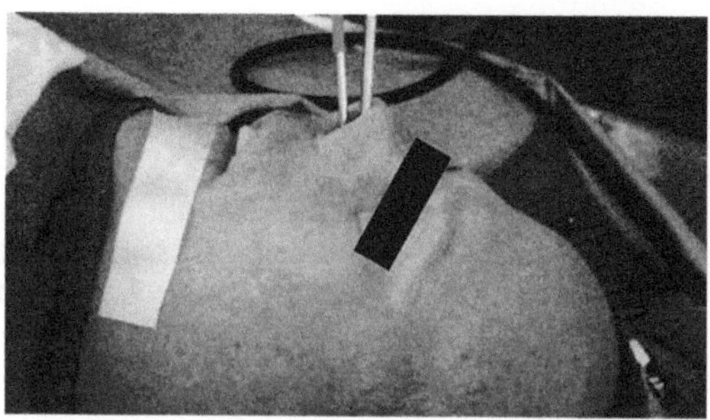

Fig. 4. Lighted guidewire in the maxillary sinus. (*Courtesy of* Acclarent, Inc, Menlo Park, CA; with permission.)

Entellus Medical uses a balloon to dilate the maxillary os through a transantral approach. A side-cutting trocar is placed through the maxillary sinus. A 0.5 mm fiber-optic telescope is passed through a dual lumen sheath where a 5.0 mm or 7.0 mm balloon is passed through the second lumen. Once the natural os is identified, the balloon is directed into the ostium and ethmoid infundibulum and dilated to 12 atmospheres of pressure.

Complications of this procedure are similar to a maxillary sinoscopy described earlier. These complications include facial numbness, tooth numbness, facial swelling, and oroantral fistula. Soft-tissue infections can occur in the cheek as a result, seeding the cheek upon trocar placement or removal. This complication can be managed by premedicating patients with antibiotics before the procedure. Failure to identify the maxillary os is a potential complication. The balloon remodeling antrostomy therapy (BREATHE) study reported a two (3.4%) failures in identifying the natural os.[18] **Fig. 5** shows the view of the natural os during a transantral approach (Entellus Medical). This result is likely to occur when placement of the trocar is not lateral enough. In the authors' experience, careful placement of the trocar allows for a good trajectory for the balloon catheter. Also in the BREATHE 1 study, two (3.4%) subjects had tooth numbness and one (1.7%) subject had facial numbness. In all, the rate of adverse incidents was quite low.[18]

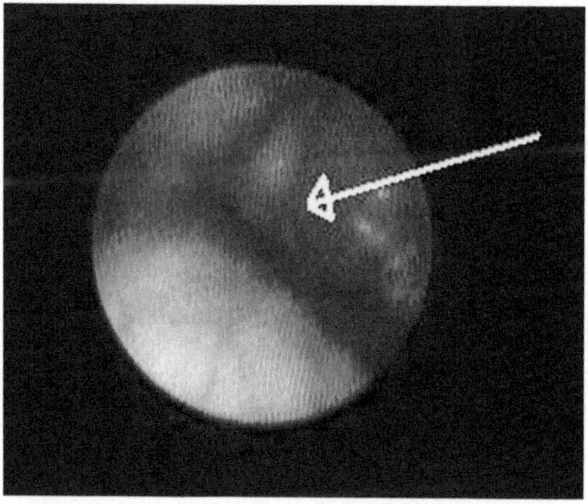

Fig. 5. View of the maxillary ostia during transantral approach, arrow is pointing to the os. Note that the view is of limited clarity. (Entellus procedure.)

MINIMALLY INVASIVE SINUS TECHNIQUE

Minimally invasive sinus technique was first described by Setliff and was described as surgery that maintains landmarks and spaces.[19] It involves complete removal of the uncinate process and exposing the inferior aspect of the agger nasi,[20] which allows for visualization of the maxillary sinus ostium but is not manipulated. Because the ostium is not enlarged, some feel that ventilation is not enough to treat the diseased sinus.[21] Scarring in 2% of cases was the most common complication of the middle meatus. Failure of the procedure regardless of cause can be managed with endoscopic middle meatal antrostomy. Catalano reported a 5.9% revision rate but did not report a revision procedure.[20]

To conclude, maxillary sinus surgery can greatly improve patients' symptoms and disease process. The authors encourage the surgeon to take great care in ensuring sound surgical principles. Understanding the potential areas in which surgery can fail will help tremendously in preventing complications.

REFERENCES

1. Hulett KJ, Stankiewicz AJ. Primary sinus surgery. In: Cummings C, Haughey B, Thomas J, et al, editors. Cummings otolaryngology: head and neck surgery. 4th edition. Philadelphia: Mosby; 2005.
2. Singhal D, Douglas R, Robinson S, et al. The incidence of complications using new landmarks and a modified technique of canine fossa puncture. Am J Rhinol 2007;21:316–9.
3. Robinson S, Wormald PJ. Patterns of innervation of the anterior maxilla: a cadaver study with relevance to canine fossa puncture of the maxillary sinus. Laryngoscope 2005;115:1785–8.
4. Cutler JL, Duncavage JA, Metheny K, et al. Results of Caldwell-Luc after failed endoscopic middle meatus antrostomy in patients with chronic sinusitis. Laryngoscope 2003;113:2148–50.
5. Matheny KE, Duncavage JA. Contemporary indications for the Caldwell Luc procedure. Curr Opin Otolaryngol Head Neck Surg 2003;11(1):23–6.
6. Defreitas J, Lucente FE. The Caldwell-Luc procedure: institutional review of 670 cases: 1975-1985. Laryngoscope 1988;98:1297–300.
7. Chastain JB, Sindwani R. Anatomy of the orbit, lacirmal apparatus and lateral nasal wall. Otolaryngol Clin North Am 2006;39:855–64.
8. Coleman JR, Duncavage JA. Extended middle meatal antrostomy: the treatment of circular flow. Laryngoscope 1996;106:1214–7.
9. Cho DT, Hwang PH. Results of endoscopic maxillary mega-antrostomy in recalcitrant maxillary sinusitis. Am J Rhinol 2008;22:658–62.
10. Chhabra N, Houser SM. The diagnosis and management of empty nose syndrome. Otolaryngol Clin North Am 2009;42:311–30.
11. Kennedy DL, Zinreich AJ, Kuhm F, et al. Endoscopic middle meatal antrostomy: theory, technique, and patency. Laryngoscope 1987;97(8 Pt Suppl 43):1–9.
12. Salam MA, Cable HR. Middle meatal antrostomy: long term patency and results in chronic maxillary sinusitis. A prospective study. Clin Otolaryngol 1993;18:135–8.
13. Albu S, Tomescu E. Small and large middle meatus antrostomies in the treatment of chronic maxillary sinusitis. Otolaryngol Head Neck Surg 2004;131:542–7.
14. Bolger WE, Crown CL, Church CA, et al. Safety and outcomes of balloon catheter sinusotomy: a multicenter 24-week analysis in 115 patients. Otolaryngol Head Neck Surg 2007;137(1):10–20.

15. Kim E, Cutler JL. Balloon dilatation of the paranasal sinuses: a tool in sinus surgery. Otolaryngol Clin North Am 2009;42:847–56.
16. Weiss RL, Church CA, Kuhn FA, et al. Long-term outcome analysis of balloon catheter sinusotomy: two-year follow-up. Otolaryngol Head Neck Surg 2008; 139:S38–46.
17. Levine H, Sertich AP, Hoisington DR, et al. Multicenter registry of balloon catheter sinusotomy outcomes for 1036 patients. Ann Otol Rhinol Laryngol 2008;117(4): 265–70.
18. Stankiewicz J, Tami T, Truitt T, et al. Transantral, endoscopically guided balloon dilatation of the osteomeatal complex for chronic rhinosinusitis under local anesthesia. Am J Rhinol Allergy 2009;23:321–7.
19. Setliff RC. Minimally invasive sinus surgery: the rational and the technique. Otolaryngol Clin North Am 1996;29:115–24.
20. Catalano PJ. The minimally invasive sinus technique: theory and practice. Otolaryngol Clin North Am 2004;37(2):401–9.
21. Chiu AG, Kennedy DW. Disadvantages of minimal techniques for surgical management of chronic rhinosinusitis. Curr Opin Otolaryngol Head Neck Surg 2004;12:38–42.

Prevention and Management of Complications in Intracranial Endoscopic Skull Base Surgery

Evan R. Ransom, MD[a], Alexander G. Chiu, MD[b,*]

KEYWORDS

- Endoscopic • Transsphenoidal
- Skull base surgery • Complications

Development of minimally invasive approaches has become a significant driver across surgical specialties in recent years, with the goal of reducing patient morbidity while maintaining good outcomes. The potential trade-off between recovery times or patient satisfaction and eradication of disease is of utmost importance. Efforts to reduce perioperative morbidity and mortality have been applied with increasing sophistication in the most complex anatomic regions of the human body, including the head and neck. These efforts have resulted in an expanded role of purely endoscopic approaches to the paranasal sinuses, the anterior skull base, and the anterior cranial fossa.

The routine use of functional endoscopic sinus surgery (FESS) in the management of chronic infectious and inflammatory sinus disease has led to significant improvements in endoscopic skills and surgical technology. Application of endoscopic surgery to the treatment of sinonasal tumors was initially confined to benign lesions, such as inverted papilloma and osteomas.[1–4] Recently, endoscopic indications have expanded to include sinonasal malignancies and skull base neoplasms.[5–8] This finding has been supported by advances in surgeon experience, advances in computer-guided technology, angled drills, and proven techniques for skull base reconstruction.[9–11] Purely endoscopic resections with proper attention to oncologic margins are now possible, with the potential benefit of decreased perioperative morbidity and improved cosmesis compared with traditional open transfacial or craniofacial approaches.[8]

[a] Department of Otorhinolaryngology–Head and Neck Surgery, University of Pennsylvania, 3400 Spruce Street, Philadelphia, PA 19104, USA
[b] Rhinology and Skull Base Surgery Fellowship Program, Department of Otorhinolaryngology–Head and Neck Surgery, University of Pennsylvania, 3400 Spruce Street, Philadelphia, PA 19104, USA
* Corresponding author.
E-mail address: Alexander.Chiu@uphs.upenn.edu

Otolaryngol Clin N Am 43 (2010) 875–895
doi:10.1016/j.otc.2010.04.012 oto.theclinics.com
0030-6665/10/$ – see front matter

However, literature in this emerging field is still developing. Evidence used in surgical and perioperative management has been derived from retrospective case series. Lack of specific protocols and limited experience with perioperative management of patients with sinus disease have the potential to significantly inhibit further advances in the routine and safe application of purely endoscopic skull base techniques. In particular, cases in which intracranial extent is present, obligating the surgeon to enter the anterior cranial fossa and reconstruct the skull base, demand nothing short of a complete understanding of the critical structures encountered in the approach and the potential morbidity of this work. This article reviews the current understanding and available literature regarding the diagnosis and management of complications associated with endoscopic anterior skull base surgery.

OPERATIVE PROCEDURES

As endoscopic skull base surgery has become feasible and widespread, otorhinolaryngologists have become increasingly involved. This involvement has expanded the required knowledge base of this specialty, particularly with regard to neurologic and endocrinologic issues in the perioperative period. Given that prevention is the best strategy for management of complications in any surgery, a review of the extended endoscopic approaches is an important first step and allows for an anatomic understanding of the clinical data. A brief summary of each of the common extended endoscopic approaches is included in this article and forms the basis for the detailed discussion of complications, prevention, and management decisions that follows.

Endoscopic Transsphenoidal Approach

The endoscopic transsphenoidal approach (TSA) represents a natural extension or modification of the traditional microscope-assisted TSA. By obviating complete nasal septal detachment and sublabial or columellar incisions, the surgeon may potentially reduce the incidence of rhinologic or cosmetic sequelae, such as septal perforation, nasal obstruction, palate or dental anesthesia, and obvious scars.[12] Data regarding the efficacy and safety of endoscopic TSA have been almost uniformly supportive, showing adequate and safe tumor resection.[13,14] Direct comparisons of microscopic and endoscopic approaches have been less common and have had differing results. Some investigators have shown reduced operative time, hospital stay, and patient-reported postoperative discomfort.[12,15] A lower incidence of lumbar drain requirement and postoperative cerebrospinal fluid (CSF) leak has also been found in a study, relative to traditional sublabial and transseptal approaches.[16]

As it is most commonly performed, the endoscopic approach to the sella is made via a partial posterior septectomy followed by a wide bilateral opening of the sphenoid rostrum. Connecting the ostia of each sphenoid sinus and then removing the bone inferiorly to the level of the sphenoid sinus floor places the underside of the bony sella turcica and clival recess in direct view. An appreciation of the lateral extent of the sphenoid sinus and the thickness of the bony covering of the internal carotid artery (ICA) and optic nerve is crucial. Tumor resection is then accomplished by removal of the thin bone of the sella and gentle dissection of the adenomatous portion of the gland from the normal residual adenohypophysis anteriorly and neurohypophysis posteriorly. If the arachnoid is sufficiently damaged, a CSF leak may be present and should be repaired with a multilayer technique.[17,18]

Transcribriform Approach

The transcribriform approach is used for lesions involving the midline anterior skull base, which is anterior to the sphenoid rostrum at the level of the cribriform plate of the ethmoid bone. This extremely thin bony roof separates the ethmoid air cells from the anterior cranial fossa and contains the olfactory fillae as they extend inferiorly from the olfactory bulbs. Lesions in this area include paranasal sinus tumors with skull base or transcranial extension, such as esthesioneuroblastomas, adenocarcinomas, squamous cell carcinomas, or mucosal melanomas among others.[6,19–22]

In contrast to the TSA, transcribriform approaches require significant paranasal sinus work either for initial debulking, as in tumor resections, or to adequately expose lesions primarily at the bony skull base. A variety of adjunct procedures may be required for oncologic concerns. These procedures include opening of the paranasal sinuses to ensure complete circumferential tumor-free margins, with the addition of endoscopic medial maxillectomy for cases with significant inferior and lateral extent. Maxillectomy may necessitate complete removal of the lamina papyracea for gross tumor involvement or as a margin in the case of malignancy. Hemostasis is crucial when working with the orbital contents. The proportion of nasal septum that must be removed is variable but is frequently substantial. Unilateral or bilateral middle turbinectomies are also required in most cases.

Anterior skull base lesions with a minimal extent of paranasal sinus or lying entirely within the anterior cranial fossa require wide opening of the ethmoid air cells, ligation of the anterior ethmoid arteries, partial septectomy, and careful skeletonizing of the ethmoid roof. Image guidance is helpful in such cases and aids the surgeon to identify the extent of the lesion and delineate the portion of bony skull base to be removed (like a trapdoor for olfactory or tuberculum meningiomas). In cases in which there is significant intracranial disease, preoperative magnetic resonance imaging (MRI) is used to assess parenchymal involvement, although the difference between displacement and invasion of the pia mater may be subtle. With pial invasion, microneurosurgical techniques are required for resection and thus increase the risk for neurovascular complications. To date, resections of frontal lobe lesions have been limited to minimal corticectomy; deeper involvement is an indication for a traditional open approach via craniotomy.

Anteriorly, the cribriform plate terminates at the posterior wall of the frontal sinus. When the lesion or margin of resection reaches this point, additional complex paranasal sinus work is required to ensure a functional and safe frontal sinus. An endoscopic modified Lothrop procedure (Draf III) is performed, resulting in a common, large frontal sinus outflow tract. Resection of the mass and reconstruction of the skull base may then proceed posteriorly from the common frontal recess.

Transplanum-Transtuberculum Approach

For lesions involving or overlying the planum sphenoidale and tuberculum sellae, a transplanum-transtuberculum approach is used. The initial steps are similar to an endoscopic TSA, but after the wide sphenoidotomy, entry through the skull base is accomplished more superiorly and anteriorly. Removal of the bone anterior to the sella turcica results in exposure of the optic chiasm and pituitary stalk, requiring careful dissection and thoughtful use of electrocautery. Significant morbidity may follow the minutest manipulation of these structures or their fragile vascular supply, which may be encountered directly in the operative field or on the tumor surface. In addition, care should be taken to avoid entry into the cavernous sinus, which may result in persistent venous bleeding and significantly compromise visualization.

Durotomy in this area creates a high-volume, high-flow CSF leak by opening the suprasellar or chiasmatic cistern. This condition is further complicated by the abnormal 3-dimensional geometry of the resulting defect, which is somewhat trapezoidal but with a bend in the middle. Reconstruction typically relies on a flat plane and a layered technique, as in the cribriform area. This added dimension makes skull base repair complex and tenuous, although pedicled septal mucosa rotation flaps have been used with frequent success.[23,24]

Tuberculum sellae and olfactory groove meningioma are the most common lesions that have been treated via a transplanum-transtuberculum approach.[25–27] Other lesions may be treated via a modified transplanum-transtuberculum approach to achieve suprachiasmatic control, including Rathke cleft cysts and craniopharyngiomas.

Transclival Approach

The clivus is the midline bony structure of variable thickness formed by the sphenoid and occipital bones, which lies inferior to the sella and slopes to the foramen magnum. The transclival approach is used in the case of clival mass lesions, most commonly including chordomas but may also include chondrosarcomas and other rare tumors.[28–31] Because of its more inferior location, less paranasal sinus work is required in this approach. The theoretical risk of CSF leak is also reduced significantly, because the ethmoid roof, planum sphenoidale, and sella are generally avoided. Entry into the CSF space at this level would require passage through the entire bone and entry into the prepontine cistern or craniocervical junction or the dissection of sella turcica, in addition.

Circumferential dissection around a clival tumor may proceed from within the sphenoid sinus, with removal of the posterior and inferior sinus walls. For smaller or more inferior lesions, minimal sphenoid work may be required or a nasopharyngeal approach could be used. In the case of a larger or more superior lesion, the transclival approach has been combined with endoscopic TSA.[28,29]

Endoscopic Approach to the Petrous Apex

Minimally invasive approaches to the petrous apex are also possible via the anterior corridor through the sphenoid sinus and have been used primarily for endoscopic treatment of cystic and inflammatory lesions, such as cholesterol granuloma and petrous apicitis.[32] After creation of a wide sphenoidotomy, identification of the anterior wall of the cystic lesion is achieved with image guidance, noting also the relative position of the optic nerve and ICA. These lesions may then be opened widely and allowed to drain via the sphenoid sinus into the nasopharynx, occasionally with the aid of a temporary Silastic stent (Dow Corning, Midland, MI, USA). Some investigators have used this approach for solid lesions as well, including smaller chordomas and chondrosarcomas.[32] Accurate and continually updated image guidance with careful intraoperative mapping of the petrous portion of the ICA is essential in this approach. For larger lesions, specific anatomic considerations of the temporal bone may become important or a combined endoscopic anterior and traditional lateral skull base procedure may be necessary.

REVIEW OF COMPLICATIONS

The anterior skull base is a complex anatomic region, which contains crucial sensory and neurovascular structures in extremely close proximity. The breadth and severity of potential perioperative complications of endoscopic surgery is thus significant. Overall, major complication rates in endoscopic approaches are consistently reported as less than 10%, with some smaller series reporting around 20%.[6,8,21,33–35] Perioperative deaths are exceedingly rare in endoscopic skull base approaches, with only 3 reported in the literature to date.[21,26,36] This rarity represents a significant improvement over the reported perioperative morbidity and mortality of traditional open craniofacial resection, which was 35% to 50% and 5% to 10%, respectively.[37–44] In addition, a meta-analysis showed the perioperative mortality rate for endoscopic TSA as 0.24%.[45] Although the different types of lesions and the extent of dissection make it impossible to compare endoscopic TSA and extended endoscopic approaches, the reported morbidity and mortality data are encouraging. Lastly, the inherent bias in morbidity and mortality statistics, which result from surgeon preference and from factors intrinsic to specific lesions (eg, size, lateral extent, parenchymal involvement), must be acknowledged. These differences make direct comparisons of open and endoscopic approaches difficult and encourage cautious interpretation of clinical series.

In this section, the cause, incidence, and basic management of potential complications in endoscopic skull base surgery are reviewed in reference to the relevant skull base and neuroanatomy. The discussion is organized by anatomic location or organ system, with reference to specific approaches where applicable.

Sinonasal Complications

All endonasal surgery inherently involves the risk for nasal mucosa injury and postoperative bleeding. Synechiae occur when opposing mucosal surfaces are abraded or lacerated and are commonly formed between the septum and turbinates, particularly in endoscopic TSA in which the turbinates remain in the operative corridor. Postoperative airway obstruction attributable to anterior adhesions is experienced as greater inspiratory resistance or change in nasal airflow direction.[46] As with most complications of nasal surgery, prevention of adhesions by careful surgical technique is the best strategy. Epistaxis, the most common postoperative complication of FESS, also occurs after endoscopic skull base surgery. This complication should be treated with packing or cautery according to severity, after endoscopic localization of the source. Significant epistaxis should be taken seriously, because it may indicate a major vessel bleed or intracranial bleed.[26]

A variable extent of paranasal sinus work is required in endoscopic endonasal approaches, frequently including ethmoidectomy, sphenoidotomy, and frontal sinusotomy. Although these surgical procedures are used for access of margins, they also affect the function of the sinuses. Similar to standard FESS, disruption of the sinus mucosa, obstruction of the sinus outflow, or the retained bony fragments and debris may result in sinusitis. A severe case of chronic frontal sinusitis after endoscopic resection was described by Unger and colleagues[47] and required FESS and subsequent osteoplastic flap. The incidence of acute or chronic rhinosinusitis after endoscopic anterior skull base surgery is not known, although patient-specific factors, including previous history of sinus disease or allergy, may predict postoperative difficulty. This feature underscores the importance of meticulous technique during the intranasal portion of the approach.

Not only particularly in the frontal sinus but also in the ethmoid region, obstruction of sinus outflow with continued mucus production may result in a mucocele. As this material accumulates, increased pressure within the cell results in an expansile lesion of the sinus with bony remodeling. Treatment involves endoscopic drainage and wide opening of the involved sinus. Although not directly reported in most studies, Nicolai and colleagues[21] noted 2 mucoceles in 134 cases (1.5%). With mucocele formation in the area of a previously resected neoplasm, directed biopsies should be done to rule out residual or recurrent tumor. Mucoceles of any origin may recur, although endoscopic approaches are proved effective even in the most complicated lesions.[48]

Finally, atrophic rhinitis is a significant concern when the paranasal sinus approach to the skull base requires removal of a large portion of the mucosal surface. Atrophic rhinitis is a condition characterized by thick crusting, persistent rhinorrhea, foul smell or taste, and a paradoxic sensation of nasal airway obstruction.[49] Although atrophic rhinitis is more common with resection of the inferior turbinates, it may also occur in cases with bilateral middle turbinectomy and subtotal septectomy. Alterations in sinonasal physiology may predispose the patient to bacterial rhinitis with distinct flora such as *Klebsiella ozaenae*.[49,50] Chronic crusting and poor nasal function has been reported in at least one-third of patients undergoing endoscopic skull base surgery, although the incidence may be even higher, because many studies do not comment on this issue.[30,51,52] Postoperative external beam radiation therapy may increase the likelihood of atrophic rhinitis in this group by delaying mucosal healing and promoting atrophy of glandular elements and cilia.[50,53] Symptomatic improvement is achieved by routine humidification, nasal irrigations, improved nasal hygiene, and topical antibiotics, but no curative treatment exists for this complication.

Orbital and Optic Nerve Complications

Orbital hematoma is a familiar and fortunately rare complication of FESS, with a reported incidence of less than 1%, and thus it is a potential complication in endoscopic skull base approaches.[54,55] Vascular injury leads to bleeding within the orbit, resulting in proptosis, elevated pressures, and subsequent ischemic damage of the optic nerve and retina.[56] This injury may be venous, frequently from the orbital fat, or arterial, in the case of anterior or posterior ethmoid artery injury. If a developing orbital hematoma is suspected, elevated intraocular pressure (normally 10–20 mm Hg) confirms the diagnosis. Initial conservative measures include massage, administration of mannitol, and intravenous steroids. With rapidly expanding hematoma or pressures greater than 40 mm Hg, the surgeon must urgently decompress the orbit via lateral canthotomy.[56] Identification and control of the source of hemorrhage may then be proceeded.

Although the incidence of orbital hematoma in endoscopic skull base surgery is not defined, it is likely similar to or somewhat less than in FESS. One case has been reported in the literature on endoscopic skull base surgery.[35] In endoscopic approaches in which orbital work is required, this generally entails removal of a significant portion of the lamina papyracea and exposure of the periorbita. Bleeding due to this exposure is more easily appreciated than that resulting from inadvertent puncture, as in FESS. In addition, optic nerve ischemia is less likely to occur in cases in which the lamina has been removed, because hematoma expands into the nasal cavity rather than building pressure within the orbit proper. Particularly in transcribriform approaches, early ligation of the anterior or posterior ethmoid arteries may be indicated.

The optic nerve may be injured directly, accidentally by surgical instrumentation, or indirectly, as was discussed in the case of orbital hematoma earlier. A thorough review of the current literature on endoscopic skull base failed to reveal a case of permanent blindness secondary to direct optic nerve injury, although the risk should be assumed to be equal to or greater than in FESS in cases in which posterior ethmoidectomy, wide sphenoidotomy, and wide exposure of the optic nerve or chiasm is required (**Fig. 1**). Careful review of the preoperative imaging reveals anatomic variations that may place the optic nerve at greater risk, including Onodi cells (present in 10% of the population) and a dehiscent optic nerve in the sphenoid sinus (present in 4%).[57–59] One case of blindness attributed to vascular injury has been reported after resection of a multiply recurrent and multiply operated craniopharyngioma.[60] No proven treatment exists for restoring vision after optic nerve transection. For incomplete injury, including inadvertent bipolar cautery, some investigators have advocated intravenous steroids and optic nerve decompression, although evidence of efficacy is lacking.[58]

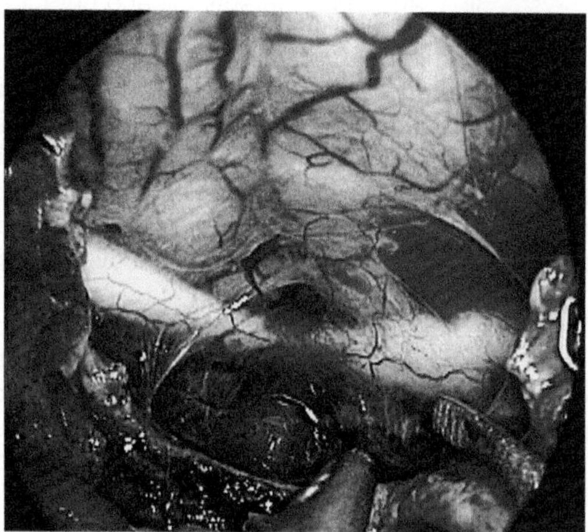

Fig. 1. Endoscopic view of the optic chiasm after purely endoscopic resection of a tuberculum sellae meningioma. The pituitary stalk is visible in the background.

Medial rectus injury is a severe but rare complication of FESS, reported in less than 0.5% of cases.[54] The incidence of this complication in endoscopic skull base surgery is not known, but a review of the current literature did not find a reported case. The mechanism of injury typically involves direct penetration of the lamina papyracea and periorbita, with subsequent contusion, disruption, or transection of muscle fibers. This injury results in eye movement abnormalities, including diplopia and strabismus. Medial rectus injury occurs most frequently in ethmoidectomy, given the thinness of the lamina and its proximity to the ethmoid air cells. Anatomic variants in this region and use of powered instruments seem to increase the risk and severity of injuries.[54,61] Treatment of medial rectus injury is extremely difficult and requires an oculoplastic expert. Depending on the degree of muscle loss, reapproximation, transposition grafts, and more advanced techniques have been used.[61,62] Results are however poor in many cases.

Ophthalmoplegia

Extraocular movement deficiency may also complicate endoscopic skull base approaches as the result of injury to the abducens or oculomotor nerve. These cranial nerves, along with the trochlear nerve and first division of the trigeminal nerve, traverse the cavernous sinus and, in some extended parasellar approaches, may be found in the endoscopic operative field.[63] During dissection, these nerves may be accidentally stretched, cauterized, or transected. The abducens nerve is most commonly affected, resulting in the typical ipsilateral lateral gaze palsy. This injury has been reported in the resection of parasellar, suprasellar, and clival lesions.[28,64,65] However, many midline skull base lesions present with oculomotor abnormalities, most, but not all, of which improve after surgery.[29,60]

Hyposmia and Anosmia

Decreased sense of smell is a common occurrence after endoscopic skull base surgery. In the immediate postoperative period, most patients have some degree of hyposmia secondary to nasal packing. True hyposmia is evident after packing removal and debridement. Although hyposmia is frequently transient after TSA or transclival approaches, transcribriform and transplanum-transtuberculum approaches may lead to permanent hyposmia or anosmia. These approaches involve extensive removal of the nasal septum, superior turbinate, or cribriform plate, with concomitant injury to or excision of the olfactory fillae. In the case of esthesioneuroblastoma, some investigators have argued for routine excision of the olfactory bulbs even in absence of gross involvement, given the cause of the tumor.[66] This excision obviously results in anosmia, and although this result is expected, patients must be counseled to avoid an unpleasant surprise postoperatively. Other investigators have posited avoidance of anosmia as an advantage of endoscopic approaches over craniofacial resection.[6]

Infectious Complications

Acute bacterial sinusitis may be common after endoscopic skull base surgery, particularly, given the degree of mucosal disruption and presence of foreign bodies (packing) in the resection cavity. For example, Unger and colleagues[47] reported acute sinusitis in 4 of 14 (29%) patients who underwent endoscopic resection and adjuvant Gamma Knife (Elekta Inc, Stockholm, Sweden) radiation therapy for esthesioneuroblastoma. Batra and colleagues[67] reported 15 cases of acute sinusitis after 200 TSAs (7.5%), including 10 cases of sphenoid sinusitis—five of which required revision surgery. Acute sinusitis must be treated quickly and aggressively, to avoid ascending infection and compromise of the healing–skull base reconstruction. Whenever possible, culture should be taken under endoscopic guidance before initiation of broad-spectrum empiric antibiotics. Subsequently, coverage may be tailored to culture results and sensitivities.

Intracranial infection may result from contamination during endoscopic skull base surgery or ascending infection via the skull base defect. Postoperative meningitis is relatively rare, with only a handful of cases reported.[19,21,34,60] Some of the larger series report an incidence of less than 1%.[6,21] Although the small number of cases makes statistical analysis impossible at this point, it is noteworthy that no cases of meningitis have been reported in the literature on transclival approaches.[28–31] Lack of cases of meningitis is likely because of the infrequency of dural disruption in this area and the location of the resection bed in the posterior-most aspect of the sinonasal cavity.

Localized suppurative infection may also complicate endoscopic skull base approaches in the form of epidural abscess, subdural empyema, or intraparenchymal abscess. These are rare events because sterile technique and perioperative antibiotics dramatically reduce the risk in immunocompetent patients. Frontal lobe abscess has been reported in 2 cases, from different investigators, each after endoscopic resection of a large transcranial esthesioneuroblastoma.[35,47] A high degree of suspicion is required in the case of smaller collections, because computed tomography (CT) may be nondiagnostic in up to 30% of cases.[68] Culture results typically reveal methicillin-resistant *Staphylococcus aureus*, gram-negative rods, or polymicrobial infections.[69] This complication requires formal craniotomy for drainage and possible revision of the skull base reconstruction, in addition to culture-specific intravenous antibiotics with CSF penetration. All grossly infected allograft materials should be removed at the time of surgery.

Neurovascular Injury, Hemorrhage, and Permanent Deficits

Injury of the ICA or the delicate intracranial vessels at the anterior skull base is perhaps the most feared operative complication in endoscopic surgery. Morbidity in such cases may range from blindness to pituitary apoplexy to stroke with permanent neurologic sequelae. Gentle dissection, judicious use of cautery, and traditional microneurosurgical technique are required to reduce vascular injury. Modern hemostatic agents, such as fibrin glue, concentrated thrombin, and microfibrillar collagen, are invaluable.

In addition, employment of the "2 nostrils 4 hands" technique provides for constant and stable visualization by allowing the primary surgeon to use both hands, while the second surgeon holds the endoscope and a second suction device.[70]

Intraoperative injury of the ICA is a rare but potentially lethal complication in endoscopic skull base surgery. Only two cases have been reported to date.[28,31] The first involved a recurrent, previously operated, and irradiated chordoma. ICA rupture was contained endonasally, without craniotomy or neurointerventional procedures, and no long-term dysfunction resulted. The second case occurred during resection of a clival chordoma with cavernous sinus extension[28] and was also controlled endoscopically; however, a pseudoaneurysm developed and required postoperative endovascular treatment. No permanent deficits resulted, although this case highlights the need for delayed postoperative angiography to rule out or treat a potentially dangerous pseudoaneurysm.

In endoscopic approaches including intracranial work, particularly in the parasellar region and with transplanum-transtuberculum approaches, injury of the circle of Willis is possible (**Fig. 2**). Tearing of the anterior cerebral artery or anterior communicating artery may result in significant subarachnoid hemorrhage (SAH), intraparenchymal hemorrhage (IPH), or intraventricular hemorrhage (IVH). Ability to control bleeding in these vessels endonasally in the event of laceration or rupture may mean life or death for the patient, and most investigators stress the need for significant experience before tackling lesions with significant intracranial extension. Although each case should involve preoperative consent and preparation for potential conversion to open craniotomy, in reality this would take too much time in the event of an intracranial arterial bleeding.

Review of the literature reveals four cases of significant ICH, with two cases each involving tuberculum sellae meningiomas and clival chordomas. In the first case, the

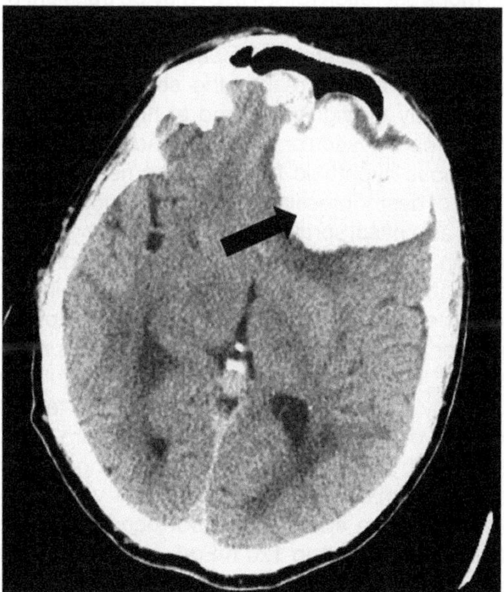

Fig. 2. Noncontrast head CT scan in the axial plane, demonstrating a left frontopolar intraparenchymal hemorrhage after endoscopic marsupialization of a large, erosive frontal sinus mucopyocele (*arrow*).

patient had developed a postoperative CSF leak, which required a trial of lumbar drainage and 3 subsequent endoscopic repairs.[36] After the final surgery, the patient's condition unexpectedly and rapidly declined. CT scan demonstrated a severe IVH of the third and fourth ventricle, and the patient expired. In the second case, a delayed postoperative bleed from a frontopolar artery pseudoaneurysm presented as epistaxis,[26] which resulted in IPH and necessitated a frontal craniotomy for control followed by embolization, and the patient was left with permanent cognitive deficit and hemiparesis. In the third case, a brainstem hemorrhage after resection of a clival chordoma was reported by Stippler and colleagues,[31] resulting in quadriparesis and lower cranial nerve deficits. In the fourth case, a diffuse SAH occurred after chordomas resection in the series by Zhang and colleagues.[71]

Neuroendocrine and Electrolyte Derangement

Postoperative neuroendocrine derangement may complicate any surgery of the anterior and middle skull base and may be difficult to manage. These disorders result from surgical manipulation of the pituitary gland or sacrifice of a portion of its vasculature. This fact is well known in the neurosurgical community and has been a staple of postoperative care for patients with pituitary adenoma.[45,72] In its most extreme form, injury may result in panhypopituitarism, with the requirement of lifelong hormone supplementation in some patients. Although more common in open procedures, this may occur in even minimally invasive surgery of the sella or parasellar and suprasellar regions.[26,60,73,74] Partial anterior pituitary dysfunction is also possible and frequently results in deficiency in systemic cortisol levels secondary to decreased adrenocorticotropic hormone secretion.

Isolated neurohypophyseal dysfunction is more common than panhypopituitarism and leads to either diabetes insipidus (DI) or, less commonly, the syndrome of inappropriate antidiuretic hormone secretion (SIADH). DI may be transient or permanent and is the result of deficient antidiuretic hormone (ADH, also called vasopressin) secretion. DI manifests as increased output of dilute urine (specific gravity <1.005) and concomitant hypovolemia. Loss of free water increases the serum sodium concentration. The resulting hypernatremia may be significant and at higher levels can lead to mental status change, seizures, cardiovascular collapse, and significant decline. Treatment initially involves intravenous hypotonic fluid but may necessitate extrinsic hormone replacement in the form of desmopressin, a synthetic analogue of ADH, which is delivered subcutaneously or as a nasal spray. DI with or without hypocortisolemia has been particularly prevalent in endoscopic resection of craniopharyngiomas, although preoperative endocrine abnormalities are also more common in these patients.[60,75,76] In some cases, DI may be permanent, requiring lifelong therapy.[72,77]

SIADH after surgery for pituitary adenoma in the sella or suprasellar compartments has been described.[78,79] SIADH after other endoscopic skull base approaches is exceedingly rare, with only 1 case presented in the literature to date.[80] SIADH results from continued secretion of ADH despite decreasing serum sodium concentration, which is normally detected by the hypothalamus as a change in osmolality. However, renal excretion of sodium is maintained and the urine is very concentrated. Patients are generally euvolemic. Diffuse edema does not occur, and urine output may be normal to low. Sodium levels less than 120 mEq/L are characterized by nausea and vomiting, headache, drowsiness, and stupor. As sodium concentration declines further, generalized seizures become a significant concern. SIADH must be distinguished from cerebral salt wasting, in which hyponatremia results from increased renal excretion of sodium rather than from increased free water retention.[79] This increased excretion of sodium leads to hypovolemia with increased urine output and therefore should not be managed with fluid restriction.

CSF Leak and Pneumocephalus

Reported postoperative CSF leak rates have been widely divergent to date, although review of the literature suggests that leak rates decrease over time. Some series have reported notably high rates, in the range of 40%, whereas others have reported no leaks.[6,26] At least part of this variance is related to imprecise terminology reflecting the extent of the surgery. It is expected that resection of sinonasal tumors that extend to the skull base but do not directly involve the bone or dura result in fewer CSF leaks than in cases with true transcranial or intracranial work. However, this distinction is frequently unclear in the literature, thus making interpretation and comparison of results somewhat less straightforward. In recent years, with improved surgical techniques, reconstructive algorithms, and available materials, CSF leak rates in transcranial endoscopic approaches have decreased dramatically. Most investigators now report postoperative CSF leak in less than 20% of cases with bony skull base and dural entry.[21,34,35,60,75]

In planning the skull base reconstruction, it is important to consider the geometry and location of the defect, as well as the pathologic condition. Close review of the endoscopic literature shows that leak rates are widely divergent across anatomic locations. The lowest incidence of postoperative leak is found in transcribriform cases, the highest rates were reported in the transplanum-transtuberculum approach, and very low to intermediate rates were reported in the transclival approach.[25,26,28,29,31,35,52] In addition, CSF-leak risk seems to be greater after resection of craniopharyngiomas.[28,60,76] In each case, familiarity with a variety of reconstructive materials and local flaps, such as the pedicled septal mucosa rotation flap (Hadad Bassagasteguy flap), provides the best opportunity for success of the primary repair.[11,23]

Extensive surgery around the sella and planum sphenoidale results in a wide opening of the suprasellar or chiasmatic cistern. This space holds a relatively large volume of CSF, particularly when compared with the minimal amount in the subarachnoid space under the frontal lobes, where communication is created during transcribriform approaches. In addition, repairs in this area have a complex geometry, where the force of gravity acts against the surgeon's efforts at watertight closure. Lastly, whereas repair of the cribriform plate may be assisted by the weight of the frontal lobes on the reconstruction, no such support mechanism is possible from within the sphenoid sinus or the sella. Repair of the skull base defect by this approach is therefore prone to failure. This fact is evidenced by the significant postoperative CSF leak rate encountered by other surgeons using this approach, including 62% in the meningioma series by Gardner and colleagues[26] and 33% in the series by de Divitiis and colleagues.[25] Studies involving extended TSA or suprasellar work have reported postoperative CSF leak rates of 10% to 30%.[28,60,75]

Reconstruction failure most often presents as CSF leak but may also result in pneumocephalus. Regardless of the surgical approach, opening of the cranial vault always results in the trapping of a small amount of air. In some cases, however, this volume may expand postoperatively, usually in conjunction with a CSF leak. Significant gas volumes may lead to tension pneumocephalus, in which intracranial structures are compressed, blood flow is inhibited, and herniation is possible. Tension pneumocephalus is a very rare complication of endoscopic skull base surgery but has been reported in 1 case, although no craniotomy was required.[34] Tension pneumocephalus in endoscopic approaches could potentially result from a 1-way valve effect at the site of a dehiscent skull base reconstruction (**Fig. 3**). Pressure changes during nasal inspiration, coughing, or sneezing may overcome the dehiscent repair, entering the intracranial space. This air then becomes trapped by the increasing pressure on repair from the inside.

Historically, surgeons performing craniofacial resections would place a tracheostomy to divert airflow from the nose and pharynx, thus eliminating the possibility of tension pneumocephalus. Although this is no longer the standard of care and adds excessive morbidity to minimally invasive surgery, the thought is instructive. Present practice involves extensive packing to support the skull base repair and blocking airflow in the superior nasal cavity. Multiple materials and arrangements are available, including nasopharyngeal airways, epistaxis balloons or tampons, urinary catheters, and topical hemostatic agents. It is important to leave at least some packing in place for approximately a week after surgery and to limit debridement in the early postoperative period. Some investigators have raised concerns about delayed CSF leak and pneumocephalus after early packing removal or overly aggressive debridement.

Lumbar Drain Placement and Complications

In addition to complications arising directly from the surgical approach, skull base surgeons have noted the potential for patient morbidity associated with lumbar drains. In fact, these concerns have led to decreased prospective use of lumbar drains by multiple groups.[6,29,75] Potential complications include overdrainage with the possibility of herniation, infection of the catheter, retained catheter fragments on removal, and persistent lumbar leak with spinal headaches requiring blood patch. The combined incidence of major and minor lumbar drain complications in endoscopic skull base surgery was found to be greater than 13%.[81] Studies have shown that CSF leak rates vary significantly according to location, with defects in the sella or planum sphenoidale showing the highest leak rates. These facts, along with improved techniques for skull base reconstruction, support a management paradigm of limited

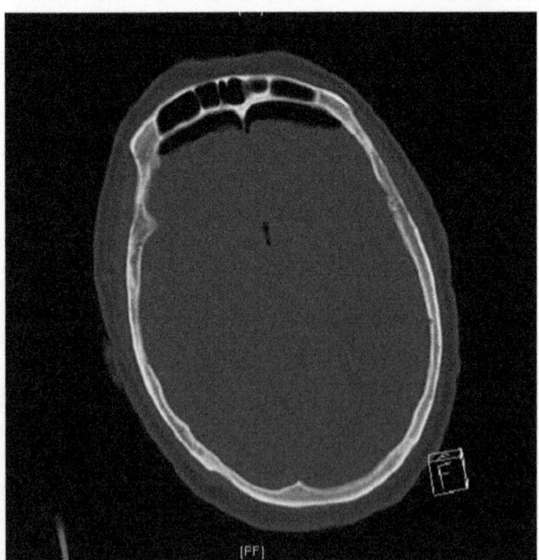

Fig. 3. Noncontrast head CT showing moderate pneumocephalus after partial dehiscence of the skull base repair in a patient undergoing endoscopic intracranial resection.

lumbar drainage, reserving drain placement for cases with problematic skull base reconstruction or postoperative leaks only.

Conversion to Craniotomy or Delayed Open Approach

It is an understood risk that, with an endoscopic approach to a skull base lesion, conversion to craniotomy may be required to ensure adequate resection. Intraoperative decision to abandon a purely endoscopic approach has been presented in an article, although this patient was excluded from the study.[35] The realization (either intraoperatively or in the immediate postoperative period) that craniotomy is needed for adequate resection has been reported in a handful of cases.[6,52,60] In some of these cases, modification of the purely endoscopic plan to a combined cranioendoscopic approach would make adequate and safe resection possible.[6,21] Some cases require partial resection and subsequent anterior or lateral open approach.[32,60] This discussion underscores the multidisciplinary nature of endoscopic skull base surgery, because neurosurgical support is critical in these rare cases.

PERIOPERATIVE MANAGEMENT AND PREVENTION

A comprehensive management strategy, including preoperative studies, prophylaxis, and postoperative monitoring is the best way to avoid complications in endoscopic skull base surgery. In this section, a brief overview of the perioperative protocol used in the management of these patients is provided. A flow diagram is included for reference (**Fig. 4**).

Preoperative Studies

In addition to routine laboratory tests and age-appropriate preoperative workup, all patients undergoing endoscopic skull base surgery should have a diagnostic CT scan and MRI. CT is essential for a preoperative review of the approach, including bony landmarks and relationships, extent of pneumatization of the sinuses and skull base, and areas of dehiscence with potential for injury. If the diagnostic scan is not compatible with the intraoperative image-guidance system, a separate image-guidance protocol CT is necessary. MRI is required for detailed examination of the intracranial contents and extent of the pathologic condition, and may also be useful in delineating tumor and inspissated secretions in the paranasal sinuses. Gadolinium-enhanced images are necessary to identify dural enhancement and parenchymal involvement.

In patients with preoperative endocrinopathies, relevant laboratory studies should be undertaken and appropriate treatment should be initiated. For example, in patients with cortisol deficiency, stress-dose corticosteroids are indicated for surgery. Also, patients with existing DI require a different perioperative fluid management and possibly desmopressin. Finally, in all patients with preoperative visual field deficits or limited extraocular movements, ophthalmologic examination should be documented and formal visual field testing is often required.

Consent Issues

In obtaining consent for endoscopic skull base surgery, a minimally invasive option for a complex disease can be offered. However, as this article demonstrates, significant complications are still possible and deserve a complete review. As with open surgery, this discussion should be tailored to the specific nature of the skull base lesion and the details of the approach. Review of the literature has confirmed that the particular location of skull base surgery and the extent of the transcranial work required determine the overall risks of the proposed surgery. Lastly, all patients with significant intracranial

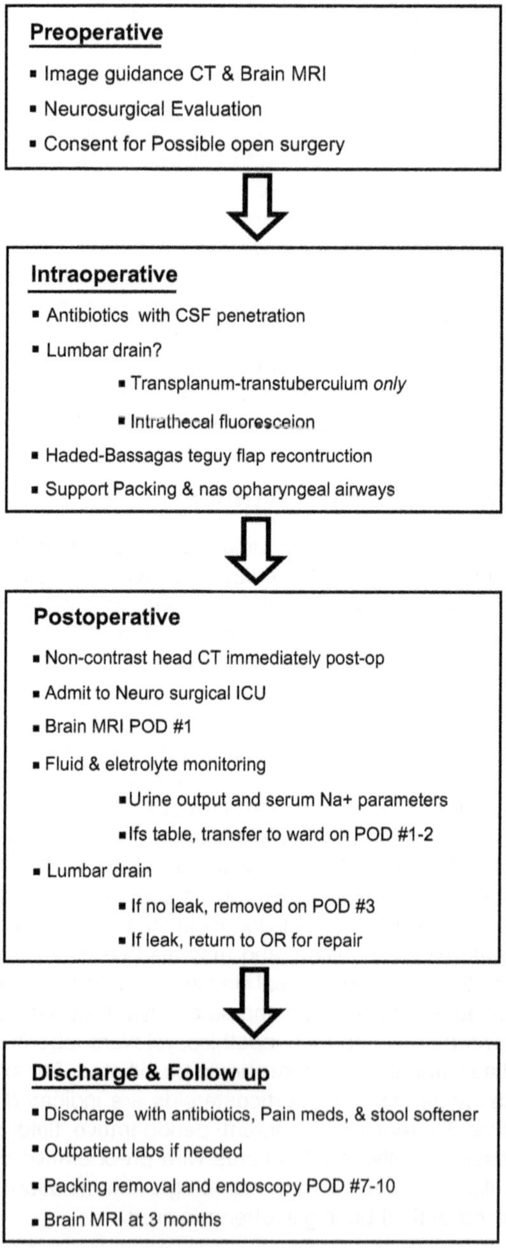

Preoperative

- Image guidance CT & Brain MRI
- Neurosurgical Evaluation
- Consent for Possible open surgery

Intraoperative

- Antibiotics with CSF penetration
- Lumbar drain?
  - Transplanum-transtuberculum *only*
  - Intrathecal fluoresceion
- Haded-Bassagas teguy flap recontruction
- Support Packing & nas opharyngeal airways

Postoperative

- Non-contrast head CT immediately post-op
- Admit to Neuro surgical ICU
- Brain MRI POD #1
- Fluid & eletrolyte monitoring
  - Urine output and serum Na+ parameters
  - Ifs table, transfer to ward on POD #1-2
- Lumbar drain
  - If no leak, removed on POD #3
  - If leak, return to OR for repair

Discharge & Follow up

- Discharge with antibiotics, Pain meds, & stool softener
- Outpatient labs if needed
- Packing removal and endoscopy POD #7-10
- Brain MRI at 3 months

Fig. 4. Perioperative management protocol for endoscopic skull base surgery.

lesions should be counseled about the possible need for craniotomy, in the case of inability to achieve complete resection or certain rare complications.

Lumbar Drains

The decision regarding the prospective use of lumbar drainage depends on the specific pathologic condition and approach involved in each case. At present, there is a move away from routine use of lumbar drains for endoscopic skull base surgery, based on the demonstrated improvements in skull base reconstruction and concerns about complications associated with drains. The authors recommend prospective (intraoperative) lumbar drain placement only in transtuberculum-transplanum approaches. In all other cases, drains are placed for mild postoperative leaks. If CSF rhinorrhea persists for 48 hours after surgery, despite lumbar drainage, then the patient is taken back to the operating room for revision of the skull base repair.

Skull Base Repair

Skull base reconstruction is undertaken with a pedicled nasoseptal flap (Hadad-Bassagasteguy flap) whenever possible (**Fig. 5**A).[23] This flap is secured in place with fibrin glue and the cavity is packed with Gelfoam (Pfizer Inc, New York, NY, USA),

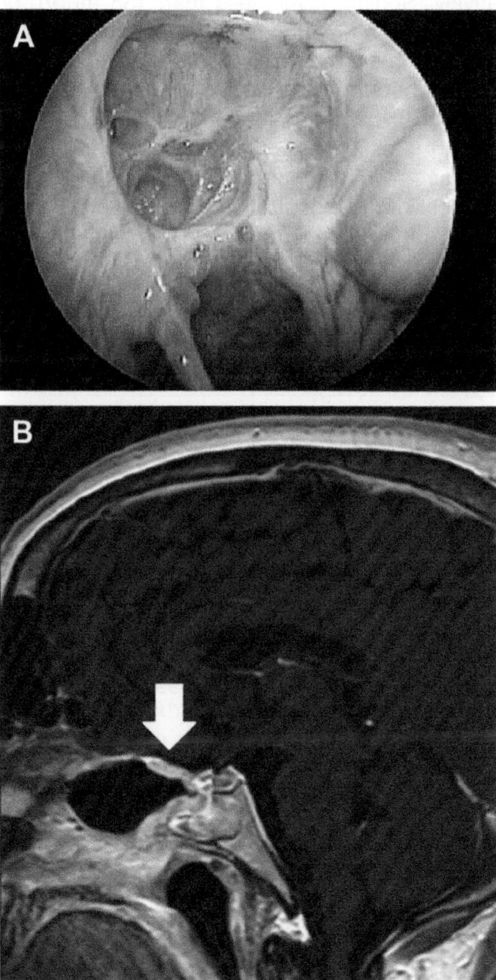

Fig. 5. (*A*) Endoscopic view of a well-healed nasoseptal mucosa rotation flap for skull base repair after a transplanum-transtuberculum approach. (*B*) Three-month postoperative T1 MRI in the midsagittal plane, showing the healed nasoseptal flap reconstruction and well-aerated sinonasal cavity (*arrow*).

microfibrillar collagen, or free abdominal fat depending on the size of the defect and the length of the flap rotation. Reconstruction is further supported with middle meatal spacers (epistaxis tampons secured in a finger of a nonlatex glove) and bilateral nasal trumpets while the patient is admitted. In cases in which the use of nasoseptal flap or pedicled inferior turbinate flap is not possible, the authors prefer a multilayer technique, which includes a lyophilized dural substitute and fibrin glue (see **Fig. 5**B).

Postoperative Issues

All patients undergoing an endoscopic intracranial approach are admitted to the neurosurgical intensive care unit (ICU) at least overnight. Deep vein thrombosis prophylaxis and perioperative antibiotics with blood-brain barrier penetration are standard. During the immediate postoperative period, careful attention to the patient's volume status, electrolyte levels, and urine output is critical. Serum electrolytes are assayed postoperatively. Sodium levels less than 135 mEq/L or greater than 145 mEq/L trigger a protocol for frequently repeated measurements. In addition, urine output less than 30 mL/h or more than 150 mL/h prompt immediate laboratory draws. Frequency of follow-up laboratory tests is then determined by the specific results. Patients experiencing significant hyponatremia are started on seizure prophylaxis.

Postoperative imaging is essential to rule out intracranial bleeding or significant pneumocephalus, and a routine noncontrast head CT scan is performed immediately after surgery. Assessment of the extent of surgical resection is also critical and may determine the need for further procedures and adjuvant therapies. MRI with and without gadolinium is performed within 24 hours in cases of tumor resection. By postoperative day 1, most patients are ready to leave the ICU. Transfer to the surgical floor occurs after the MRI is complete.

Discharge and Follow-up

Hospital discharge is considered as early as postoperative day 3 for patients who have had a smooth postoperative course, who did not show any signs or symptoms of CSF leak or infection, and who have been out of bed and ambulating. Nasal trumpets are removed at hospital discharge, but the remainder of the packing is left in place until the first postoperative visit. All patients are educated as to the signs and symptoms of CSF leak and meningitis and are encouraged to contact the surgeon's staff with any concerns. Strenuous activity is restricted (including lifting of objects heavier than 4.5 kg), although ambulation is highly encouraged.

After 7 to 10 days of surgery, patients return for removal of the residual packing and endoscopic assessment of the reconstruction. Aggressive sinonasal debridement is absolutely avoided, with removal of only loose crusts and clot. Antibiotic therapy is instituted immediately for all postoperative signs or symptoms of sinusitis. Routine sinonasal irrigation is prohibited until the skull base is completely healed, although patients are encouraged to use a humidifier.

SUMMARY AND FUTURE DIRECTIONS

Minimally invasive surgery is often perceived as minimal risk surgery, which is a serious misconception. Purely endoscopic skull base surgery can be safe and effective. However, even in the smoothest and most satisfying operation, significant complications are possible. The authors believe that there is significant and growing potential for endoscopic anterior skull base surgery and that rhinologists and head and neck surgeons will play an integral part in its development. However, familiarity with the potential complications and perioperative issues involved in these procedures is essential.

Although a randomized clinical trial in this patient population is precluded for epidemiologic and ethical reasons, the existing literature supports the overall safety and efficacy of endoscopic approaches.[8,45] However, further prospective collection of clinical information and rigorous analysis of treatment paradigms and outcomes is still needed. Indeed, as more patients are treated, important questions about the optimum patient management will become answerable. Multi-institutional assessment of predictors of endoscopic success, determination of complication rates according to surgical approach, and analysis of the health-related quality of life of patients undergoing endoscopic resections contribute significantly to the literature in the growing multidisciplinary field of skull base surgery.

REFERENCES

1. Poetker DM, Toohill RJ, Loehrl TA, et al. Endoscopic management of sinonasal tumors: a preliminary report. Am J Rhinol 2005;19:307.
2. Stankiewicz JA, Girgis SJ. Endoscopic surgical treatment of nasal and paranasal sinus inverted papilloma. Otolaryngol Head Neck Surg 1993;109:988.
3. Tomenzoli D, Castelnuovo P, Pagella F, et al. Different endoscopic surgical strategies in the management of inverted papilloma of the sinonasal tract: experience with 47 patients. Laryngoscope 2004;114:193.
4. Waitz G, Wigand ME. Results of endoscopic sinus surgery for the treatment of inverted papillomas. Laryngoscope 1992;102:917.
5. Chen MK. Minimally invasive endoscopic resection of sinonasal malignancies and skull base surgery. Acta Otolaryngol 2006;126:981.
6. Lund V, Howard DJ, Wei WI. Endoscopic resection of malignant tumors of the nose and sinuses. Am J Rhinol 2007;21:89.
7. Podboj J, Smid L. Endoscopic surgery with curative intent for malignant tumors of the nose and paranasal sinuses. Eur J Surg Oncol 2007;33:1081.
8. Snyderman CH, Carrau RL, Kassam AB, et al. Endoscopic skull base surgery: principles of endonasal oncological surgery. J Surg Oncol 2008;97:658.
9. Harvey RJ, Nogueira JF, Schlosser RJ, et al. Closure of large skull base defects after endoscopic transnasal craniotomy. Clinical article. J Neurosurg 2009;111:371.
10. Leong JL, Citardi MJ, Batra PS. Reconstruction of skull base defects after minimally invasive endoscopic resection of anterior skull base neoplasms. Am J Rhinol 2006;20:476.
11. Snyderman CH, Kassam AB, Carrau R, et al. Endoscopic reconstruction of cranial base defects following endonasal skull base surgery. Skull Base 2007;17:73.
12. Koren I, Hadar T, Rappaport ZH, et al. Endoscopic transnasal transsphenoidal microsurgery versus the sublabial approach for the treatment of pituitary tumors: endonasal complications. Laryngoscope 1999;109:1838.
13. Dehdashti AR, Ganna A, Karabatsou K, et al. Pure endoscopic endonasal approach for pituitary adenomas: early surgical results in 200 patients and comparison with previous microsurgical series. Neurosurgery 2008;62:1006.
14. Gondim JA, Schops M, de Almeida JP, et al. Endoscopic endonasal transsphenoidal surgery: surgical results of 228 pituitary adenomas treated in a pituitary center. Pituitary 2010;13:68–77.
15. Higgins TS, Courtemanche C, Karakla D, et al. Analysis of transnasal endoscopic versus transseptal microscopic approach for excision of pituitary tumors. Am J Rhinol 2008;22:649.

16. Neal JG, Patel SJ, Kulbersh JS, et al. Comparison of techniques for transsphenoidal pituitary surgery. Am J Rhinol 2007;21:203.
17. Cavallo LM, Messina A, Esposito F, et al. Skull base reconstruction in the extended endoscopic transsphenoidal approach for suprasellar lesions. J Neurosurg 2007;107:713.
18. Tabaee A, Anand VK, Brown SM, et al. Algorithm for reconstruction after endoscopic pituitary and skull base surgery. Laryngoscope 2007;117:1133.
19. Batra PS, Luong A, Kanowitz SJ, et al. Outcomes of minimally invasive endoscopic resection of anterior skull base neoplasms. Laryngoscope 2010;120:9–16.
20. Bogaerts S, Vander Poorten V, Nuyts S, et al. Results of endoscopic resection followed by radiotherapy for primarily diagnosed adenocarcinomas of the paranasal sinuses. Head Neck 2008;30:728.
21. Nicolai P, Battaglia P, Bignami M, et al. Endoscopic surgery for malignant tumors of the sinonasal tract and adjacent skull base: a 10-year experience. Am J Rhinol 2008;22:308.
22. Shipchandler TZ, Batra PS, Citardi MJ, et al. Outcomes for endoscopic resection of sinonasal squamous cell carcinoma. Laryngoscope 2005;115:1983.
23. Hadad G, Bassagasteguy L, Carrau RL, et al. A novel reconstructive technique after endoscopic expanded endonasal approaches: vascular pedicle nasoseptal flap. Laryngoscope 2006;116:1882.
24. Kassam AB, Thomas A, Carrau RL, et al. Endoscopic reconstruction of the cranial base using a pedicled nasoseptal flap. Neurosurgery 2008;63:ONS44.
25. de Divitiis E, Cavallo LM, Esposito F, et al. Extended endoscopic transsphenoidal approach for tuberculum sellae meningiomas. Neurosurgery 2008;62:1192.
26. Gardner PA, Kassam AB, Thomas A, et al. Endoscopic endonasal resection of anterior cranial base meningiomas. Neurosurgery 2008;63:36.
27. Presutti L, Trani M, Alicandri-Ciufelli M, et al. Exclusive endoscopic removal of a planum sphenoidale meningioma: a case report. Minim Invasive Neurosurg 2008;51:51.
28. Frank G, Sciarretta V, Calbucci F, et al. The endoscopic transnasal transsphenoidal approach for the treatment of cranial base chordomas and chondrosarcomas. Neurosurgery 2006;59:ONS50.
29. Fraser JF, Nyquist GG, Moore N, et al. Endoscopic endonasal transclival resection of chordomas: operative technique, clinical outcome, and review of the literature. J Neurosurg 2010;112(5):1061–9.
30. Solares CA, Fakhri S, Batra PS, et al. Transnasal endoscopic resection of lesions of the clivus: a preliminary report. Laryngoscope 2005;115:1917.
31. Stippler M, Gardner PA, Snyderman CH, et al. Endoscopic endonasal approach for clival chordomas. Neurosurgery 2009;64:268.
32. Zanation AM, Snyderman CH, Carrau RL, et al. Endoscopic endonasal surgery for petrous apex lesions. Laryngoscope 2009;119:19.
33. Batra PS, Citardi MJ, Worley S, et al. Resection of anterior skull base tumors: comparison of combined traditional and endoscopic techniques. Am J Rhinol 2005;19:521.
34. Carrau RL, Kassam AB, Snyderman CH, et al. Endoscopic transnasal anterior skull base resection for the treatment of sinonasal malignancies. Oper Tech Otolaryngol Head Neck Surg 2006;17:102.
35. Dave SP, Bared A, Casiano RR. Surgical outcomes and safety of transnasal endoscopic resection for anterior skull tumors. Otolaryngol Head Neck Surg 2007;136:920.

36. de Divitiis E, Cavallo LM, Esposito F, et al. Extended endoscopic transsphenoidal approach for tuberculum sellae meningiomas. Neurosurgery 2007;61:229.
37. Cantu G, Riccio S, Bimbi G, et al. Craniofacial resection for malignant tumours involving the anterior skull base. Eur Arch Otorhinolaryngol 2006;263:647.
38. Dias FL, Sa GM, Kligerman J, et al. Complications of anterior craniofacial resection. Head Neck 1999;21:12.
39. Fukuda K, Saeki N, Mine S, et al. Evaluation of outcome and QOL in patients with craniofacial resection for malignant tumors involving the anterior skull base. Neurol Res 2000;22:545.
40. Ganly I, Patel SG, Singh B, et al. Complications of craniofacial resection for malignant tumors of the skull base: report of an International Collaborative Study. Head Neck 2005;27:445.
41. Ganly I, Patel SG, Singh B, et al. Craniofacial resection for malignant paranasal sinus tumors: report of an International Collaborative Study. Head Neck 2005;27:575.
42. Patel SG, Singh B, Polluri A, et al. Craniofacial surgery for malignant skull base tumors: report of an international collaborative study. Cancer 2003;98:1179.
43. Sakashita T, Oridate N, Homma A, et al. Complications of skull base surgery: an analysis of 30 cases. Skull Base 2009;19:127.
44. Van Tuyl R, Gussack GS. Prognostic factors in craniofacial surgery. Laryngoscope 1991;101:240.
45. Tabaee A, Anand VK, Barron Y, et al. Endoscopic pituitary surgery: a systematic review and meta-analysis. J Neurosurg 2009;111:545.
46. Rettinger G, Kirsche H. Complications in septoplasty. Facial Plast Surg 2006; 22:289.
47. Unger F, Haselsberger K, Walch C, et al. Combined endoscopic surgery and radiosurgery as treatment modality for olfactory neuroblastoma (esthesioneuroblastoma). Acta Neurochir (Wien) 2005;147:595.
48. Har-El G. Endoscopic management of 108 sinus mucoceles. Laryngoscope 2001;111:2131.
49. Dutt SN, Kameswaran M. The aetiology and management of atrophic rhinitis. J Laryngol Otol 2005;119:843.
50. Moore EJ, Kern EB. Atrophic rhinitis: a review of 242 cases. Am J Rhinol 2001; 15:355.
51. Castelnuovo PG, Delu G, Sberze F, et al. Esthesioneuroblastoma: endonasal endoscopic treatment. Skull Base 2006;16:25.
52. Folbe A, Herzallah I, Duvvuri U, et al. Endoscopic endonasal resection of esthesioneuroblastoma: a multicenter study. Am J Rhinol Allergy 2009;23:91.
53. Lou PJ, Chen WP, Tai CC. Delayed irradiation effects on nasal epithelium in patients with nasopharyngeal carcinoma. An ultrastructural study. Ann Otol Rhinol Laryngol 1999;108:474.
54. Corey JP, Bumsted R, Panje W, et al. Orbital complications in functional endoscopic sinus surgery. Otolaryngol Head Neck Surg 1993;109:814.
55. May M, Levine HL, Mester SJ, et al. Complications of endoscopic sinus surgery: analysis of 2108 patients—incidence and prevention. Laryngoscope 1994;104:1080.
56. Welch KC, Palmer JN. Intraoperative emergencies during endoscopic sinus surgery: CSF leak and orbital hematoma. Otolaryngol Clin North Am 2008;41:581.
57. Arslan H, Aydinlioglu A, Bozkurt M, et al. Anatomic variations of the paranasal sinuses: CT examination for endoscopic sinus surgery. Auris Nasus Larynx 1999;26:39.

58. Bhatti MT, Stankiewicz JA. Ophthalmic complications of endoscopic sinus surgery. Surv Ophthalmol 2003;48:389.
59. Dessi P, Moulin G, Castro F, et al. Protrusion of the optic nerve into the ethmoid and sphenoid sinus: prospective study of 150 CT studies. Neuroradiology 1994;36:515.
60. Dehdashti AR, Ganna A, Witterick I, et al. Expanded endoscopic endonasal approach for anterior cranial base and suprasellar lesions: indications and limitations. Neurosurgery 2009;64:677.
61. Huang CM, Meyer DR, Patrinely JR, et al. Medial rectus muscle injuries associated with functional endoscopic sinus surgery: characterization and management. Ophthal Plast Reconstr Surg 2003;19:25.
62. Penne RB, Flanagan JC, Stefanyszyn MA, et al. Ocular motility disorders secondary to sinus surgery. Ophthal Plast Reconstr Surg 1993;9:53.
63. Jho HD, Ha HG. Endoscopic endonasal skull base surgery: part 2–the cavernous sinus. Minim Invasive Neurosurg 2004;47:9.
64. Hwang PY, Ho CL. Neuronavigation using an image-guided endoscopic transnasal-sphenoethmoidal approach to clival chordomas. Neurosurgery 2007; 61:212.
65. Jho HD, Ha HG. Endoscopic endonasal skull base surgery: part 3–the clivus and posterior fossa. Minim Invasive Neurosurg 2004;47:16.
66. Har-El G, Casiano RR. Endoscopic management of anterior skull base tumors. Otolaryngol Clin North Am 2005;38:133.
67. Batra PS, Citardi MJ, Lanza DC. Isolated sphenoid sinusitis after transsphenoidal hypophysectomy. Am J Rhinol 2005;19:185.
68. Hlavin ML, Kaminski HJ, Fenstermaker RA, et al. Intracranial suppuration: a modern decade of postoperative subdural empyema and epidural abscess. Neurosurgery 1994;34:974.
69. Dashti SR, Baharvahdat H, Spetzler RF, et al. Operative intracranial infection following craniotomy. Neurosurg Focus 2008;24:E10.
70. Castelnuovo P, Pistochini A, Locatelli D. Different surgical approaches to the sellar region: focusing on the "two nostrils four hands technique". Rhinology 2006;44:2.
71. Zhang Q, Kong F, Yan B, et al. Endoscopic endonasal surgery for clival chordoma and chondrosarcoma. ORL J Otorhinolaryngol Relat Spec 2008;70:124.
72. Fatemi N, Dusick JR, Mattozo C, et al. Pituitary hormonal loss and recovery after transsphenoidal adenoma removal. Neurosurgery 2008;63:709.
73. de Divitiis E, Cappabianca P, Cavallo LM, et al. Extended endoscopic transsphenoidal approach for extrasellar craniopharyngiomas. Neurosurgery 2007; 61:219.
74. Honegger J, Buchfelder M, Fahlbusch R. Surgical treatment of craniopharyngiomas: endocrinological results. J Neurosurg 1999;90:251.
75. Laufer I, Anand VK, Schwartz TH. Endoscopic, endonasal extended transsphenoidal, transplanum transtuberculum approach for resection of suprasellar lesions. J Neurosurg 2007;106:400.
76. Stamm AC, Vellutini E, Harvey RJ, et al. Endoscopic transnasal craniotomy and the resection of craniopharyngioma. Laryngoscope 2008;118:1142.
77. Dusick JR, Fatemi N, Mattozo C, et al. Pituitary function after endonasal surgery for nonadenomatous parasellar tumors: Rathke's cleft cysts, craniopharyngiomas, and meningiomas. Surg Neurol 2008;70:482.
78. Kristof RA, Rother M, Neuloh G, et al. Incidence, clinical manifestations, and course of water and electrolyte metabolism disturbances following transsphenoidal

pituitary adenoma surgery: a prospective observational study. J Neurosurg 2009; 111:555.
79. Taylor SL, Tyrrell JB, Wilson CB. Delayed onset of hyponatremia after transsphenoidal surgery for pituitary adenomas. Neurosurgery 1995;37:649.
80. Ransom ER, Lee J, Lee JYK, et al. Endoscopic transcranial and intracranial resection: case series and design of a perioperative management protocol. Presented at the American Rhinologic Society Meeting. San Diego (CA), October 2009.
81. Ransom ER, Palmer JN, Kennedy DW, et al. Assessing risk/benefit of lumbar drains in endoscopic skull base surgery. Presented at the American Rhinologic Society Meeting. Las Vegas (NV), April 2010.

Complications and Management of Septoplasty

Amy S. Ketcham, MD, Joseph K. Han, MD*

KEYWORDS

- Septoplasty • Complications • Nasal septum
- Endoscopic septoplasty • Septal perforation
- Septal hematoma • Saddle nose • Cerebrospinal fluid leak

Septoplasty is one of the most common and earliest-learned otolaryngologic operations. A deviated nasal septum requiring septoplasty to improve the nasal airway may result from traumatic injury, iatrogenic injury, congenital deformation, or as a complication of a severe nasal infection. In many cases, patients have no obvious cause for their septal deviation. Other reasons to perform septoplasty include the treatment of facial pain caused by contact of the septum with the lateral nasal wall and improvement of intraoperative visualization during distribution of topical nasal sprays after endoscopic sinus surgery (ESS).[1] Given the number of people affected by nasal obstruction caused by septal deviation, continued evaluation of the effectiveness, complications, management, and modifications of modern septoplasty is warranted.

Generally, nasal airflow is not only decreased on the side of the septal deviation but also on the contralateral side. The reason for this phenomenon is compensatory inferior turbinate hypertrophy. As a result, inferior turbinate reduction is frequently performed at the same time as septoplasty to maximize improvement in nasal airflow. Some complications from inferior turbinate reduction are reviewed in this article.

Septoplasty has traditionally been performed as an open procedure working through hemitransfixion incisions just caudal to the septum. Mucoperichondrial flaps are raised bilaterally and the offending cartilage and bone is selectively removed. Historically, maximal resection of the bony and cartilaginous septum has been performed to ensure a midline septum after septoplasty. Maximal excision, however, prevents septal cartilage use in future procedures and may also be associated with an increased incidence of postoperative cosmetic deformities. As a result, other

Disclosures: No funding or additional support was given in support of this paper.
Department of Otolaryngology and Head and Neck Surgery, Eastern Virginia Medical School, 600 Gresham Drive, Suite 1100, Norfolk, VA 23507, USA
* Corresponding author.
E-mail address: hanjk@evms.edu

Otolaryngol Clin N Am 43 (2010) 897–904
doi:10.1016/j.otc.2010.04.013 oto.theclinics.com
0030-6665/10/$ – see front matter

techniques, such as scarification remodeling, have arisen to preserve as much of the septum as possible while still straightening it.[2] In this procedure, Doyle splints may be placed to provide support during the postoperative period while the perichondrium reattaches to the nasal septal cartilage in its new straightened position.[2]

PAIN AND POSTOPERATIVE DISCOMFORT

Some have advocated postoperative use of decongestant nasal sprays, such as xylometazoline hydrochloride, in hopes that these sprays would aid in pain control and decrease postoperative congestion, rhinorrhea, and hyposmia. Unfortunately, Humphreys and colleagues[3] found that this decongestant actually increased pain and had no advantages over nasal saline irrigation. Measures, such as cold compresses, elevation of the head of the bed, and avoidance of straining, may help decrease postoperative swelling, congestion, and discomfort in the immediate postoperative period.

BLEEDING

Intraoperative bleeding and postoperative epistaxis are of particular concern in septoplasty given the high vascularity of the intranasal mucosa. Surgically speaking, one should make every attempt to dissect in the avascular submucoperichondrial and submucoperiosteal plans. The addition of low concentrations of epinephrine to the local anesthetic used in hydrodissection of the mucoperichondrial flaps during preparation for surgery appears to effectively induce vasoconstriction of the mucosa; it also greatly aids in prevention of a bloody surgical field. Although using epinephrine in this manner has been found to raise systolic blood pressure significantly in some patients,[4] in the authors' experience epinephrine may be used safely and effectively in many patients during septoplasty. Intraoperative bleeding may also be decreased by the anesthesiologist's careful attention to the blood pressure parameters. This topic is addressed in detail by Timperly and Harvey elsewhere in this issue.[5]

Topical vasoconstrictors can be used to minimize or even arrest intraoperative bleeding. Oxymetazoline may be effective in some cases and its risk profile is minimal. However, some patients may require more vasoconstriction than oxymetazoline can provide. Topical 1:2000 epinephrine and topical 4% cocaine may be used with greater effect. These agents may cause cardiac complications if improperly used.[5] A systematic literature review by Higgins and colleagues[6] addresses the issue of the safety and efficacy of topical vasoconstrictors in nasal procedures. Although oxymetazoline is the safest agent, it also appears to be the least effective. Cocaine and epinephrine both yield good vasoconstriction but are associated with case reports of cardiac complications, including myocardial infarction and cardiogenic shock. Use of halothane as an anesthetic in combination with cocaine and epinephrine should be avoided. Topical cocaine and epinephrine should be used judiciously in patients with a known history of cardiac disease.

Nasal packing has been traditionally used to prevent significant postoperative epistaxis and septal hematomas. Given the patient discomfort and minor complications associated with packing and its removal, many have sought alternatives. One randomized, controlled trial showed no difference in postoperative bleeding between nasal packing and fibrin sealant without packing.[7] Another randomized, controlled trial found that placing septal quilting sutures and performing routine postoperative nasal care was associated with the same rate of postoperative bleeding, septal hematomas, adhesions, and infections as in patients with nasal packing. In other words, packing not only failed to decrease the rate of complications it was intended to prevent but it was also associated with increased postoperative pain and discomfort.[8] For this reason, many surgeons have either abandoned or significantly modified their use of postoperative packing.

Quilting sutures have been used in lieu of nasal packing since 1984. The sutures help to re-approximate the mucoperichondrial flaps and prevent a dead space where blood can accumulate. Typically, absorbable sutures, such as chromic or Vicryl, are used for this purpose. Using a curved needle instead of the traditional straight needle may also decrease mucosal trauma.[9] Many recommend placing small stab incisions in the septal mucosa to create drainage ports for any blood that may collect. Still others support the application of fibrin sealant to aid in hemostasis and prevent postoperative epistaxis.[10] After considering the previously mentioned techniques for acquiring hemostasis and preventing postoperative bleeding, the standard recommendations still remain true: patients should avoid aspirin, nonsteroidal antiinflammatory drugs, anticoagulants, and strenuous activity for 2 weeks after surgery, whenever possible.

CEREBROSPINAL FLUID RHINORRHEA

In rare cases, a defect in the cribriform plate caused during septoplasty may lead to a cerebrospinal fluid (CSF) leak. Such defects may be created by angling dissecting forceps more superiorly than posteriorly during submucoperiosteal elevation. Another etiology may be multidirectional forces exerted on the perpendicular plate of the ethmoid during attempts to grasp and remove part of the bony ethmoid plate. Either error will be exacerbated by a variation in anatomy that brings the cribriform plate closer to the ethmoid air cells.[10,11] To prevent this major complication, detailed knowledge of patients' anatomy and the proper use of dissection technique with sharp removal of the septum and elimination of multidirectional forces are required.[11] Preoperative CT scans can be helpful in delineating the anatomy at risk. Generally speaking, it is prudent to pay particularly careful attention to any septal bone removal posterior to the anterior attachment of the middle turbinate. In the event that a CSF leak is created, it may be repaired endoscopically with a fascial graft and fibrin glue. In some cases, simple application of fibrin glue over the bony disruption and approximation of the nonporous mucosal flaps by the fracture site with quilting sutures is sufficient to repair the CSF leak.

OCULAR COMPLICATIONS

In rare instances, ocular complications may occur secondary to the inferior turbinate reduction that is often performed along with septoplasty. Typically these complications are associated with violation of the medial orbital wall or orbital floor.[12] There is, however, one case report involving medial rectus palsy caused by inferior turbinate radiofrequency ablation in which the orbit remained completely intact.[12] In this case, the damage was likely caused by improper distribution of radiofrequency. Close intraoperative attention to patients' anatomy will help prevent such complications.

TOXIC SHOCK SYNDROME AND OTHER INFECTIOUS COMPLICATIONS

The rate of local infection and septal abscess after septoplasty ranges from 0.4% to 12.0%.[13–15] The routine use of antibiotics has not been found to change the rate of infection.[10]

The rate of toxic shock syndrome (TSS) after septoplasty is estimated at 0.0165%. TSS is fatal in 10% of patients who contract it.[16] It is indeed understandable how postoperative infections occur in the nose because 19% to 55% of individuals in good health grow *Staphylococcus aureus* in cultures taken from their nasal passages.[17] A transient intraoperative bacteremia has been seen in patients undergoing septoplasty and septorhinoplasty, however, this has not been correlated to rates of postoperative infection or toxic shock syndrome.[17] One case of *S aureus* endocarditis and one case of osteomyelitis have been reported after septoplasty.[18,19]

To develop toxic shock syndrome, patients must not only be colonized with endotoxin-producing *Staphylococcus aureus* but also have an inability to mount an immune response against endotoxin; a nasal environment conducive to colony growth (neutral pH and aerobic); and a violated mucosa.[20] All these conditions are possible during septoplasty. Postoperatively, nasal packing increases the risk for TSS, largely by providing an ideal environment for bacterial growth. The specific type of packing may or may not contribute to risk. One incidence of TSS after Gelfoam packing[20] and one after silicone Doyle splints[21] have been reported.

NASAL SEPTAL PERFORATION

The rate of nasal septal perforation after septoplasty ranges from 1.6% to 6.7%.[2,15,22–26] Higher rates of perforation are seen when inferior turbinate reduction is performed in combination with septoplasty.[26] Devascularization of septal mucosa may lead to postoperative septal perforations. If significant electrocautery is used on the septum during attempts to obtain intraoperative hemostasis, mucosal compromise may result. Underlying cartilage may subsequently be deprived of nutrients and a perforation may develop. Bilateral mucosal rents may also lead to septal perforation if the rents appose one another after the cartilage is resected. Yet another reason for septal perforation involves the placement of quilting sutures or sutures to maintain septal splint placement. If the suture is tight enough to cause ischemia and necrosis of the surrounding area, a perforation may result. In some patients, local mucosal trauma caused by intranasal steroid and nasal saline sprays is enough to cause a perforation. Treatments for septal perforations include appropriate postoperative nasal care with saline and bacitracin or petroleum jelly, a septal button, or eventual operative repair.[10] When an iatrogenic perforation is created during surgery, it can often be repaired intraoperatively. Several techniques exist for this repair and range from re-suturing the area to interposition of an autologous or artificial graft.

SADDLE NOSE DEFORMITY AND SUPRATIP DEPRESSION

The overall rate of significant change in the cosmetic appearance of the nose after septoplasty has been quoted between 0.4% to 3.4%.[15,27] The most commonly cited cosmetic defects arising from septoplasty are saddle nose deformity and supratip depression. In addition to these, the nose may become deviated, the tip bulbous or de-projected, the columella retracted, or the alar cartilage collapsed. These results stem from a weak dorsal strut or a displaced caudal septum.[27] The dorsal strut may not be sufficient to support the normal nasal anatomy after septoplasty if less than 10 to 15 mm of cartilage is left.

Minor cosmetic alterations may actually occur after septoplasty as much as 40% of the time, but these minor changes are seldom noted; the highest rate of major change has been quoted at 4%.[22]Daudia found that there is no correlation between objective quantification of cosmetic changes using facial analysis and subjective patient opinion.[22] This data leads one to believe that minor changes in tip projection; columellar retraction; and supratip depression (defined as <3 mm) could be considered acceptable. However, major changes, such as an obvious saddle nose deformity, are not intrinsic to the procedure and should be avoided.

One of the main causes of the saddle nose deformity is over-resection of cartilage. The key to prevention of the saddle nose deformity is preservation of adequate dorsal and caudal struts.

Once over-resection and weakening of these struts has occurred, not only has the cosmetic, and often functional, status of the nose been altered but several simple means of repair have also been eliminated by removing cartilage that could have been used in a revision septoplasty.[14] A mobile, dislocated nasal septum will often lead to a saddle nose deformity. Raeessi and colleagues have described a temporary tension suture placed through the mucoperichondrial flaps and septal cartilage to distribute force and lend support to the septum without causing depression of the nasal dorsum. They have found this to be an effective way to prevent saddle nose even when left with a dislocated septum after cartilage resection.[14]

Given the fact that cosmetic changes, whether significant or not, often result from septoplasty, Bateman and Woolford recommend preoperative photo-documentation for more accurate comparison, analysis, and informed preoperative and postoperative comparisons and planning.[28]

One reason for persistent nasal tip depression or altered symmetry may be failure to address caudal septal deviation during septoplasty.[29] The swinging-door technique has been used to disarticulate the caudal septum and replace it centrally on the maxillary crest. Various fixation sutures may also be used. Lawson and Westreich describe a modified Goldman technique where a 5-0 polydioxanone suture figure-of-eight suture is used to fix the septum in position.[29] Other rhinoplasty cartilage grafting techniques may be used to reshape the nose as needed. Rhinoplasty may be required to correct cosmetic defects arising from septoplasty. Spreader grafts or onlay grafts may be used to reshape the depressed crooked nasal dorsum if needed.[2]

MISCELLANEOUS COMPLICATIONS

Although not a direct complication of septoplasty itself, empty nose syndrome may result from inferior turbinate reduction performed along with septoplasty. It is characterized by a feeling of nasal congestion and decreased nasal airflow when in fact the nasal passages are wide open. The etiology of this sensation is over-resection of nasal mucosa over the inferior turbinates and septum such that nasal airflow is disrupted and does not contact the degree of mucosa it did previously. To alleviate this sensation, surgery may be required to project the turbinates or lateral nasal wall further into the nasal airway where airflow will then be sensed and registered.

Several other alterations in sensation may also occur postoperatively. First, anosmia may develop in patients post-septoplasty because of damage to the olfactory nerves. The rate of developing such a problem ranges between 0.3% to 2.9%.[15,30,31] There is no treatment for this complication, however, some sense of smell generally returns with time. Another change in sensation following septoplasty is palate denervation. This problem may occur if the long sphenopalatine nerve or greater palatine nerve were damaged intraoperatively during removal of the maxillary crest or posterior bony septum, respectively. The final post-septoplasty sensory change is dental anesthesia. MacDougall and Sanderson found that 50% of submucous resection septoplasties and 14% of conservative septoplasties resulted in dental anesthesia.[32] This complication occurs as a result of damaging the nasopalatine nerve intraoperatively.[33] Difficult visualization caused by severity of nasal septal deviation, possibly in combination with inexperience, can lead to perforation of the mucoperichondrial flap and inadvertent resection of the anterior head of the middle turbinate. This initial error may lead to further errors because of the decreased visualization resulting from increased bleeding. Bateman's review suggested that level of training influences complications after septoplasty.[28] The study stated that resident surgeons created more mucosal tears and perforations than attending physicians, but this information did not correlate with a greater overall complication rate.[28]

TECHNIQUES

Traditionally, septoplasty has been performed under general anesthesia, but septoplasty with local anesthesia and sedation have also been reported. According to Fedok and colleagues,[34] operative times may be slightly shorter, hospital admissions fewer, and postoperative nausea, emesis, and epistaxis reduced if general anesthetic is avoided.

Endoscopic septoplasty has arisen as the most significant modification of the traditional septoplasty. It may be performed in one of two ways: limited endoscopic or endoscopic traditional. Limited endoscopic septoplasty is ideal to address septal spurs or isolated posterior septal deviations. A vertical incision is made in the septal mucosa directly anterior to the defect to be addressed and a limited mucoperichondrial or mucoperiosteal flap is elevated with endoscopic guidance. Nasal endoscopic irrigation and a suction freer are crucial to maintaining optimal visualization during this procedure. Only rarely is closure of the mucosal incision needed. For more extensive or severe septal deviations or for better access during ESS, an endoscopic traditional septoplasty can be performed. A hemitransfixion or Killian incision is made and the same steps of a traditional septoplasty are performed under endoscopic guidance. After selective cartilage and bone resection is performed, the nasal endoscope can be used to assess the nasal passage. After the mucosal incision is closed with a dissolvable suture, a septal quilting stitch is placed throughout the operated septum to approximate the mucosal flap and to repair any mucosal injury.

Endoscopic septoplasty is ideal for posterior septal deviations because visualization is traditionally most difficult posteriorly. The endoscope easily passes beyond areas of anterior obstruction and can visualize and guide the removal of posterior obstruction.[33] Nasal endoscopy provides a magnified view of the operative field. This improved visualization allows for proper elevation of the submucoperichondrial flap in the correct plane, thereby minimizing bleeding. The improved picture can also help prevent and identify mucosal tears. Use of a powered burr can additionally aid in removal of isolated pathologic areas of the septum, thus minimizing trauma and preventing tissue over-resection.[35]

Visualization is unquestionably better with endoscopic septoplasty, especially in cases of difficult anatomy, such as revision septoplasties and significant posterior septal deviations. However, this strength is also a pitfall of the procedure. A tendency to lose one's frame of reference by focusing only on the area of interest may lead to a more superior and posterior dissection than intended, which creates a risk for violating the cribriform plate and causing a CSF leak. Thankfully, repair of such a defect with a simple mucosal graft or suture is easily performed using the endoscope and instruments already on the field.

SUMMARY

Regardless of the type of septoplasty performed, postoperative complications remain largely the same. No significant differences in complication rates or outcomes have been reported despite the theoretical advantages already discussed. As a result, the procedure most appropriate for a particular patient's anatomy and that with which the surgeon is most comfortable and skilled should be performed. Meticulous attention to detail in identifying the appropriate anatomy and maintaining good visualization is the key to a safe and effective septoplasty.

REFERENCES

1. Laguna D, Lopez-Cortijo C, Millan I, et al. Blood loss in endoscopic sinus surgery: assessment of variables. J Otolaryngol 2008;37(3):324–30.
2. Kantas I, Balatsouras D, Papadakis C, et al. Aesthetic reconstruction of a crooked nose via extracorporeal septoplasty. J Otolaryngol 2008;37(2):154–9.
3. Humphreys M, Grant D, McKean S, et al. Xylometazoline hydrochloride 0.1 per cent versus physiological saline in nasal surgical aftercare: a randomized, single-blinded, comparative clinical trial. J Laryngol Otol 2009;123:85–90.
4. Thevasagayam M, Jindal M, Allsop P, et al. Does epinephrine infiltration in septoplasty make any difference? Eur Arch Otorhinolaryngol 2007;264:1175–8.
5. Orlandi RR, Warrier S, Han JK. Concentrated topical epinephrine is safe in endoscopic sinus surgery. Am J Rhinol Allergy 2010;24:140–2.
6. Higgins T, Hwang P, Han JK, et al. Systematic literature review of topical vasoconstrictors in endoscopic sinus surgery. Laryngoscope, submitted for publication.
7. Vaiman M, Sarfaty S, Shlamkovich N, et al. Fibrin sealant: alternative to nasal packing in endonasal operations. A prospective randomized study. Isr Med Assoc J 2005;7:571–4.
8. Awan M, Iqbal M. Nasal packing after septoplasty: a randomized comparison of packing versus no packing in 88 patients. Ear Nose Throat J 2008;87(11):624–7.
9. Hari C, Marnane C, Wormald P. Quilting sutures for nasal septum. J Laryngol Otol 2008;122(5):522–3.
10. Bloom J, Kaplan S, Bleir B, et al. Septoplasty complications: avoidance and management. Otolaryngol Clin North Am 2009;42:463–81.
11. Onerci T, Ayhan K, Ogretmenoglu O. Two consecutive cases of cerebrospinal fluid rhinorrhea after septoplasty operation. Am J Otolaryngol 2004;25(5):354–6.
12. Atighchi S, Alimohammadi S, Baradaranfar M, et al. Temporary adduction deficit after nasal septoplasty and radiofrequency ablation of the inferior turbinate. J Neuroophthalmol 2009;29(1):29–32.
13. Makitie A, Aaltonen L-M, Hytonen M, et al. Postoperative infection following nasal septoplasty. Acta Otolaryngol Suppl 2000;543:165–6.
14. Raeessi M, Farhadi M, Shirazi A, et al. A new technique during septoplasty to prevent saddle nose. Clin Otolaryngol 2008;33(2):123–6.
15. Yanagisawa E, Ho S. Unintended middle turbinectomy during septoplasty. Ear Nose Throat J 1998;77(5):368.
16. Jacobson J, Kasworm E, Crass B, et al. Nasal carriage of toxigenic *Staphylococcus aureus* and prevalence of serum antibody to toxic shock syndrome toxin 1 in Utah. J Infect Dis 1986;153:356–9.
17. Okur E, Yildirim I, Aral M, et al. Bacteremia during open septorhinoplasty. Am J Rhinol 2006;20(1):36–9.
18. Cohen B, Johnson J, Raff M. Septoplasty complicated by staphylococcal spinal osteomyelitis. Arch Intern Med 1985;145:556–7.
19. Coursey D. Staphylococcal endocarditis following septorhinoplasty. Arch Otolaryngol 1974;99:454–5.
20. Keller J, Evan K, Wetmore R. Toxic shock syndrome after closed reduction of a nasal fracture. Otolaryngol Head Neck Surg 1999;120(4):569–70.

21. Moser N, Hood C, Ervin D. Toxic shock syndrome in a patient using bilateral silicone nasal splints. Otolaryngol Head Neck Surg 1995;113:632–3.
22. Daudia A, Alkhaddour U, Sithole J, et al. A prospective objective study of the cosmetic sequelae of nasal septal surgery. Acta Otolaryngol 2006;126:1201–5.
23. Phillipps J. The cosmetic effects of submucous resection. Clin Otolaryngol 1991; 16:179–81.
24. Low W, Willatt D. Submucous resection for deviated nasal septum: a critical appraisal. Singapore Med J 1992;33:617–9.
25. Bohlin L, Dahlqvist A. Nasal airway resistance and complications following functional septoplasty. A ten years' follow-up study. Rhinology 1994;32:195–7.
26. Haraldsson P-O, Nordemar H, Anggard A. Long term results after septal sur gery - Submucous resection versus septoplasty. ORL J Otorhinolaryngol Relat Spec 1987;49:218–22.
27. Yeo N-K, Jang Y. Rhinoplasty to correct nasal deformities in post-septoplasty patients. Am J Rhinol 2009;23(5):540–5.
28. Bateman N, Woolford T. Informed consent for septal surgery: the evidence-base. J Laryngol Otol 2003;117:186–9.
29. Lawson W, Westreich R. Correction of caudal deflections of the nasal septum with a modified Goldman septoplasty technique: how we do it. Ear Nose Throat J 2007;86(10):617–20.
30. Fiser A. Changes of olfaction due to aesthetic and functional nose surgery. Acta Otorhinolaryngol Belg 1990;44:457–60.
31. Kimmelman C. The risk to olfaction from nasal surgery. Laryngoscope 1994;104: 981–8.
32. MacDougall G, Sanderson R. Altered dental sensation following intranasal surgery. J Laryngol Otol 1993;107:1011–3.
33. Sautter N, Smith T. Endoscopic septoplasty. Otolaryngol Clin North Am 2009;42: 253–60.
34. Fedok F, Rerraro R, Kingsley C, et al. Operative times, postanesthesia recovery times, and complications during sinonasal surgery using general anesthesia and local anesthesia with sedation. Otolaryngol Head Neck Surg 2000;122: 560–6.
35. Becker D, Park S, Toriumi D. Powered Instrumentation for rhinoplasty and septoplasty. Otolaryngol Clin North Am 1999;32(4):683–93.

Medicolegal Issues in Endoscopic Sinus Surgery

Ankit M. Patel, MD[a,*], Thomas E. Still Esq, JD[b], Winston Vaughan, MD[c,d]

KEYWORDS

• Endoscopic sinus surgery • Medicolegal • Malpractice • Lawsuit

OVERVIEW

"Few issues in health care spark as much ire and angst as medical malpractice litigation."[1] The current malpractice climate in the United States has fueled much debate and emotion on the part of attorneys as well as physicians. Physicians may feel pressure, real or perceived, to order additional testing or take additional steps to document for fear of litigation, adding to the cost of health care delivery.

Frivolous lawsuits comprise approximately 37% of malpractice cases, accounting for about 15% of the system's cost.[2] Studies have shown that the great majority of patients who sustain a medical injury as a result of negligence do not sue.[3,4] However, lawsuits, whether appropriate or frivolous, are viewed as an assault on the character and competence of the physician. For psychologic, monetary, and patient safety reasons, the malpractice system has tremendous effect on physicians and society.

Functional endoscopic sinus surgery (FESS), due to its location adjacent to the orbit and beneath the skull base and its proximity to the optic nerve and carotid artery, is a procedure fraught with potentially catastrophic complications.[5] Sinusitis is the most common diagnosis involved in otolaryngology lawsuits. From 1985 to 2005, rhinology claims represented 70% of the total indemnity compensation for otolaryngology claims.[6]

[a] ENT Surgical Consultants, 2201 Glenwood Avenue, Joliet, IL 60435, USA
[b] Hinshaw Law Firm, Hinshaw, Draa, Marsh, Still & Hinshaw, 12901 Saratoga Avenue, Saratoga, CA 95070, USA
[c] California Sinus Centers, 3351 El Camino Real, Suite 200, Atherton, CA 94027, USA
[d] Department of Otolaryngology-Head & Neck Surgery, Stanford University Medical Center, 801 Welch Road, Stanford, CA 94305-5739, USA
* Corresponding author.
E-mail address: ankitpatel1@yahoo.com

Otolaryngol Clin N Am 43 (2010) 905–914
doi:10.1016/j.otc.2010.04.014
oto.theclinics.com

ANATOMY OF A LAWSUIT

Malpractice law is part of personal-injury tort law. To win a lawsuit, the plaintiff must "prove that the defendant owed a duty of care to the plaintiff, that the defendant breached this duty by failing to adhere to the standard of care expected, and that this breach of duty caused an injury to the plaintiff."[1,7,8] Typically, the standard of care and causation must be determined by testimony of expert witness. In theory, the mere occurrence of a complication should not result in loss of a lawsuit, if the physician was following the standard of care. The reality, however, is that the occurrence of a disastrous injury is predictive of payment to the plaintiff regardless of whether the standard of care was met.[2,9]

MALPRACTICE AND RHINOLOGY

Endoscopic sinus surgery is one of the most litigated surgeries in otolaryngology. It can also be the most expensive in terms of judgments. The 3 most common complications listed in FESS lawsuits are intracranial complications (including cerebrospinal fluid [CSF] leak), orbital injury (including blindness), and anosmia (**Box 1**).[10]

In Lynn-Macrae and colleagues'[8] review of 41 cases from 1989 to 2003, they found that the average award to plaintiffs in FESS cases was $751,000, with a range of $61,000 to $2.87 million. The highest awards were in cases of CSF leak, anosmia, blindness, wrongful death, and intractable pain. The following allegations were noted in Lynn-Macrae and colleagues' review: 76% of cases alleged negligent technique; 37%, lack of informed consent; 5%, wrongful death; 27%, surgery not indicated; and 7%, failure to diagnose. Multiple allegations are often present within a case. About 41% of cases were won by plaintiff, whereas 56% of cases were successfully defended by the physician. Lydiatt and Sewell[10] similarly found that in 62% of cases, the physician defendant won the case, with plaintiffs winning 23% of cases that went to court, whereas 15% of cases were settled. In the study by Lydiatt and Sewell, the median judgment was $650,000, with a median settlement of $575,000. The range of awards given was from $16,000 to $25 million. FESS complications, sinonasal cancer, and misdiagnosis were the most common cases seen in their analysis of sinonasal lawsuits.

INFORMED CONSENT

Failure to obtain a patient's informed consent before sinus surgery is malpractice. A patient has the legal right to consent, or refuse consent, to any recommended treatment or procedure and the right to sufficient information to make a knowledgeable and informed decision about a proposed procedure. Informed consent is not simply a form or the signature of the patient on the operative permit. It is the process of

Box 1
Most common complications cited in rhinology lawsuits

- Intracranial complications (CSF leak, brain injury, meningitis, hemorrhage)
- Orbital injuries (blindness, diplopia)
- Anosmia
- Atrophic rhinitis
- Death
- Failure to diagnose or delayed diagnosis of cancer.

discussion between patient and provider as well as the documentation of that process and the patient's agreement to proceed with treatment. Physicians must describe the recommended treatment or procedure and disclose the benefits, risks, potential complications, and alternatives to the proposed treatment, nontreatment, or procedure (**Box 2**). The surgeon's emphasis should be on the discussion with the patient, not just a signed piece of paper. Several studies have been published on informed consent in endoscopic sinus surgery.[11–14]

The legal standard for informed consent is typically the reasonable patient or reasonable physician standard, outlined as follows: what would the typical physician discuss about the intervention (the reasonable physician standard) and what would the average patient need to know to make an informed decision (the reasonable patient standard).[15,16] In the United States, the applicable legal standard for judging the adequacy of informed consent is determined at the state level. As to the reasonable patient standard, Vaughan and colleagues[12] found that patients want to know not only the common risks and complications in FESS but also the rare, high-morbidity risks. FESS risks are outlined in **Box 3**. Most otolaryngologists counsel patients regarding the risk of CSF leak and orbital injury, but Wolf and colleagues[11] found that only 40% of otolaryngologists disclosed the risk of anosmia as a possible complication of FESS. Anosmia should be discussed as a potential risk during the informed consent process. Documentation of the extent of smell and taste should be done before performing FESS.

A full and open discussion should take place with the patient and all questions should be answered. This process must be documented. Care should be taken to ensure that the patient understands the recommendations and risks associated with endoscopic sinus surgery. Questions such as "Do you understand? Should I draw you a diagram? Would you like me to repeat that? Do you have any other questions or concerns that we haven't addressed?" can help the patient and guide the speed and level of detail that the surgeon provides. A preprinted handout for the patient to review may also generate questions ahead of time and be helpful as an adjunct to the consent discussion (**Fig. 1**). It is advisable to have the patient sign the handout.

In addition, the American Academy of Otolaryngology–Head and Neck Surgery has videos available, describing common expectations and risks associated with various surgeries, including FESS. These educational materials, together with the physician's discussion, enhance patient education as well as thoroughly document the informed consent process.

Box 2
Informed consent from the American Medical Association

- Patient's diagnosis, if known
- Nature and purpose of proposed treatment
- Risks and benefits of treatment
- Alternatives
- Risks and benefits of alternative treatments
- Risks and benefits of not proceeding with the suggested treatment

Data from AMA Patient Physician Relationship Topics. Informed consent. Available at: http://www.ama-assn.org/ama/pub/physician-resources/legal-topics/patient-physicianrelationship-topics/informed-consent.shtml; accessed January 10 2010.

Box 3
Some risks and expectations of endoscopic sinus surgery

- Bleeding, infection, synechiae
- Lacrimal duct injury
- Atrophic rhinitis
- Skull base or intracranial injury: CSF leak, intracranial hemorrhage, brain damage, pneumocephalus, meningitis/abscess
- Orbital injury: blindness, diplopia, orbital hematoma, subcutaneous emphysema
- Anosmia or hyposmia
- Death, stroke, heart attack, or other unexpected problems associated with anesthesia
- Need for postoperative nasal endoscopy, debridement, and long-term care
- Potential need for future surgeries and medicines

APPROACH TO THE DIFFICULT PATIENT AND DISCLOSURE OF MEDICAL ERRORS

The dissatisfied patient is more likely to sue the physician. Establishing rapport and open communication, preferably on more than 1 visit before surgery, is a vital step that the sinus surgeon can take to reduce litigation risk. Three factors in particular have been cited in studies as risk factors for litigation. Poor physician communication and interpersonal skills, withholding information, and the impression that the physician is rushed and uninterested in patient concerns are all associated with higher risk of litigation.[17]

Perhaps the most important strategy is preoperative prevention of dissatisfaction. A critical part of caring for patients with sinus problems is management of expectations. The physician should not promise cure. Endoscopic sinus surgery is meant to improve quality of life and reduce frequency of infection but does not completely eliminate sinus problems forever. Patient education is paramount in this regard. Establishing rapport on more than 1 patient visit is helpful in building a good patient-doctor relationship.

If only 1 visit is required preoperatively then the physician or a member of the physician's team should call the patient to answer any further questions before surgery. A phone call can help put the patient at ease and let the patient feel confident that the surgeon is their advocate. This communication can be done in the evening, which allows the patient to feel safe in their home, with enough time to ask questions about their surgery.

In addition, the surgeons should be mindful of how they communicate. During consultation, the physician should sit down with the patient and ensure that there is sufficient time available to speak with the patient, without feeling rushed. The same applies when breaking bad news to a patient or family member. Bruera and colleagues[18] found in their study of 168 patients with cancer that when delivering bad news, physicians who sit were viewed as significantly more compassionate than physicians who stand. The need to have sinus surgery, or any surgery for that matter, is considered bad news by many patients. A common patient complaint is that the physician did not take the time to listen or that the patient felt his or her needs were being ignored. Appropriate communication and communication style reduce this risk.

Prevention of complications is equally important, and familiarity with anatomy is critical. Other articles have addressed techniques of FESS, but a few points bear repeating. At all times, the surgeon should be clear on the anatomic location and landmarks during surgery, without solely relying on image guidance or surgical navigation technology. The typical margin of error of navigation systems is 1 to 2 mm,[19] yet the

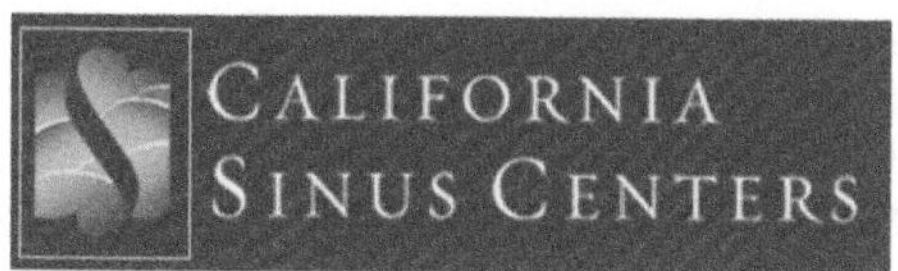

POSSIBLE RISKS AND COMPLICATIONS
RELATED TO FUNCTIONAL ENDOSCOPIC SINUS SURGERY

All surgical procedures have risks, benefits, alternatives and complications. The following possible risks and complications have been discussed with the patient regarding this surgical procedure to include but not limited to:

1. **Bleeding-Mild to moderate bleeding is expected up to 48 hours after surgery.**
2. **Infection**
3. **Injury to tear duct or sac resulting in tearing of the eyes. This may require further surgery**
4. **Need for frequent post-surgical visits for cleaning, to help prevent the disease from recurring.**
5. **May have an external scar if external approach is used.**
6. **Drainage of brain spinal fluid from the nose may occur. Further surgery may be needed.**
7. **Numbness of the teeth/cheek or near any external cuts.**
8. **Reactions to anesthesia.**
9. **Blindness or near vision changes. The patient should call the ENT clinic immediately if vision decreases.**
10. **Meningitis- (Brain infection)-Symptoms include: Stiff painful neck, increase in temperature and headache.**
11. **Voice change due to airflow changes between nose and mouth.**
12. **Change in sense of smell and/or taste.**
13. **Unexpected cardiac, pulmonary or kidney changes from anesthesia or medications given during surgery.**
14. **Need for future medical (like antibiotics) and surgical care.**

Other alternatives have been discussed with the patient (including no surgery with monitoring, continued medical management) and he/she has agreed to this procedure.

____

____

Patient / Guardian signature **Date / Time**

Thank You !

Fig. 1. California Sinus Centers' FESS informed consent form. (*Courtesy of* the California Sinus Centers, Atherton, CA, USA; with permission.)

skull base and lamina papyracea are only 0.1 mm thick. Also, surgical instrumentation is typically 3 to 5 mm in thickness. Overreliance on surgical navigation can result in significant complications.

If the field is too bloody, topical vasoconstrictive agents should be used to allow safe surgery. If hemostasis and appropriate visualization cannot be obtained, the surgeon should stop and consider a staged procedure. The surgeon's own experience and knowledge of his or her own limitations should be kept in mind for performing a safe, conservative surgery. If the situation requires, the surgeon should not hesitate to refer the patient to a more experienced surgeon.

If, despite the above measures, a complication does occur or a patient is unhappy then the physician should take extra care and time speaking with the patient in the postoperative period. The surgeon should take time to listen and should be empathetic to patient concerns and complaints. The surgeon should be accessible to the patient; whether this means providing pager access, cell phone access, or overbooking extra time at the end of the day to give undivided attention to the patient. The patient should not feel abandoned; the patient who feels alone is more likely to sue. Also, the family should be engaged, because if the patient is critically ill, it will be the family who will decide whether or not to seek litigation. When a complication does occur, it should be discussed openly and frankly with the family without admitting guilt or wrongdoing. An apology without stating guilt is comforting to the family and does not compromise defense of a future potential lawsuit. In fact, the apology itself along with compassionate care can be a deterrent to lawsuit (**Box 4**).

AREAS FOR CAUTION

In general, do not promise cure or dramatic improvement with endoscopic sinus surgery. Be sure to counsel patients regarding sense of smell, telling that surgery may improve or worsen it. Be conservative with nasal surgery, preserving turbinates (inferior and middle) to avoid atrophic rhinitis, unusual airflow patterns, or empty nose syndrome.

Be cautious when operating on patients for facial pain. Migraine, allergy, and atypical facial pain may mimic sinusitis, and surgery does not likely improve pain over the long term in this patient population. Another area for caution is mirror-image reversal of computed tomographic (CT) scan images.[20] With the advent of picture archiving and communication systems (PACS), images can become reversed with the simple press of a button by a CT technician. Always confirm sidedness with examination and endoscopy. Confirming the side of a septal deviation or placing a radiopaque marker is a simple method to corroborate the correct side. Mirror reversals are

Box 4
How to disclose an error or complication

- Inform the patient or family that an error occurred: "Remember we talked about the thin wall..."
- Explain how and why it occurred: "While opening the upper sinus we..."
- Describe how the problem was corrected: "We used tissue from the lower nose and surgical glue to..."
- Provide emotional support to the patient: "I know this is a difficult time. Here is my cell phone number/e-mail if you need to reach me. We will work together to..."
- Apologize without placing blame or attributing legal fault: "I feel bad that this has happened..." or "I am sorry that this happened..."

more common on coronal images. Therefore, for surgical cases, axial and coronal views should be reviewed and used in the operating room.

Signs of potential postoperative complications must be taken seriously. Uncontrolled pain and headache can be warning signs of orbital or intracranial injury. Patients with such complications should be seen and evaluated and should not be just treated over the phone. If indicated, CT of head and sinus should be performed. Also, uncontrolled bleeding (eg, due to injury to anterior ethmoid artery) can be a warning sign of intracranial bleeding or injury. Preoperatively, any unilateral friable nasal mass should be considered cancerous until proven otherwise. Bony unilateral erosion likewise is suspicious for malignancy. Unilateral nasal masses or polyps also should be imaged and reviewed carefully to rule out encephalocele or vascular structure. Magnetic resonance imaging can be helpful in this regard.

Often used in preoperative medical management, fluoroquinolones have black box warnings from the Food and Drug Administration regarding tendonopathy and tendon rupture. These are more common in patients older than 60 years, in patients taking oral corticosteroids, and in patients with kidney, heart, or lung transplants. If possible, fluoroquinolones should be avoided in these patient populations (**Box 5**).[21]

DOCUMENTATION AND PATIENT EDUCATION

Your sinus surgery and patient care plan must always be based on the simple and time-tested principle– first, do no harm. Second, document your care and treatment– before, during, and after surgery. The physician record is the main source of evidence and can be one's best defense during malpractice cases. All notes should be signed, dated, and timed. Phone conversations, correspondence by mail, videos watched, educational information from web sites, e-mails, and written educational materials distributed to the patient should all be documented in the medical record. Radiologic findings should be reviewed with patients and their families, showing actual images when possible, and this discussion should be documented.

Document the informed consent discussion and that the proposed procedure, the benefits, complications, and risks were discussed "including but not limited to…." Any recommendations or instructions given to the patient should be documented along with documentation of proper maximal medical therapy and results before surgery. Missed or canceled appointments should be noted in the chart, as well as any attempts to contact the patient to reschedule. The physician's office staff should have a process in place so that these procedures are followed routinely. In addition, the physician's office should have a mechanism to ensure that all tests ordered by the physician are reviewed.

Box 5
Areas for caution

- Do not promise cure or dramatic improvement
- Be conservative with turbinates; both middle and inferior
- Counsel patients regarding risk of anosmia with FESS
- Mirror reversal of CT images
- Uncontrolled pain, bleeding, or headache in the postoperative period
- Unilateral nasal masses
- Quinolones in elderly patients or patients with concomitant oral steroid use

If a patient refuses (informed refusal) a recommended medical treatment, the refusal should be documented in the chart. The risks associated with refusing the treatment should be stated. To add further importance to the refusal, the patient can be asked to countersign the note. Alternatively, the physician may dictate the note concerning patient refusal in the examination room with the patient listening.

Detailed and honest operative reports should be dictated within 24 hours of surgery. Appropriate surgical indications must exist and should be documented in the chart. This step is important because surgery done for improper reasons is difficult to defend in the event of major complications.

DO NOT ALTER THE MEDICAL RECORD

When there is a bad outcome, a physician or staff member may be tempted to go back and alter or modify the existing medical record on the misguided belief that they can improve the chart and thereby better defend themselves in the event of future litigation. The medical record should *never* be falsely altered. Criminal liability, loss of licensure, and loss of insurance coverage may result due to this action. Altering the medical record can destroy the physician's chances of successfully defending malpractice action. The original medical record may already have been secured by the plaintiff's attorney, through patient request or subpoena, before the physician going back to alter the medical record, thereby setting the stage for the fraudulent changes to be subsequently revealed to the unsuspecting surgeon at deposition or trial. In addition, handwriting experts readily detect these falsifications. If a late entry must be made, it should be noted as a late entry and signed, timed, and dated as such.

GETTING SERVED WITH LEGAL PAPERS

Receiving legal papers detailing a lien, requesting a deposition, or threatening an impending lawsuit can be a very stressful experience. A few points of advice for the physicians are worth mentioning. Do not discuss the case with other physicians if threatened with a lawsuit. Any discussion of the case with individuals other than their own attorneys or insurance carrier is not confidential but rather discoverable information. Incriminating details or opinions from other physicians can be used against the defendant in a court of law. The exception to this rule is in a peer review proceeding, such as a morbidity and mortality conference, which is protected information. Notify the malpractice insurance carrier if legal papers stating the intent to sue have been received. This notification activates coverage for the incident. Likewise, in high-risk cases with poor outcomes, the insurance carrier or risk management department should be contacted expediently (**Box 6**).

Box 6
When to notify malpractice insurance carrier

- During receipt or service of legal documents
- During rare and/or serious complications and unanticipated results
- When patient complains of dissatisfaction
- When statement comes from patient with intent to seek legal advice or sue
- When patient requests medical records, following a complication

When faced with a lawsuit, keep in touch with the malpractice insurance carrier and defense attorney to stay on top of the case and keep up with any deadlines. Do *not* directly contact the patient or the patient's attorney under any circumstances. Rather, all communications should be handled through the malpractice coverage and/or the defense attorney. If the advice of an attorney is needed for any reason, ask the insurance carrier or a trusted colleague to obtain reputable counsel.

SUMMARY

Endoscopic sinus surgery is commonly litigated due to the potentially disastrous nature of its associated complications. Patient education with appropriate management of expectations, a good patient-doctor relationship, open communication, documentation, and appropriate disclosure are ways to reduce a surgeon's medicolegal risk. If matters reach the point of litigation or if serious complications occur, the physicians should soon notify their insurance carrier and seek competent legal representation.

REFERENCES

1. Studdert DM, Mello MM, Brennan TA. Medical malpractice. N Engl J Med 2004; 350:283–92.
2. Studdert DM, Mello MM, Gawande AA. Claims, errors, and compensation payments in medical malpractice litigation. N Engl J Med 2006;354(19):2024–33.
3. Localio AR, Lawthers AG, Brennan TA, et al. Relationship between malpractice claims and adverse events due to negligence: results of the Harvard Medical Practice Study III. N Engl J Med 1991;325:245–51.
4. Studdert DM, Thomas EJ, Burstin HR, et al. Negligent care and malpractice claiming behavior in Utah and Colorado. Med Care 2000;38:250–60.
5. Stankiewicz J. Complications of endoscopic sinus surgery. Otolaryngol Clin North Am 1989;22:749–58.
6. Dawson DE, Kraus EM. Medical malpractice and rhinology. Am J Rhinol 2007;21: 584–90.
7. Keeton WP, Dobbs DB, Keeton RE, et al. Prosser and Keeton on the law of torts. 5th edition. St Paul (MN): West Publishing; 1984.
8. Lynn-Macrae AG, Lynn-Macrae RA, Emani J, et al. Medicolegal analysis of injury during endoscopic sinus surgery. Laryngoscope 2004;114:1492–5.
9. Brennan TA, Sox CM, Burstin HR. Relation between negligent adverse events and the outcomes of medical-malpractice litigation. N Engl J Med 1996;335:1963–7.
10. Lydiatt DD, Sewell RK. Medical malpractice and sinonasal disease. Otolaryngol Head Neck Surg 2008;139:677–81.
11. Wolf JS, Malekzadeh S, Berry JA, et al. Informed consent in functional endoscopic sinus surgery. Laryngoscope 2002;112:774–8.
12. Bowden MT, Church CA, Chiu AG, et al. Informed consent in functional endoscopic sinus surgery: the patient's perspective. Otolaryngol Head Neck Surg 2004;131:126–32.
13. Wolf JS, Chiu AG, Palmer JN, et al. Informed consent in endoscopic sinus surgery: the patient perspective. Laryngoscope 2005;115:492–4.
14. Taylor RJ, Chiu AG, Palmer JN, et al. Informed consent in sinus surgery: link between demographics and patient desires. Laryngoscope 2005;115:826–31.
15. Informed consent. Gale encyclopedia of surgery. Available at: http://www.answers.com/topic/informed-consent. Accessed January 10, 2010.

16. Berg JW, Lidz PS, Appelbaum LS, et al. Informed consent: legal theory and clinical practice. 2nd edition. London: Oxford University Press; 2001.
17. Klimo GF, Daum WJ, Brinker MR, et al. Orthopedic medical malpractice: an attorney's perspective. Am J Orthop 2000;29(2):93–7.
18. Bruera E, Palmer JL, Pace E, et al. A randomized, controlled trial of physician postures when breaking bad news to cancer patients. Palliat Med 2007;21(6): 501–5.
19. Knott PD, Batra PS, Citardi MJ. Computer aided surgery: concepts and applications in rhinology. Otolaryngol Clin North Am 2006;39:503–22.
20. Schmidt D, Odland R. Mirror-image reversal of coronal computed tomography scans. Laryngoscope 2004;114(9):1562–5.
21. Levaquin important safety information. Available at: http://www.levaquin.com/levaquin. Accessed January 10, 2010.

Informed Consent Process and Patient Communication After Complications in Sinus Surgery

Eugene P. Snissarenko, MD, Christopher A. Church, MD*

KEYWORDS

• Consent • Complication • Sinus

INFORMED CONSENT PROCESS

As the paranasal sinuses are in intimate relationship with the orbit and anterior cranial fossa, sinonasal surgery has always been a potential source of complications. Moreover, the continued evolution of endoscopic techniques, as well as medicolegal developments, has made the situation even more complex. In their review of 152 malpractice suits in sinonasal cases, Lydiatt and Sewell[1] found that 26% alleged lack of informed consent, with 48% receiving a plaintiff award. Similarly, a review by Lynn-Macrae and colleagues[2] of 41 suits involving endoscopic sinus surgery (ESS) found that 37% alleged lack of informed consent. Clearly, informed consent and communication with patients before and after surgery are of paramount importance to the rhinologic surgeon.

What Is Informed Consent?

As Miles[3] has observed, there is moral, legal, and social agreement that patients should participate in decision making about medical treatment and direct their medical care. The moral view is based on respect for personal autonomy and the belief that a person's subjective view of the condition, options, and prognosis should shape one's medial decision making. Legally, this view is supported by the right to privacy and the right to be secure in one's person. The social view is affirmed by the desire of contemporary Western society to be fully informed about medical conditions and therapeutic options and to be allowed to make treatment decisions for themselves.

Department of Otolaryngology–Head and Neck Surgery, Loma Linda University School of Medicine, 11234 Anderson Street, Suite 2588, Loma Linda, CA 92354, USA
* Corresponding author.
E-mail address: cchurch@llu.edu

Otolaryngol Clin N Am 43 (2010) 915–927
doi:10.1016/j.otc.2010.04.015
0030-6665/10/$ – see front matter

The idea of informed consent has evolved over the past century. Today, informed consent consists of explaining to alert, competent patients the nature of their illness or disability balanced against the risks and benefits of the recommended treatment. Approval is then sought from the patient to proceed. Truly valid consent is most likely achieved through effective personal communication within the physician-patient covenant, as opposed to the simple signing of a legal consent form. Even in cases of surrogate consent for patients who are unable to comprehend treatment decisions, informed consent is a communication process. The presumption in favor of prolonging life and the difficulty of decision making for these patients should not lead the clinician to discount discoverable information about how a patient would weigh the burdens and benefits of therapy in choosing a treatment course.[4]

Three criteria must be satisfied for a consent or refusal to be valid. First, adequate information must be presented. In the United States, the legal requirements for informed consent contents are controlled at the state level. Some states support the view that it is necessary to inform the patient of risks that reasonable prudent physicians would disclose to their patient, whereas other states have enacted the "prudent patient standard," in which the physician must disclose all risks that a reasonable prudent patient would consider material to the decision to undergo or refuse a particular procedure.[5] It is the physician's responsibility to provide material information regarding treatment issues in clear, jargon-free language, which includes information about the patient's medical condition and likely course with and without the preferred treatment as well as availability and effect of alternative therapies. In addition to prognostic information, the physician should help patients to anticipate and plan for their disability. As the patient's values, goals, and fears are identified, the physician should encourage the patient to ask questions to clarify the treatment issues related to these values. The personal nature of material information means that the informing physician must listen with the ear of a counselor rather than merely comprehensively list the effects of treatment.

Second, the communication process must be free of coercion. The patient should choose the treatment voluntarily rather than acquiescing to a necessary or inevitable course of action. This decision can be compromised by presentation of incomplete or biased information. It can also be compromised when patients are compelled by unnecessary institutional policies. A physician, however, has a right and sometimes an obligation to make recommendations, but these recommendations must not be manipulative (by disclosing biased facts) or coercive.

Third, the patient must be competent to consent or refuse. In regard to informed consent for medical procedures, emphasis is generally placed on *capacity,* which is a much more clinical and task-specific idea, than the more global legal concept of *competence*. Although there is no gold standard definition of capacity or competence, most ethicists agree that at minimum, the patient must be able to understand that a decision must be made and the relevant options and consequences that attend that decision. Furthermore, they should be able to reason about the alternatives and effectively communicate with caregivers regarding the decision. The fact that the patient needs to apply their own values in their reasoning process leaves considerable ambiguity in the process.

Obtaining informed consent is a legal standard for practice and an incompletely realized ethical ideal. The courtroom process has emphasized the aspect of consent that pertains to informing patients of the risks and uncertainties of a single medical treatment and stressed the importance of documented evidence of a patient's consent. Moreover, the definition of consent that has emerged from malpractice actions has led some physicians to conclude that informed consent is a legal ritual that is satisfied by simply obtaining the patient's signature.[3] Most physicians are acutely aware of the difficulty in achieving the ideal of informed consent in clinical practice because of differences in understanding of medical facts between physician and patient, the emotional impact of the diagnosis, and the patient's unique world views, preferences, and values.

Informed Consent for ESS

As an elective surgical procedure, ESS can present a unique challenge in achieving informed consent. Consideration must be given to many issues, including which complications are discussed with patients, which complication rates are quoted, who obtains the consent, and the circumstances under which consent is obtained. The impact of cultural and demographic differences must be appreciated. Finally, the informed consent process as perceived by the patient and the effectiveness of the process must be considered.

Discussion of Complications

Although there is no set standard in regard to which complications are to be discussed, a frequently quoted rule of thumb has been to discuss complications specific to a procedure that occur in more than 1% of cases or are considered catastrophic in nature.[6–8] In ESS, the rates of complication are generally lower than this figure, a common example being orbital ecchymosis, which occurs in only about 0.44% of cases.[8] However, the severe and incapacitating nature of the potential complications of ESS requires their discussion, especially because the procedure is not being performed for a life-threatening condition. Wolf and colleagues[7] reported that approximately 60% of surveyed physicians believed that an incidence of 1% is significant enough to warrant discussion; however, 69% of patients wanted to know of complications with an incidence of more than 0.1%.[5]

When discussing complications with a patient, it is unclear whether one should present one's personal incidence of a complication or that found in the literature. Wolf and colleagues[7] found that 19% of surveyed US physicians described their personal incidence, 37.5% quoted that found in the literature, and 35% used both. However, nearly half of respondents of a similar survey in England did not quote any figures, with 33% of surgeons quoting their own series for complication rates, 11% quoting national rates, and 10% quoting both. The researchers suggested that quotation of one's individual figures and results would be preferable, as it would be a better reflection of actual experience, whereas national rates are only estimates of practice.[8] Kennedy and colleagues[9] in a 1994 survey found that physicians who discussed potential complications were more likely to have encountered those complications. They speculate that this tendency may be because once surgeons experience a complication, they are more likely to discuss it with their subsequent patients or simply because physicians who are forthcoming with their patients are also likely to be forthcoming in reporting their complications.

How Much Information Is Enough?

Morally and legally, medical practitioners have an obligation to their patients to attempt to explain a procedure, to offer the therapeutic options, and to specify possible risks and complications. Some, especially in North America, believe that the best way to meet these requirements, especially in the face of the increasingly educated patient, is to provide an exhaustive list of all possible complications. There is concern, however, that patients might be burdened with unwanted information and that such information may increase the patient's anxiety. This controversy highlights the irreconcilable conflict between medical paternalism and patient autonomy in the informed consent process.[6]

Kerrigan and colleagues[10] specifically addressed the issue of the amount of information presented and patient anxiety and found that a very detailed account of what might go wrong does not increase patient anxiety significantly but has the advantage of allowing the patient to make a fully informed choice before consent, thus reducing the potential for subsequent litigation.

Stanley and colleagues[11] likewise found that patient anxiety levels were unaltered by the increase in the amount of information they were given. Bowden and colleagues[12] noted that although a thorough discussion of potential complications frequently provoked anxiety, this rarely resulted in cancellation of surgery.

Clearly, the manner in which potential complications are discussed may have significant effect on patient anxiety. Simply providing a list of potential complications and their incidence rates is inadequate. Common courtesy demands an explanation in layman's terms of what the patient would experience with each complication, along with discussion of how that complication would be managed. The look of terror on the face of a patient preparing for ESS who has just been described a skull base violation will often vanish with additional information: "Should this happen, I will repair the damaged area during the surgery. This has about a 95% success rate in my experience and rarely causes any long-term problems."

Who Should Obtain Consent?

There is also debate as to who should obtain informed consent from a patient. Previous studies found that surgeons consistently overestimate the mortality risk of elective surgery. It was also found, however, that when informed consent was obtained by nurses, medical students, or residents, there was greater inaccuracy of risk estimation than when obtained by attending physicians, suggesting that attending physicians are the most appropriate members of the surgical team to discuss informed consent.[13] Nevertheless, the American College of Surgeons stated that the surgeon who is "responsible for obtaining informed consent from the patient...need not personally obtain the patient's signature on the consent form".[14]

In a recent study by Houghton and colleagues,[15] data for informed consent of 100 consecutive patients were analyzed. In all of the cases, consent was obtained by a junior doctor, who was unlikely to be performing the surgery. Even though most patients were satisfied with the explanation of the operation given to them and considered themselves fully informed, 45% believed that the doctor who signed the consent form with them would be performing the procedure and the majority felt that this should be the standard of practice. When junior doctors obtaining the consents were interviewed, approximately one-third of them admitted to obtaining consent for procedures of which they had little understanding and more than half of them thought that the surgeon who performed the surgery should sign the consent form. Looking at these data, it is reasonable to conclude that if the act of signing the consent form is to be more meaningful, it should be signed by the surgeon who is going to perform the operation.

Cultural Differences

Is the discussion of informed consent different between different health systems or cultures? In Great Britain, material risk is identified as an incidence of 10%, with a risk of 1% for complications that are vital to the informed consent choice, such as death, paralysis, or blindness.[11] In the United States, no such standards have been set.

Interpretations of informed consent requirements vary greatly among cultures in terms of content and whether this should be verbal or in writing. Generally, a consent form is not signed in France, Sweden, or the Netherlands, although practitioners are advised to register in general terms in the notes that such a discussion took place. The amount of information provided ranges from relatively little to every specific and general complication. In Germany, it is necessary to discuss not only the complications of the operation but also rarities such as cardiac arrest resulting from the use of local anesthesia and even the potential side effects of a blood transfusion.[6]

Studies have also examined patients' views of informed consent based on racial, educational, and socioeconomic backgrounds. Taylor and colleagues[16] reported on the link between demographics and patient desires regarding informed consent in ESS. They found that younger, white, and more educated patients wished to know about complications at the lowest risk levels, regardless of severity. With regards to specific complications, black patients and those with less formal education were less interested in being informed about the potential risks of orbital complications, cerebrospinal fluid (CSF) leak, or possible need for revision surgery. Women wished to discuss more frequently than men such complications as bleeding and infections.

Informed Consent in ESS: Patient Perspective

What are patients' expectations on informed consent prior to ESS? In comparing patient responses with physician responses, it is apparent that physicians do an excellent job of discussing complications that are specifically related to ESS. More than 95% of physicians discuss risks such as CSF leak, eye injury, and bleeding, whereas only 72% to 83% of patients would want to be informed of these complications.[7] For general complications pertaining to all surgeries (myocardial infarction or cerebrovascular accident), only 8% to 18% of physicians inform patients of these preoperatively, whereas the majority of patients would want to be informed of them. This low rate might be explained by the fact that most of the surgeons expect that the anesthesia staff would discuss these during a separate informed consent discussion.[5]

There is discrepancy in the literature regarding patients' desire to know all possible complications. Bowden and colleagues[12] reported that more than 85% of patients wished to be informed of all potential complications, regardless of the incidence of these complications. Wolf and colleagues,[7] however, found that only 44% of patients wanted to be informed of all potential complications, whereas Burns and colleagues[17] stated this figure as 73%. Adhikari and Pradhananga[18] found that 90% of patients in their study expected that all known complications would be discussed. Differences in study design, size of the study, and geographic regions can attribute to this discrepancy; however, it is notable that a significant percentage of patients expect their surgeon to inform them about even rare complications.

In the time of widespread availability of information through the Internet and other means of media, it would be naive to think that patients solely rely on their doctors for providing them with information regarding their upcoming procedure. Burns and colleagues[17] reported that two-thirds of patients in their study had sought information elsewhere before signing their consent form, including relatives, friends, and the Internet, which reflects an increased awareness and interest of patients in their own treatment and a desire to become more involved in the decision-making process. It may also show that information provided by surgeons may not meet the expectations of today's informed patient and that doctors need to adjust their standards of a "prudent patient."

What do patients see as the purpose of informed consent? Cassileth and colleagues[19] reported that 80% of patients studied viewed consent forms as a protection for the physician. They suggested that the legalistic and adversarial overtones of the consent form may appear inconsistent to the patient who has a fundamental orientation to and preference for a doctor-patient relation based on trust. Dawes and colleagues[20] found that three-quarters of patients studied viewed the consent form as a legal document and felt obliged to sign the form, especially when they underwent a brief, unstructured, purely formal consent process.

Effectiveness of Informed Consent

Several studies have evaluated patients' recollection of the contents of informed consent for ESS. Even though most patients are satisfied with the information given by doctors before surgery, the majority of them (56%–77%) could not list even a single complication, even after a relatively short time period.[17,18] This observation is consistent with studies of information retention in other surgical specialties. Godwin assessed recall 6 days after reduction mammoplasty and found that although 97% of patients felt that the procedure of obtaining consent was adequate, the average number of retained facts was 3 of 12.[21] Adhikari and Pradhananga[18] found that low educational status, increasing time since consent, and patients' lack of enthusiasm were factors related to poor recall.

Taking into consideration that for elective surgeries considerable time can elapse between informed consent and the actual procedure, it has been suggested that patients may benefit from written consent documents that would serve as "aide-mémoire" and improve patients' understanding of their condition and treatment as well as compliance.[17,21] Stanley and colleagues,[11] however, found that providing additional written information did not improve their patients' understanding of the risks and complications of surgery.

Visual aids may also be helpful because of the fact that informed consent communications are sometimes too complex and difficult for many patients to grasp despite the fact that many patients may report understanding the information.[21] The correlation between educational background and the patient's ability to recall complications may also support the use of visual materials.[19]

Bedridden patients are less able to recall information than patients in a better physical condition. Cassileth and colleagues[19] found that as patients become increasingly ill, their sense of control over their own destinies may give way to intensified dependence on their physicians, and this dependence may result in poorer attention to, interest in, and recall of information about consent.

When evaluating the causes of poor retention of information after informed consent, one must consider both patient and surgeon factors. From the patient's point of view, especially after procedures with high satisfaction rates such as ESS, it is difficult to recall what could have gone wrong with the operation. Another reason for poor recall could be related to the stress of a hospital admission. The patient is often bombarded with questions from the surgeon, anesthetist, and nursing staff. Too much information can have a confusing effect on the patient. The doctor needs to act as the patient's adviser, counselor, advocate, and support. Two-way discussions and complex questions are possible with the articulate patient. Some elements of trust must exist that doctors give accurate information to the best of their ability. There would be no need to ask questions or seek medical advice if the patient had all the answers. With pressure on the surgeon to cover all risks, they tread a fine line between informing patients and confusing them with too much information.[21]

Valid Informed Consent: a Process, Not a Signature

Meaningful communication and negotiation are absolute necessities in the patient-physician relationship. Successfully imparting the professional's insights enables patients to make a truly informed decision about their care. Providing only technical services to a patient is inadequate and reduces the patient-physician relationship to a mere contract.[22]

The ethical imperative for the practice of informed consent is the principle of respect for self-determination. Medical professionals may become insensitive to the fact that invasive and sometimes dangerous interventions are exceptional. Patients accept loss of privacy; painful, uncomfortable, and anxiety-introducing procedures; sharing of intimate information; and sometimes risks to life that are not part of normal human experience. To be sure such acceptance is usually understood by a patient as in his or her health interest, but the sacrifices are not routine. Respect for the autonomy of another is practiced by gaining the other's reasoned and deliberate agreement for tests, treatments, and invasive procedures.

This process can be enhanced by giving the patient a sense of control during the consent interview. Dawes and colleagues[20] described the so-called structured interview techniques when an informational sheet is used to guide the interview with patients before they sign the consent form. These materials are designed to explain why the operation was being done and what it involves, to list and explain complications, to explain how the patient would feel after the operation, and to explain the chance of success and any alternative treatment. When the information sheet was read with patients before they signed the consent form and then given to them so that they could read it on their own, it resulted in patients feeling less obliged to sign the consent, more likely to think that they had been involved in the decision to operate, and less likely to consider the interview a formality. Furthermore, despite the fact that patients interviewed with the information sheet–guided technique were given a much more comprehensive description of their surgery, anxiety was not increased.[23] Techniques such as these may provide patients with a greater feeling of autonomy about the decision to operate. They also may feel more confident to refuse treatment because they feel less dependent on the doctor to make the final decision. This may also enable patients to be more accepting of an unexpected outcome.

Surgeons have obligations of education. Anxiety is ever present and is reduced by helping the patient to know what to expect and by responding to particular concerns. The educational process is not limited to the preoperative period. Daily instruction and clarification of anticipated problems and their prevention will often be needed during recovery. Written instructions, including means of access for calls and appointments and notes about activity, diet, and wound care, are more useful aids to patients than the brief oral instructions.[22]

Informed consent must be understood as a process, not as an event. The goals of informed consent are impossible to satisfy in a single sitting but are accomplished through an ongoing educational process beginning at the first visit and extending through recovery. Practicing the skill of placing oneself in the patient's shoes allows the ESS surgeon to meet the demands of informed consent and to account for variations in personality and circumstance.

PATIENT COMMUNICATION AFTER COMPLICATIONS

Complications Are Inevitable

All sinus surgeons will eventually encounter complications associated with ESS, regardless of how careful they are. Although there is a learning curve with ESS, even experienced surgeons can incur complications. Unexpected outcomes can be extremely distressing to patients and their families. Often, this may be as much the result of fear of the unknown, unexpected disability and treatment, as it is from actual physical symptoms. Complications are distressing for the surgeon as well. Aside from concern for the patient's suffering, the professional's management of the situation can be influenced by damage to one's self-image and fear of retribution. Wu[24] describes the physician as the "second victim" in these situations. Unfortunately, no training is usually provided in medical school or residency on how to communicate with patients after a surgical complication, and for most physicians, the first such conversation occurs without guidance.[25]

Litigious Nature of ESS

ESS is highly litigious. The complex anatomy of the nose and sinuses and the contiguity to vital structures as well as unpredictable changes caused by disease make operating in this area inherently and unavoidably demanding, with significant potential risks to the patient. The development of sophisticated technologies and instruments for ESS has been responsible for a dramatic increase in the number of otolaryngologists performing sinus surgery and in the number of cases performed. This expansion was accompanied by an increase in malpractice lawsuits.[26]

Another possible reason for litigation after ESS complications is that patient's expectations sometimes exceed what can reasonably be delivered by the appropriate operation, even when performed by a skilled, competent surgeon.[4] Although surgical complications may never be easy for patients and their families to accept, those occurring in elective, outpatient procedures may be the most difficult.

The practice of settling disputes by litigation is cultural tradition in the United States. The injured, angry patient seeks monetary compensation to right the real or perceived wrong. Once a dispute has become polarized and enters the legal system, resolution by mutual agreement of the parties involved is rare. Moreover, the compensation demanded frequently escalates to levels that are not, by any rational explanation, correlate with the alleged wrongful act.[4]

Appropriate Level of Communication

Effective physician communication after complications in ESS is essential for optimal outcomes and patient satisfaction. Although most surgeons acknowledge this, it is still surprising how often contact with patients and their family is severely limited or even cut off once a complication has been discovered. This behavior may be unintentional or may simply be the perception of the patient. It may represent a fear on the surgeon's part of exacerbating a situation that he or she is resigned that litigation will result. It may also represent a legitimate desire to transfer the patient to another facility where a higher level of care is available. The opposite approach is occasionally seen as well, in which a surgeon is so overly attentive that the patient feels smothered. This approach can easily be mistaken for insincerity and imply to the patient that the physician is trying to simply pacify them, rather than being genuinely concerned about their well-being.

The appropriate level of communication is achieved by understanding the patient's desires and fears after a complication has occurred. Recognizing the fear of the unknown that patients likely experience and combating it with education about the complication and its management is key. Patients may fear abandonment by their physicians or may fear that they have been taken advantage of. Recognizing and responding to the patient's legitimate sense of entitlement to increased access to the surgeon and his staff will go far to alleviate patient fears.

Disclosure

There is basic intellectual agreement within the medical profession that telling patients the truth, including the truth about medical mistakes, constitutes a professional obligation for physicians. However, the nature of the practice of disclosure, what is meant by the phrase "telling the truth" in cases of medical error, continues to be among the most highly contested and emotionally fraught issues within conversations on patient safety.

Some have suggested that disclosure of complications, particularly errors that did not result in symptoms likely to be noticed by the patient, may only serve to increase the chances of litigation. However, a greater risk may result from failure to disclose a complication. As Witman and colleagues[27] found, patients are less likely to seek litigation if physicians honestly and directly disclose events, rather than if patients learn of their occurrence through other means. Moreover, Kraman and Hamm[28] studied a full disclosure risk management policy at the Veterans Administration Hospital in Lexington, Kentucky, and found positive economic outcomes for such an approach.

Several studies have found that an extremely high percentage of (92%–98%) patients expect to be told about any and all complications, whereas a much lower percentage (60%) of physicians felt the same.[27,29] This discrepancy may become a significant impediment in the physician-patient relationship.

Disclosure should occur as soon as reasonably possible after a complication is recognized, even if all the details of the incident are yet to be determined. A delay in disclosure may be perceived as lack of concern, ineptitude, or obfuscation on the part of the physician. Emphasizing to the patient and family that communication is an ongoing process and that the surgeon will keep them informed of new information in a timely manner will serve to reduce negative perceptions.

It is important that the ESS surgeon not delegate the disclosure of the complication to another member of the medical team. Circumstances may dictate that other personnel become involved, but having the surgeon discuss the complication, prognosis, and plan with the patient and family members reassures that the person in whom they have put their trust is in control of the situation.

The details of what to discuss in the disclosure conversation are extremely important. Surgeons should strive to present only factual information, avoiding the tendency to speculate about causes and prognosis. Assuring the patient that this is an ongoing process may serve to reduce patient anxiety.

Communication

Effective communication requires physicians to be able to understand patients' perceptions of illness. This is never truer than after a surgical complication has occurred. Unfortunately, communication between physicians and patients is often deficient. Studies show that agreement between the physician and the patient about the principal problem can be achieved only in half of the encounters at primary care centers. Otolaryngology practices are certainly not different. Patients from lower socioeconomic groups tend to agree less often with their doctors about basic aspects of their medical care than do patients from higher socioeconomic groups.[30] Duffy and colleagues[31] found that although physicians performed a physical examination of the areas relevant to patients' illness in 97% of encounters, they ascertained the patients' emotional response to illness in only 35% of encounters and asked the patients what they understood about the illness in only 27%.

If poor communication can undermine physician-patient relations even during the good outcome of treatment, it can only complicate the devastating result of unwanted outcomes. Anger, miscommunication, ignoring the patient's family, and a patient's perception that he or she has been regarded or treated disrespectfully by the surgeon are some of the factors that may influence patients to seek legal recourse in the case of an undesirable event. Studies have repeatedly shown that the quality of medical care alone is a poor predictor of patient satisfaction with their health care and that the rapport between physicians and their patients is a principal determinant of patients' evaluation of their treatment. Moore and colleagues[32] compared patients with postprocedural complications who were exposed to positive doctor-patient relations with those exposed to negative relations. Positive doctor-patient relations increased patients' perceptions of physician competence, decreased their perceptions of physician responsibility for an adverse medical outcome, and reduced their expressed intentions to file malpractice claims against the physician and the hospital.

Without the benefit of the physician's perspective, patients may equate unanticipated outcomes with errors. To remedy this disconnect, a primary goal for the surgeon after a complication is education. An understanding of the medical facts of the case and options for management allows the patient to attain something of the physician's perspective and thereby a sense of control over the situation.

One of the challenges in communication after ESS complications can be interaction with the patient's family. Many times, family members, who have not developed the trust-based relationship with the surgeon that the patient has, may be even more angry and hostile than the patient who has suffered the unfavorable outcome. Taking the time to sit with the patient's family and answer questions can be immensely helpful; however, the physician must balance the desire to satisfy the family with the legal requirement to protect the patient's health information. A practical step to help with this problem is to routinely ask every patient before surgery, "Who would you like me to discuss your case with afterward?" Even with the patient's verbal consent to speak with his family, every attempt should be made to discuss all details with the patient directly. In cases where the patient is incapacitated and there are a large number of family members, having a designated person to discuss care with can be extremely helpful.

Access to the physician and staff is a key factor in combating patient fears and frustrations, as well as in improving compliance. Within limits, it is reasonable to grant additional access to these patients compared with other patients. Knowing how to contact the physician or their designate at any time (including nights and weekends) reduces fear of abandonment. Prompt return of voicemail and email communications (along with appropriate documentation of such) shows genuine concern for patients and their problem.

Educating office staff about questions and issues that the patient might have, as well as giving colleagues who provide call coverage a "heads up," allows them to provide attention to detail, which again demonstrates the surgeon's concern and competence. Careful attention to billing practices can also avoid adding insult to injury. Initially forgiving patients may change their mind after being sent to collections.

Apology

One of the debates surrounding communication with patients after complications is the idea of an apology. Clearly, patients desire an apology after an adverse outcome.[33] Many physicians, attorneys, and risk management experts have expressed concern that a physician apology is an admission of guilt and an open invitation to litigation.[34] Others, however, suggest that offering a sincere expression of apology may actually decrease the likelihood of legal action, and when polled, jurors respond favorably to physician apologies and tend to be sympathetic to the physician.[35] Recently, several states crafted and adopted "I'm sorry" laws, which offer varying degrees of legal protection for expressions of sympathy and even admissions of fault after incidents of harm, including medical mistakes. The words "I'm sorry" can mean two different things, depending on the context, but either way, they are important for the patient to hear. Saying "I'm sorry that your father died" communicates empathy, even though it doesn't necessarily acknowledge any mistake on the physician's part. "I'm sorry that I killed your father," however, does.[36]

It is important to distinguish apology from disclosure. Although both often go hand-in-hand, there are important differences. Disclosure is an ethical right, whereas apology is a therapeutic necessity that shows humanity and remorse and that may help patients with forgiveness and emotional healing.[37]

An insincere apology is worse than no apology at all. Specifically acknowledging the event and the pain that was caused is critical. One of the best ways to demonstrate that the surgeon is taking the patient's injury seriously is to participate in a root-cause analysis of the event. A very real concern of patients and their families is that nothing will be learned from their complication and that others might needlessly suffer the same fate.

SUMMARY

Informed consent and communication with a patient after a complication are intricate, often complex processes that require much effort and trust. Although there is no single best method for achieving optimal outcomes in these areas, success can be achieved adhering to the golden rule: "Whatever you want men to do to you, you also do to them..." As the rule implies, this is an active process, one that can be understood only through the eyes of a healer who is ready to serve.

REFERENCES

1. Lydiatt DD, Sewell RK. Medical malpractice and sinonasal disease. Otolaryngol Head Neck Surg 2008;139:677–81.
2. Lynn-Macrae AG, Lynn-Macrae RA, Emani J, et al. Medicolegal analysis of injury during endoscopic sinus surgery. Laryngoscope 2004;114:1492–5.
3. Miles SH. Informed consent: an ideal and a standard of practice. In: Stultz BM, Dere WH, editors. Practical care of the ambulatory patient. Philadelphia: WB Saunders Co; 1989. p. 553–7.
4. Kidder TM. Malpractice considerations in endoscopic sinus surgery. Curr Opin Otolaryngol Head Neck Surg 2002;10:14–8.
5. Wolf JS, Chiu AG, Palmer JN, et al. Informed consent in endoscopic sinus surgery: the patient perspective. Laryngoscope 2005;115:492–4.
6. Lund VJ, Wright A, Yiotakis J. Complications and medicolegal aspects of endoscopic sinus surgery. J R Soc Med 1997;90:422–8.
7. Wolf JS, Malekzadeh S, Berry J, et al. Informed consent in functional endoscopic sinus surgery. Laryngoscope 2002;112:774–8.
8. Sharp HR, Crutchfield L, Rowe-Jones JM, et al. Major complications and consent prior to endoscopic sinus surgery. Clin Otolaryngol 2001;26:33–8.
9. Kennedy DW, Shaman P, Han W, et al. Complications of ethmoidectomy: a survey of fellows of the American Academy of Otolaryngology-Head and Neck Surgery. Otolaryngol Head Neck Surg 1994;111:589–99.
10. Kerrigan DD, Thevasagayam RS, Woods TO, et al. Who's afraid of informed consent? BMJ 1993;306:298–300.

11. Stanley BM, Walters DJ, Maddern GJ. Informed consent: how much information is enough? Aust N Z J Surg 1998;68:788–91.
12. Bowden MT, Church CA, Chiu AG, et al. Informed consent in functional endoscopic sinus surgery: the patient's perspective. Otolaryngol Head Neck Surg 2004;131:126–32.
13. Soin B, Smellie W, Thomson H. Informed consent: a case for more education of the surgical team. Ann R Coll Surg Engl 1993;75:62–5.
14. Statement on principles underlying perioperative responsibility. American College of Surgeons. Bull Am Coll Surg 1996;81(9):39–40.
15. Houghton DJ, Williams S, Bennett JD, et al. Informed consent: patients' and junior doctors' perceptions of the consent procedure. Clin Otolaryngol 1997; 22:515–8.
16. Taylor RJ, Chiu AG, Palmer JN, et al. Informed consent in sinus surgery: link between demographics and patient desires. Laryngoscope 2005;115:826–31.
17. Burns P, Keogh I, Timon C. Informed consent: a patients' perspective. J Laryngol Otol 2005;119:19–22.
18. Adhikari P, Pradhananga RB. Patients' expectations on informed consent before ENT surgery. International Archives of Otolrhinolaryngology 2007;11:51–3.
19. Cassileth BR, Zupkis RV, Sutton-Smith K, et al. Informed consent – why are its goals imperfectly realized? N Engl J Med 1980;302:896–900.
20. Dawes PJ, O'Keefe L, Adcock S. Informed consent: using a structured interview changes patients' attitudes towards informed consent. J Laryngol Otol 1993;107: 775–9.
21. Godwin Y. Do they listen? A review of information retained by patients following consent for reduction mammoplasty. Br J Plast Surg 2000;53:121–5.
22. English DC. Valid informed consent: a process, not a signature. Am Surg 2002; 68:45–8.
23. Dawes PJ, O'Keefe L, Adcock S. Informed consent: the assessment of two structured interview approaches compared to the current approach. J Laryngol Otol 1992;106:420–4.
24. Wu AW. Medical error: the second victim. BMJ 2000;320:726–7.
25. Rosner F, Berger JT, Kark P, et al. Disclosure and prevention of medical errors. Arch Intern Med 2000;160:2089–92.
26. Rice DH. Endoscopic sinus surgery. Otolaryngol Head Neck Surg 1994;111: 100–10.
27. Witman AB, Park DM, Hardin SB. How do patients want physicians to handle mistakes? A survey of internal medicine patients in an academic setting. Arch Intern Med 1996;156:2565–9.
28. Kraman SS, Hamm G. Risk management: extreme honesty may be the best policy. Ann Intern Med 1999;131:963–7.
29. Hingorani M, Wong T, Vafidis G. Patients' and doctors' attitudes to amount of information given after unintended injury during treatment: cross sectional, questionnaire survey. BMJ 1999;318:640–1.
30. Epstein AM, Taylor WC, Seage GR. Effects of patients' socioeconomic status and physicians' training and practice on patient-doctor communication. Am J Med 1985;78:101–6.
31. Duffy DL, Hamerman D, Cohen MA. Communication skills of house officers. Ann Intern Med 1980;93:354–7.
32. Moore PJ, Adler NE, Robertson PA. Medical malpractice: the effect of doctor-patient relations on medical patient perceptions and malpractice intentions. West J Med 2000;173:244–50.

33. Vincent C, Young M, Phillips A. Why do people sue doctors? A study of patients and relatives taking legal action. Lancet 1994;343:1609–13.
34. Gallagher TH, Waterman AD, Ebers AG. Patients' and physicians' attitudes regarding disclosure of medical errors. JAMA 2003;289:1001–7.
35. Boothman RC. Apologies and a strong defense at the University of Michigan Health System. Physician Exec 2006;32(2):7–10.
36. Berlinger N. After harm: medical error and the ethics of forgiveness. Baltimore (MD): Johns Hopkins University Press; 2005.
37. Butcher L. Lawyers say "sorry" may sink you in court. Physician Exec 2006; 32(2):20–4.

Malpractice Claims in Nasal and Sinus Surgery: A Review of 15 Cases

Samuel S. Becker, MD[a,*], James A. Duncavage, MD[b]

KEYWORDS

- Rhinology • Malpractice claims
- Sample cases • Nasal surgery

Rhinology is a highly litigated area of otolaryngology. This article presents a sample of 15 malpractice claims involving surgery on the nose and paranasal sinuses provided by member companies of the Physician Insurers Association of America (PIAA). Cases are arranged in chronologic order and are summarized to include facts that might be useful to practicing otolaryngologists. These examples were selected from hundreds of cases, and are representative of several similar cases reviewed. Outcomes of malpractice claims were not available in all cases.

CASES

Case 1

An adult male patient with chronic sinusitis with polyps, and septal deviation underwent septorhinoplasty and bilateral endoscopic sinus surgery in 1991. The patient's post-operative course was notable for persistent epiphora from lacrimal duct injury, and he was referred to an ophthalmologist who performed a dacrycystorhinostomy. It was noted during the course of the malpractice claim that although lacrimal duct injury may be a known and accepted complication of sinus surgery, it was not adequately listed in the consent forms used by the surgeon.

Case 2

A pediatric male patient with nasal obstruction and chronic sinusitis underwent septoplasty, bilateral inferior turbinate reduction, adenoidectomy, and bilateral endoscopic sinus surgery in 1995. The patient developed a sinus infection 4 months postoperation. Repeat computed tomography (CT) scan revealed radiopaque material

[a] Becker Nose and Sinus Center, LLC, 2301 Evesham Road, Suite 404, Voorhees, NJ 08043, USA
[b] Division of Rhinology, Department of Otolaryngology, Vanderbilt University Medical Center, 7209 Medical Center East, South Tower, 1215 21st Avenue South, Nashville, TN 37232-8605, USA
* Corresponding author.
E-mail address: sam.s.becker@gmail.com

Otolaryngol Clin N Am 43 (2010) 929–932
doi:10.1016/j.otc.2010.04.019

consistent with a retained sponge that required a return visit to the operating room for removal and debridement.

Case 3

A pediatric female patient with a history of chronic sinusitis that persisted through multiple episodes of intravenous (IV) antibiotics underwent bilateral endoscopic maxillary antrostomies and total ethmoidectomies in 1995. Five weeks after surgery, she began to have purulent nasal drainage and fevers. She was taken back to the operating room (OR) where a 4-cm foreign body covered in purulent debris and granulation tissue was removed from the left middle meatus. Pathology report confirmed the presence of a large piece of cotton with acute inflammatory exudate.

Case 4

An adult male Chinese American patient, former smoker, with several months of epistaxis, was referred to an otolaryngologist in 1996 for further evaluation. The otolaryngologist's examination was negative, although the evaluation did not include nasal endoscopy. One year later, the patient saw another otolaryngologist and was diagnosed with invasive squamous cell carcinoma arising from the sphenoid sinus.

Case 5

An adult patient who underwent sinus surgery in 1997 complained of bilateral eye pain post-operatively and was diagnosed with bilateral corneal abrasions.

Case 6

An adult female patient underwent right sinus surgery in 1999 for a persistent lesion/cyst in the right frontal sinus. Post-operatively it was found that the radiologist had mislabeled the coronal scans and that the lesion was, in fact, in the left frontal sinus.

Case 7

An adult male patient underwent bilateral endoscopic sinus surgery in 1999. The patient had been on multiple prior courses of antibiotics, and so the treating surgeon did not prescribe an additional course of antibiotics prior to surgical intervention. The patient was noted to have a cerebrospinal fluid (CSF) leak during surgery. The leak was repaired by the surgeon intra-operatively with middle turbinate graft. The patient had a unilateral loss of vision and proptosis in the recovery room. Lateral canthotomy was performed. Orbital CT was performed on the day of surgery and there was significant intraorbital air but no obvious violation of the lamina. The patient was discharged and seen the following day in the office. The plaintiff's attorney alleged deviation from the standard of care by failure to treat the patient with a trial of appropriate antibiotics before performing surgery. Plaintiff's attorney also alleged deviation from the standard of care while performing surgery, as well as failure to immediately admit the patient to the hospital for observation of sequelae from CSF leak.

Case 8

An adult female patient underwent bilateral endoscopic total ethmoidectomy and maxillary antrostomies in 2002 for chronic sinusitis with polyposis. The surgeon noted violation/dehiscence of the lamina papyracea intra-operatively and was able to see orbital fat. This area was left undisturbed and the surgery was completed. No iatrogenic injury was noted by the surgeon during surgery. The patient was seen for her initial post-operative visit 2 days after surgery. She complained of diplopia and was noted to have an ecchymotic right eye. The surgeon stated that he would continue to follow the patient closely. The patient sought a second opinion from an ophthalmologist who ordered a CT scan. Defect of the right lamina papyracea with displacement of the right medial rectus muscle was noted. The plaintiff's attorney alleged deviation from the standard of care during surgery, with inappropriate informed consent.

Case 9

An adult male patient underwent bilateral endoscopic total ethmoidectomy, sphenoidotomies, maxillary antrostomies, and frontal recess exploration in 2002 for chronic sinusitis with polyposis. During surgery, while opening what was felt to be the frontal recess, increased bleeding and what appeared to be fat were encountered. An intra-operative biopsy of this area showed muscle fibers. Intra-operative consultation was obtained from an ophthalmologist. The patient was noted to have post-operative diplopia with disruption of the medial rectus, and subsequently underwent several ophthalmologic procedures for attempted correction of this defect. The plaintiff's attorney alleged the surgeon's performance was a deviation from the standard of care, with violation of the lamina papyracea and damage to the orbital contents.

Case 10

An adult male patient with rhinosinusitis with polyps underwent bilateral endoscopic total ethmoidectomies and maxillary antrostomies in 2002. There was no complication noted during surgery and the procedure was concluded uneventfully. On post-operative day 2, the patient was difficult to arouse. He was transferred to the emergency room and was obtunded on arrival. CT scan showed intracranial free air. The patient was taken to the OR for evacuation of the air by a neurosurgeon; however, he experienced brain herniation and significant brain damage.

Case 11

An adult female patient underwent right endoscopic sphenoidotomy in 2002 for persistent symptomatic sinusitis despite treatment with antibiotics and oral steroids. CT scan was notable for persistent opacification of the right sphenoid sinus. During surgery, the uncinate process was removed and an anterior and posterior ethmoidectomy was performed. The sphenoid sinus was entered with a straight Blakesley forceps. A culture swab was placed into the sinus and thick yellow discharge was removed, which was followed by a copious amount of arterial bleeding filling the nasal and oral cavities. Gauze was packed into the nasal cavity, nasopharynx, oral cavity, and oropharynx followed by placement of large-bore IV catheters and a Foley catheter. The patient was emergently taken for a CT scan that revealed subarachnoid hemorrhage and hydrocephalus. Angiography was also performed, which revealed a possible aneurysm. The patient was transferred to the surgical intensive care unit and prepared for clipping of the supraclivoid portion of the carotid artery. On post-operative day 1, a craniotomy was performed and 2 clips were placed on the internal carotid artery along the site of the apparent defect. On post-operative day 16, the patient had a massive stroke to the right brain and was declared dead. Post-mortem analysis revealed no aneurysm, but a defect in the lateral sphenoid wall and a laceration of the internal carotid artery.

Case 12

An adult male patient underwent bilateral endoscopic sinus surgery in 2003 for chronic rhinosinusitis. During surgery, the fovea ethmoidalis was breached and a CSF leak occurred that was repaired intra-operatively with a turbinate graft. Post-operatively the patient was informed of this complication, admitted for observation, and placed on antibiotics to prevent meningitis. The pathology report confirmed the presence of glial cells. The patient was discharged on post-operative day 2. On post-operative day 6, the patient returned for follow-up and complained of fatigue and headaches. He had no further rhinorrhea, but a complete blood count revealed an elevated white blood cell count. The patient presented to the emergency room (ER) on post-operative day 7. Lumbar puncture revealed CSF with elevated levels of white blood cells. CT scan revealed a 2-cm lesion; intracranial abscess versus cerebritis with focal edema. The patient was placed on IV antibiotics and made a good recovery. He was released to return to work 2 months after surgery.

Case 13

An adult female patient underwent septoplasty in 2003. Post-operatively she fell to the floor from the operating room table and suffered bruising on the face and head.

Case 14

An adult male patient with a history of chronic sinusitis sought treatment by an otolaryngologist in 2005. The patient was treated with Augmentin (amoxicillin and clavulanate), although his chart noted allergies to penicillin, cephalosporins, and sulfa drugs. He later presented to the ER with swelling of the lips and tongue, pruritic rash, and difficulty in breathing and swallowing. The symptoms improved with epinephrine and IV diphenhydramine (Benadryl).

Case 15

An adult male patient underwent revision right Caldwell-Luc maxillary sinus surgery in 2006. Intra-operatively, the surgeon noted that the anterior entrance into the maxillary sinus was likely too superior because of the presence of orbital fat. The surgeon did not remove this fatty tissue and proceeded to perform a second canine fossa trephination in a more inferior location; however, this opening was also found to be too superior. The surgeon then performed a traditional endonasal maxillary antrostomy using blunt and powered instrumentation. When the patient awoke in the recovery room, he had no light perception in his right eye. An ophthalmologist was immediately consulted, and a lateral canthotomy and cantholysis was performed and high-dose IV steroids given. However, the patient's vision was not restored. The pathology report noted the presence of fibro-fatty and muscle tissue. Post-operative CT scan revealed violation of the inferior orbital floor, anterior orbital hemorrhage, damage to the inferior rectus muscle, and possible contusion of the optic nerve. Ophthalmologic examination on post-operative day 3 revealed severe motility restriction, hypoglobus and enophthalmos, and ischemic retina. The patient continued to have problems with right maxillary sinusitis, and underwent additional revision maxillary sinus surgery approximately 1 year later.

Ten Pearls for Safe Endoscopic Sinus Surgery

Marc A. Tewfik, MD, MSc, FRCSC[a],
Peter-John Wormald, MD, FRCS, FRACS[a,b,*]

KEYWORDS

• Complications • Endoscopic sinus surgery
• Chronic rhinosinusitis • Nasal polyposis

Endoscopic sinus surgery (ESS) is effective in improving the symptoms of chronic rhinosinusitis and thus in ameliorating the quality of life of patients suffering from this common disease. However, one important drawback to this type of surgery remains the potential for serious complications. This is inevitably because of the proximity of critical anatomic structures such as the orbit, the internal carotid arteries, the skull base, dura, and brain.

Several risk factors exist for the occurrence of complications in ESS[1]; these can be broadly divided into anesthetic, surgeon-related, and disease-related factors. General anesthesia increases the risk of complications because of the lack of patient feedback when approaching sensitive structures like the lamina papyracea and the skull base. Right-sided surgery for a right-handed surgeon is a risk factor, as is left-sided surgery for a left-handed surgeon, because of the angle of the endoscope and instruments. Another risk factor is lack of surgeon experience, for the obvious reasons of unfamiliarity with the anatomy and use of instrumentation. Extensive sinus disease, excessive bleeding, and revision surgery, all of which can obscure or distort the sinonasal structures normally encountered during surgery, are important risk factors.

Although some of these factors are unavoidable, and the avoidance of others such as general anesthesia is impractical, there are several measures and technical points that can be used to remain safe when performing ESS. This article highlights 10 pearls that are routinely taught in our institution and have stood us in good stead. We believe that by adhering to these simple principles, ESS can be made safe and the likelihood of intraoperative complications reduced.

---

[a] Department of Otolaryngology–Head and Neck Surgery, The Queen Elizabeth Hospital, 28 Woodville Road, Woodville South, South Australia 5011, Australia
[b] Department of Otolaryngology–Head and Neck Surgery, Adelaide and Flinders Universities, Adelaide, 28 Woodville Road, Woodville South, South Australia 5011, Australia
* Corresponding author. Department of Otolaryngology–Head and Neck Surgery, The Queen Elizabeth Hospital, 28 Woodville Road, Woodville South, South Australia 5011, Australia.
E-mail address: peterj.wormald@adelaide.edu.au

Otolaryngol Clin N Am 43 (2010) 933–944
doi:10.1016/j.otc.2010.04.017
oto.theclinics.com
0030-6665/10/$ – see front matter.

IDENTIFY HIGH-RISK SITUATIONS

Before surgery can begin, preoperative imaging must be carefully scrutinized. This is done to identify anatomic variants that, if unrecognized, may lead to adverse outcomes. A high-definition helical multislice computed tomography (CT) scan of the sinuses should be obtained after an adequate trial of maximal medical therapy. Ideally, cuts should measure between 0.5 and 1 mm in the axial plane, and be reconstructed in the coronal and parasagittal planes.

Several key areas must be systematically evaluated on the preoperative CT scan. As a memory aid for performing this thorough checklist, the acronym CLOSE can be used. The "C" stands for cribriform plate, the position of which should be assessed according to the Keros classification.[2] A deeper olfactory fossa with a longer lateral wall (**Fig. 1**), such as with Keros 2 and 3, exposes a longer lateral wall of thin bone at risk of injury and leaking of cerebrospinal fluid (CSF). The angle that this lateral wall forms with the perpendicular should also be assessed, because those that are more tilted (away from the perpendicular plane) are predisposed to skull base injury during dissections of the frontal recess (**Fig. 2**). The "L" stands for lamina papyracea, which should be scanned along its entire length, looking for dehiscences or orbital fat protrusion into either the ethmoid or maxillary sinuses (**Fig. 3**). The lamina may also be in an excessively medialized position relative to the lateral nasal wall, particularly in cases of atelectasis of the maxillary sinus (**Fig. 4**A, B). This situation must be recognized before performing the uncinectomy, or anterior ethmoidectomy, as either of these steps can readily result in orbital penetration. The "O" stands for Onodi cell and optic nerve dehiscence. An Onodi cell is a posterior ethmoid cell that pneumatizes into the superolateral aspect of the sphenoid sinus, and its presence places the optic nerve at risk of injury during instrumentation of the posterior ethmoids. This cell is best detected if there is a horizontal septation within the sphenoid sinus, as seen in the first coronal CT slice in which the complete posterior bony choana can be identified (**Fig. 5**). The "S" stands for the sphenoid and skull base. The pneumatization of the sphenoid sinus needs to be assessed; if the anterior clinoid is pneumatized, the optic nerve may be in a mesentery across the roof of the sphenoid. In addition, the internal carotid arteries should be assessed for overlying bony dehiscences, a medialized trajectory, or the presence of an aneurysm. It is also important to assess the vertical

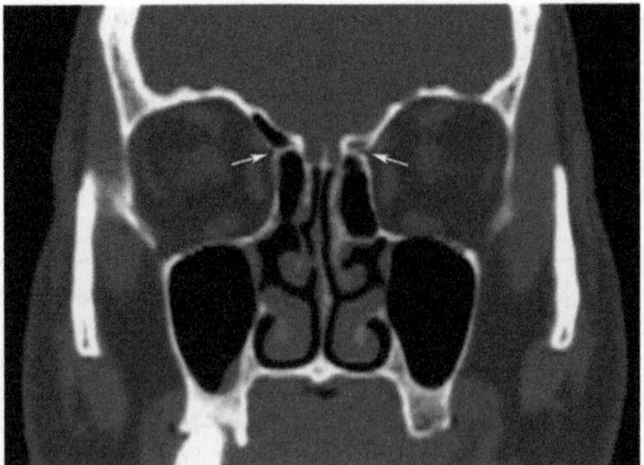

Fig. 1. CT scan of the sinuses, coronal view, demonstrating a deep olfactory fossa with a low-lying cribriform plate (Keros 2); note also the position of the anterior ethmoidal arteries (*white arrows*), hanging in bony mesenteries below the skull base, placing them at risk of injury during surgery.

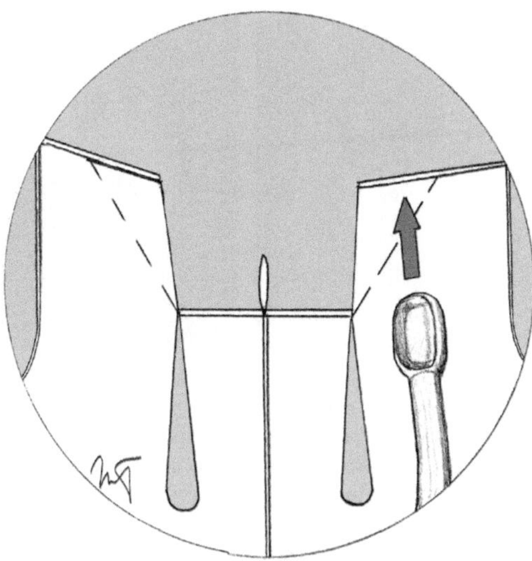

Fig. 2. Diagram of the anterior skull base, in coronal view, depicting the orientation of the lateral wall of the olfactory fossa; the more tilted away from the vertical plane that it is (*dotted line*), the greater the risk of skull base injury during dissections of the frontal recess.

height of the posterior ethmoids. If unrecognized, a very low-lying ethmoid roof may be inadvertently breached on entering the posterior ethmoids through the ground lamella. The "E" stands for the (anterior) ethmoidal artery. If the anterior ethmoidal artery is in a mesentery hanging below the skull base (see **Fig. 1**), this must be appreciated preoperatively, to avoid severing the artery as the septations on the skull base are removed.

OPTIMIZE THE SURGICAL FIELD

It is essential to reduce the amount of blood obscuring the visual field in ESS. This will allow proper visualization of the landmarks that are critically important to the safety and success of surgery. Several measures can be taken intraoperatively to reduce bleeding[3–6]; these include reverse Trendelenburg positioning, the application of topical and local vasoconstrictors,[3,6] maintaining the mean arterial pressure at around

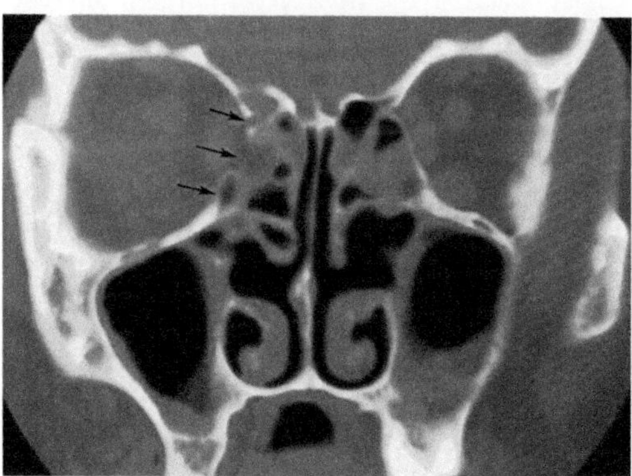

Fig. 3. CT scan of the sinuses, coronal view, demonstrating a bony defect of the right lamina payracea (*black arrows*), with prolapse of orbital tissue into the adjacent ethmoid sinus.

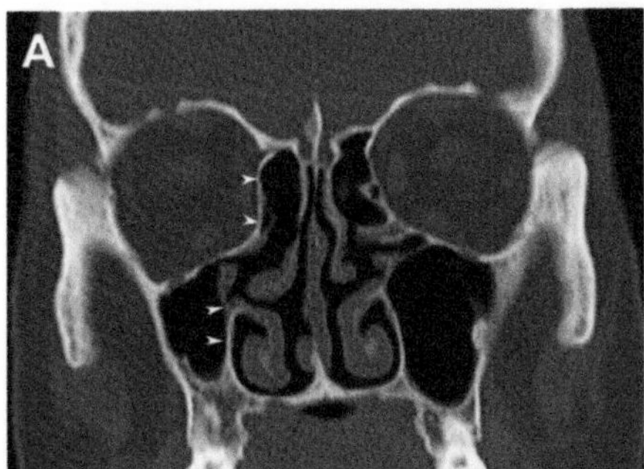

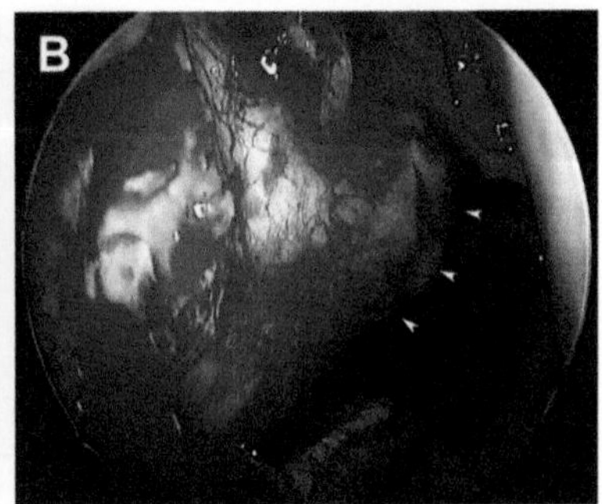

Fig. 4. (*A*) CT scan of the sinuses, coronal view, illustrating the medialized position of the right lamina payracea (*white arrows*) relative to the medial wall of the right maxillary sinus (*white arrowheads*), in the context of an atelectatic maxillary sinus. (*B*) Intraoperative view of the medialized lamina payracea (*white arrowheads*) in the same patient, following uncinectomy; note the free edge of the right uncinated process (*asterisk*). It is easy to confuse this patient's orbital wall with the anterior face of the bulla ethmoidalis, which could lead to devastating orbital injury if not recognized before surgery.

75 mm Hg and the heart rate less than 60 beats/min.[4,5] This is best achieved with total intravenous anesthesia.[4,7] A preoperative course of systemic steroids may also be beneficial[8,9] to reduce the size and vascularity of nasal polyps, thus reducing capillary bleeding during ESS. However, the optimal dose, length of treatment, and ideal groups of patients who would benefit from this treatment require further research.

There are several patient factors that predispose to increased bleeding, and thus, a poor surgical field. These should be actively sought and, if possible, dealt with preoperatively. Local factors include acute infection, inflammatory processes including the granulomatous diseases, and excess local tissue trauma during dissection. If suspected clinically, active infection of the sinuses should be treated with an appropriate course of preoperative antibiotics. Systemic comorbidities that can increase surgical bleeding include hypertension, peripheral vascular disease, and liver and renal diseases. Chronic alcohol abuse, malnutrition, and vitamin deficiencies (most notably vitamin K), can also affect coagulation, and must be explored if

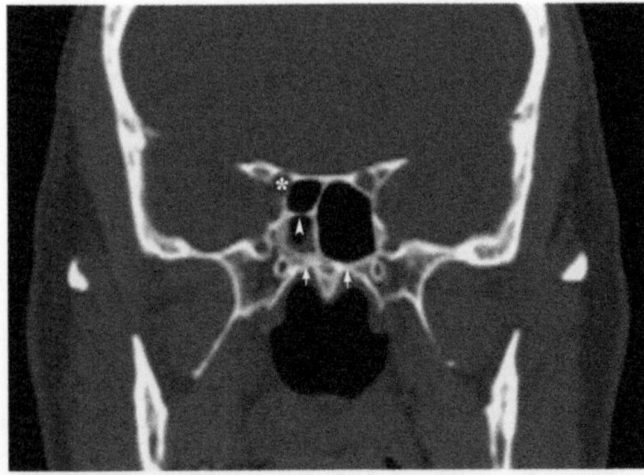

Fig. 5. CT scan of the sinuses, coronal view at the level of the sphenoid sinus, demonstrating a right Onodi cell and dehiscent right optic nerve (*asterisk*). The presence of the Onodi cell is determined by the demonstration of a horizontal bony septation (*white arrowhead*) within the sphenoid sinus, which is above the complete bony choana (*white arrows*).

suspected clinically. Bleeding diatheses such as hemophilia A or B and von Willebrand disease, require clotting factor replacement or specialized pharmacotherapy (desmopressin [DDAVP], tranexamic acid, or aminocaproic acid), and must be planned for. Medications affecting surgical field, including aspirin, nonsteroidal antiinflammatory drugs, warfarin, and antiplatelet agents, must be discontinued for an adequate length of time before surgery, in consultation with the patient's regular treating physician. Several herbal and alternative therapies, such as ginseng, ginkgo and kava, can affect coagulation pathways, and the surgeon should be aware of these. It is prudent for patients to discontinue all herbal and alternative medicines at least 7 days before surgery.

Even if all preventable causes of excessive surgical bleeding have been addressed preoperatively, cases of excessive bleeding will still be encountered during surgery. The surgeon should reflexively double-check that the patient position and anesthetic parameters are optimal. Care is taken not to suction blood away from raw mucosal edges, because this will promote further bleeding. Rather, saline irrigation is used to wash away excessive blood. Most of the bleeding that clouds the end of the endoscope occurs proximal to the position of the endoscope. The surgeon should actively seek such bleeding sites and coagulate these with the suction bipolar forceps to ensure that when the scope touches the side wall, accumulated blood does not run down the scope and contaminate the end. Suction instruments (such as the Freer dissector and curette) are used to ensure optimal visualization of the dissection in the bloody surgical field.

SAFELY REMOVE THE MIDDLE PORTION OF THE UNCINATE PROCESS

In certain patients, because of the proximity of the middle (vertical) portion of the uncinate process to the lamina papyracea, the technique used to perform the uncinectomy may place the orbit at risk of penetration. This is particularly true if a powered instrument is used on the midportion of the uncinate. To remove the uncinate flush with the frontal process of the maxilla, the microdebrider blade needs to be pushed firmly against the orbital wall in the area where the lamina papyracea is thinnest. The lamina may be dehiscent in the region directly behind the frontal process of the maxilla in some patients, significantly increasing the risk of damage to the orbit and medial rectus muscle. We therefore recommend that microdebriders be avoided in this area, and that cold steel instruments be used instead.

The swing-door technique of uncinectomy was created with the aim of safely achieving a complete removal of the midportion of the uncinate process. Briefly, the technique uses a sickle knife to make a superior cut through all 3 layers (mucosa-bone-mucosa) of the uncinate horizontally just under the axilla of the middle turbinate until the hard bone of the frontal process of maxilla is encountered. Next the pediatric backbiter is introduced into the middle meatus and the tooth of the instrument is slid into the hiatus semilunaris to engage the junction of the vertical and horizontal portions of the uncinate. Generally 3 bites of the backbiter are performed in a posterior to anterior direction to reach the frontal process, but this may be variable depending on the width of the uncinate and the size of the back-biting blade. With the final bite, the backbiter is rotated from horizontal to an angle of 45° upward to protect the nasolacrimal duct from injury. The right-angled ball probe is placed through the inferior cut behind the uncinate process and the midportion of the uncinate process is fractured anteriorly. Next, an upturned 45° through-biting Blakesley forceps is used to cut the uncinate flush with the lateral nasal wall, and the midportion of the uncinate is removed in one piece. In the original research comparing the swing-door technique with the conventional sickle knife removal of the uncinate, the rate of orbital penetration was significantly reduced.[10]

SAFELY REMOVE THE ATELECTATIC UNCINATE PROCESS

In instances when the uncinate process is in close proximity or directly apposed to the lamina papyracea, the risk of injury to the orbit is even greater. This situation may arise as a result of isolated atelectasis of the uncinate process or in combination with an atelectatic maxillary sinus or silent sinus syndrome. For this reason, modifications to the usual technique must be adopted to avoid orbital injury. The first point of note is that such situations must be detected on the preoperative imaging, as stated earlier, before an attempt is made to remove the uncinate process. A decision should be made when planning surgery on the technique that will be necessary for safe uncinectomy. As a general rule, the sickle knife should not be used in such cases because of a lack of sufficient space between the uncinate and the lamina papyracea and because the uncinate in these patients is paper thin and flaccid. If a sickle knife is used to incise the uncinate, there is a high risk that the tip of the knife will penetrate the orbit. The pediatric backbiter can be used to securely perform the superior horizontal cut in the uncinate just below the axilla of the middle turbinate, in addition to the inferior cut. The middle and horizontal portions of the uncinate process can then be removed using the usual swing-door technique described earlier.

KNOW WHERE AND HOW TO PENETRATE THE GROUND LAMELLA

As mentioned earlier, the vertical height of the posterior ethmoid cells and position of the skull base must be analyzed before the start of surgery. The concern is that the skull base may be easily violated after penetration of the vertical ground lamella, resulting in a CSF leak, optic nerve injury, or intracranial injury. Even in the absence of an abnormally low posterior ethmoid roof, injury can occur in this area if the entry into the ground lamella is performed incorrectly. Both the location and the angle of entry are important, and as **Fig. 6** illustrates, one affects the other. The superior meatus should be entered immediately adjacent to the middle turbinate, through the medial aspect of the ground lamella as it turns vertically, just anterior to its horizontal portion. The superior meatus should be clearly identified and the anterior end

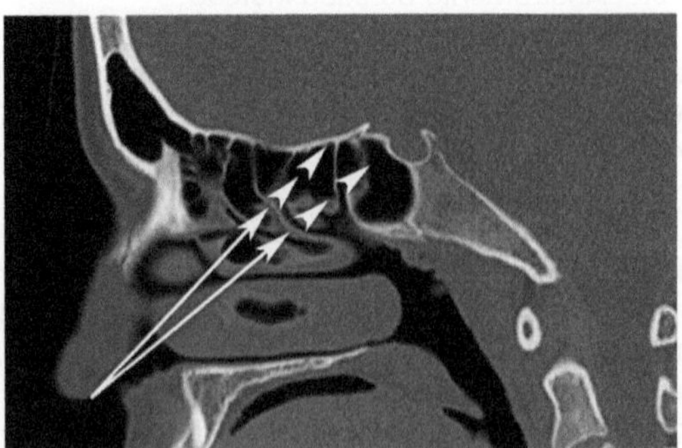

Fig. 6. CT scan of the sinuses, sagittal view, illustrating the importance of penetrating the ground lamella of the middle turbinate in the proper location, immediately anterior to its horizontal portion as it turns vertically; if the ground lamella is entered even a few millimeters too superiorly, the path of the instrument will be toward the ethmoid roof, and risk of skull base injury will be much greater.

of the superior turbinate actively sought to confirm the correct entry and current location of the dissection. If entered even just a few millimeters too superiorly, the resultant angle between the nostril and the entry point into the lamella will be such that the instrument is directed acutely toward the skull base; this is easily demonstrated in a sagittal view of the ground lamella (see **Fig. 6**). For this reason, care must be taken to penetrate into the superior meatus in an inferior and medial location, and to maintain the orientation of the scope and instrument in a relatively parallel plane to the ethmoid roof. It is also for this reason that the use of angled scopes is not recommended for the dissection of ethmoid cells along the skull base, particularly for the inexperienced surgeon. The angled view may give the surgeon a distorted perception of orientation and lead to inadvertent skull base injury.

FIND LANDMARKS WHEN IT SEEMS THERE ARE NONE

The usual anatomic landmarks used for performing ESS may be altered or obscured in several settings, including revision surgery and severe polypoid disease. These landmarks include the uncinate process, bulla ethmoidalis, ground lamella, as well as the middle and superior turbinates. In such instances, computer-aided surgical navigation systems may offer some benefit. However, beyond this, several techniques can be used to safely clear residual disease in cases with altered landmarks.

It is always prudent to clearly identify the maxillary sinus ostium as an initial landmark in primary as well as revision surgery. The 30° endoscope should be used and directed toward the lateral nasal wall for this step. In the absence of a clear free edge of the uncinate process, the insertion of the inferior turbinate can help guide the surgeon to the position of the ostium, which is located immediately superior to the midportion of this turbinate. A curved suction or right-angle ball probe can be used to palpate for the position of the ostium and to penetrate into the maxillary sinus by advancing the tip in an inferolateral (at least 45° from the horizontal) direction just above the insertion of the inferior turbinate. If the suction or probe is advanced horizontally, it is highly likely that the region of the medial wall and floor of the orbit will be damaged. The ostium is then enlarged posteriorly into the area of the fontanelle using a through-cutting Blakesley forceps, and anteriorly to clear any residual uncinate using backbiting forceps. The position of this ostium can now be used as a landmark, as can the junction of the medial orbital floor and the lamina papyracea. If this junction is followed posteriorly in a horizontal plane, this should take the dissection onto a point on the anterior face of the sphenoid, which approximates the inferior third to middle third of the sphenoid sinus (**Fig. 7**).

After confirming the presence and size of the sphenoid on the CT scan, the sphenoid should be opened widely in cases of severe disease to prevent restenosis as well as to clearly identify the position of the skull base. For the latter reason, the sphenoid should be addressed before dealing with any partially resected ethmoid cells. In the presence of a superior turbinate, the sphenoid ostium can be found medial to the inferior third of this turbinate. Other methods of locating the ostium include measuring 12 mm superior to the rim of the posterior bony choana, or measuring 7 cm from the anterior nasal spine in a plane rising 30° above the floor of the nasal cavity. If the ostium cannot be visualized, the sinus can be entered using the blunt end of a Freer elevator in the expected position of the ostium.

The frontal recess cell structure and drainage pathway should be elucidated preoperatively using multiplanar CT views of the sinuses. However, in cases of complex anatomy, exuberant disease, or previous surgery with local scarring, the drainage pathway may be difficult to localize intraoperatively. Frontal sinus mini-trephination

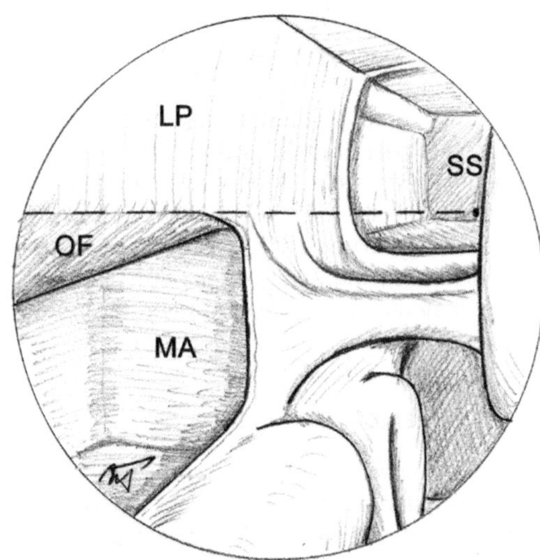

Fig. 7. Diagram of the right nasal cavity, as seen intraoperatively after wide maxillary antrostomy (MA) and complete sphenoethmoidectomy, depicting the junction of the medial orbital floor (OF) and the lamina payracea (LP), which is oriented in a horizontal plane that can be followed posteriorly toward a point approximating the inferior to middle third of the sphenoid sinus (SS).

(Medtronic ENT, Jacksonville, FL, USA) and fluorescein instillation can help in this situation by providing a stream of brightly colored fluorescein solution along the frontal sinus drainage pathway. Dissecting instruments can then be precisely placed into this corridor and the surrounding cells fractured away.

The use of computer-aided surgical navigation systems is now commonplace, and should be planned for during the preoperative workup of any patient with altered anatomic landmarks. However, these systems are merely an additional tool available to the surgeon and are only as good as the operator using them. Their danger lies in the creation of a false sense of security, which may lead inexperienced surgeons to tackle cases that are beyond their expertise. Computer-aided surgery has limitations, and these need to be recognized by the surgeon using it.

SAFELY REMOVE BONY SEPTATIONS

Certain measures can be taken to make the removal of bony septations more secure in the region of the ethmoid and sphenoid sinuses. Bone can be fractured using several instruments. Thin lamellae are easily broken using a ball probe, seeker, regular curette, or through-biting Blakesley forceps. However, in the setting of excessive bleeding, the malleable suction curette is particularly well suited, continually removing blood and allowing good visualization of the surgical field. The other benefit of a malleable instrument is that it allows the correct angle of the instrument to be selected and thus optimizes the plane of dissection of the curette.

Thicker lamellae, such as the anterior face of the sphenoid, require heavier cutting instruments such as the Hajek-Koefler or Kerrison punches. It is important to engage the distal lip of the instrument firmly onto the posterior surface of the bony septation to be removed to avoid damage to adjacent structures. The most devastating examples of such a situation are the injury of a dehiscent internal carotid artery or optic nerve during enlargement of the sphenoidotomy. To avoid these devastating complications, the initial bites should be made superiorly above the sphenoid ostium up to the skull base, and lateral to the ostium inferiorly. This results in an "L" shape when performed on the left side of the sphenoid (and the mirror image of this on the right side). At this point, the endoscope can be advanced into the sinus to verify the positions of the carotid and optic nerves before removing the remainder of the anterior face of the sphenoid.

If used properly, the Hajek-Koefler and Kerrison punches are safe options for the removal of septations in delicate areas, such as along the lamina papyracea. The risk with noncutting instruments is of penetrating through the lamina, and therefore the tip of these instruments should never be oriented directly toward the lamina papyracea during dissection, but rather held in an upright orientation parallel to the lamina.

BE THOROUGH BUT SAFE ALONG THE SKULL BASE

The fear of producing a CSF leak during clearance of ethmoid cells along the skull base causes many surgeons to leave bony septations and pockets of diseased material along the ethmoid roof. Although it is important to preserve mucosa in this region, the complete and thorough clearance of infected and inflamed material from all sinuses will allow for the best chance of achieving a successful outcome in ESS. The first step in this process is to identify the position of the anterior ethmoid artery (AEA) on preoperative imaging, and determine whether it is in a bony mesentery or running within the ethmoid roof. Intraoperatively, the AEA is usually located behind the second lamella of bone back from the frontal sinus, which often corresponds to the superior attachment of the anterior face of the bulla ethmoidalis; it should be visible after thorough clearance of the skull base. As mentioned in the previous section, bony septations can be fractured with a curette, which should be held in an upright orientation and used to apply force in a posterior to anterior direction. The risk of damaging the fovea ethmoidalis increases when instruments are pushed in a posterior direction.

The microdebrider can also be used to remove fractured bone and diseased mucosa from the ethmoid roof; however, care must be taken not to sever the AEA. One technique to prevent complete transection of the artery is to advance and withdraw the microdebrider blade at an angle toward the skull base until the excess tissue and bone has been removed (**Fig. 8**A). This will generally result in a gentle debridement and will only cause slight bleeding from shaving the artery, rather than a through and through cut if the microdebrider is passed in a posterior to anterior direction (see **Fig. 8**B). If necessary, such an injury to the artery can be easily managed with the suction bipolar diathermy.

USE AN ENDOSCOPIC-ASSISTED APPROACH FOR THE CANINE FOSSA TREPHINATION

The canine fossa trephine (CFT) is an invaluable technique for clearing material from severely diseased maxillary sinuses, particularly in patients with eosinophilic mucus, fungal disease, and Samter triad. However, if performed improperly or in a blind manner, this approach can result in injury to the anterior superior alveolar nerve (ASAN). As a result of this, an endoscopically guided technique has been developed, which allows a 5-mm hole to be accurately drilled through the anterior face of the maxilla under direct visualization, thus avoiding branches of the ASAN and decreasing the risk of damage to the ASAN to less than 5%.[11] In order to accomplish this, the canine fossa trephination kit (Medtronic ENT, Jacksonville, FL, USA) contains an endoscope sheath with a protruding blade, which allows retraction of soft tissues

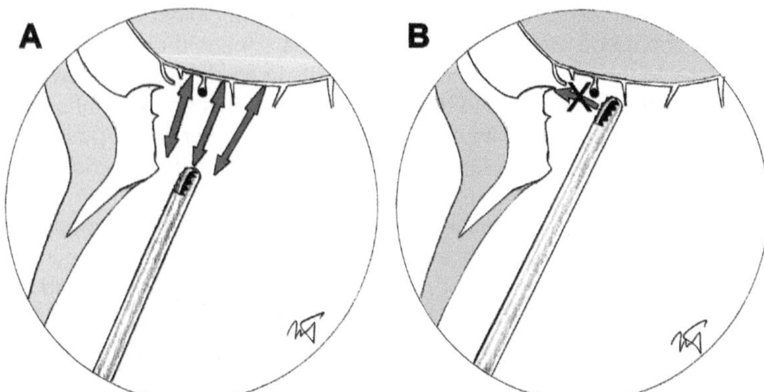

Fig. 8. (*A*) Diagram of the nasal cavity in sagittal view, depicting the proper method of using the microdebrider along the skull base, moving back and forth toward and away from the skull base; note that the AEA is hanging below the skull base in a bony mesentery. (*B*) Diagram of the nasal cavity in sagittal view, depicting the improper method of using the microdebrider along the skull base, moving from posterior to anterior, placing the AEA at risk of being completely severed.

during dissection on the anterior face of the maxilla. The kit contains a reusable drill guide and 5-mm reusable drill bit that fits the microdebrider handpiece.

Another modification to this technique that is useful in identifying nerve branches before performing the trephination is sinus transillumination.[12] This involves introducing a second 70° endoscope through the middle meatal antrostomy, to which the light source is attached, and positioning the light to face the anterior wall of the sinus from within. The resultant illumination is viewed by the external 0° endoscope, and highlights the anatomy of neural branches passing over the anterior maxilla for the identification of a safe entry point for the trephine.

Other technical points for performing the CFT include thoroughly removing any bone dust or bone fragments surrounding the trephine, to prevent postoperative granulations in the adjacent soft tissues. In addition, the position of the microdebrider blade must be confirmed visually through the maxillary ostium before activation, to avoid accidental injury to the orbit or soft tissues. Care must be taken when debriding polypoid tissue along the roof of the maxillary sinus and lamina papyracea, which should only be done after judicious ballottement of the eye to rule out orbital dehiscence.

ENSURE PROPER HEMOSTASIS

At the end of every ESS procedure, the anesthetist is asked to restore the patient's blood pressure toward the normal preoperative level while hemostasis is verified. Thorough suctioning of blood from within the sinus cavities followed by careful inspection of the nasopharynx should be performed looking for pooling of fresh blood. Most of the blood and blood clot is cleared using a straight Fraser suction. The suction is then transferred to the suction bipolar diathermy and the bleeding vessel is cauterized. A suction bipolar instrument allows simultaneous evacuation of blood from the operative field and cauterization of the bleeding points. This is important because blood rapidly dissipates heat from the tines of the bipolar and renders the diathermy less effective. In addition, blood quickly covers the bleeding vessel and the precise location of the bleeding point cannot be seen, making cautery of the vessel difficult and increasing unnecessary collateral tissue damage.

Most of the oozing (bleeding) from mucosal damage will stop spontaneously after sinus surgery. However, larger blood vessels can result in significant postoperative hemorrhage, especially if these vessels are in spasm during surgery and not dealt with at that time. Common areas of arterial bleeding after ESS that should be attentively examined are the regions supplied by large branches of the sphenopalatine artery and anterior ethmoidal artery. These regions include the anterior face of the sphenoid sinus (which is supplied by the posterior nasal/septal branch), the area of the sphenopalatine foramen especially if a middle turbinate resection has been performed, the posterior rim of an enlarged maxillary antrostomy, and the posterior end of the inferior turbinate (after a powered inferior turbinoplasty). Bleeding from branches of the anterior ethmoidal artery should be sought in the olfactory cleft below the bony "T" on the anterior skull base formed by the superior bony nasal septum as the floor of the frontal sinus is removed. After appropriately cauterizing the points of bleeding, the nasopharynx is again suctioned and inspected for pooling of fresh blood; this should be the last maneuver performed in any endoscopic sinus procedure.

SUMMARY

ESS is an excellent treatment option in the management of medically refractory chronic rhinosinusitis. Continual refinements in endoscopic technique are simultaneously allowing an expanded range of applications and a lower rate of complications for this kind of surgery. However, the potential for serious complications is ever present. The sinus surgeon must always be aware of this, and actively seek to identify high-risk situations preoperatively. The technical points presented in this article should be followed to minimize the risk of complications. However, the sinus surgeon must recognize their own limitations, and select surgical cases that are commensurate with their level of expertise.

REFERENCES

1. Stankiewicz JA. Complications of sinus surgery. In: Bailey BJ, Johnson JT, Newlands SD, editors. 4th edition, Head & neck surgery–otolaryngology, vol. 1. Philadelphia: Lippincott Williams & Wilkins; 2006. p. 477–91.
2. Keros P. [On the practical value of differences in the level of the lamina cribrosa of the ethmoid]. Z Laryngol Rhinol Otol 1962;41:809–13 [in German].
3. Wormald PJ, Athanasiadis T, Rees G, et al. An evaluation of effect of pterygopalatine fossa injection with local anesthetic and adrenalin in the control of nasal bleeding during endoscopic sinus surgery. Am J Rhinol 2005;19(3):288–92.
4. Wormald PJ, van Renen G, Perks J, et al. The effect of the total intravenous anesthesia compared with inhalational anesthesia on the surgical field during endoscopic sinus surgery. Am J Rhinol 2005;19(5):514–20.
5. Nair S, Collins M, Hung P, et al. The effect of beta-blocker premedication on the surgical field during endoscopic sinus surgery. Laryngoscope 2004;114(6): 1042–6.
6. Cohen-Kerem R, Brown S, Villasenor LV, et al. Epinephrine/Lidocaine injection vs. saline during endoscopic sinus surgery. Laryngoscope 2008;118(7):1275–81.
7. Eberhart LH, Folz BJ, Wulf H, et al. Intravenous anesthesia provides optimal surgical conditions during microscopic and endoscopic sinus surgery. Laryngoscope 2003;113(8):1369–73.
8. Wright ED, Agrawal S. Impact of perioperative systemic steroids on surgical outcomes in patients with chronic rhinosinusitis with polyposis: evaluation with

the novel Perioperative Sinus Endoscopy (POSE) scoring system. Laryngoscope 2007;117(11 Pt 2 Suppl 115):1–28.

9. Sieskiewicz A, Olszewska E, Rogowski M, et al. Preoperative corticosteroid oral therapy and intraoperative bleeding during functional endoscopic sinus surgery in patients with severe nasal polyposis: a preliminary investigation. Ann Otol Rhinol Laryngol 2006;115(7):490–4.
10. Wormald PJ, McDonogh M. The 'swing-door' technique for uncinectomy in endoscopic sinus surgery. J Laryngol Otol 1998;112(6):547–51.
11. Singhal D, Douglas R, Robinson S, et al. The incidence of complications using new landmarks and a modified technique of canine fossa puncture. Am J Rhinol 2007;21(3):316–9.
12. Tan NC, Floreani SR, Robinson S, et al. Transillumination-assisted maxillary trephination: cadaver validation of a new technique. Laryngoscope 2009;119(5):984–7.

10 Pearls for Safe Endoscopic Skull Base Surgery

Madeleine R. Schaberg, MD, MPH[a,*], Vijay K. Anand, MD[a], Theodore H. Schwartz, MD[a,b,c]

KEYWORDS

• Endoscopic skull base approaches • Intrathecal fluorescein
• Image-guided surgery • Complications

The skull base is one of the most complex anatomic locations in the human body. The introduction of the endoscopic endonasal approach for the management of lesions of the skull base has produced a paradigm shift in the way these complicated lesions are managed. The endonasal approach provides the most direct route to the anterior cranial base (including sella, cribriform plate, planum sphenoidale, and suprasellar cistern) as well as the clivus, pterygopalatine fossa, and adjacent parasagittal skull base locations. The advantages over the traditional transcranial or transfacial approaches include decreased retraction of the brain and cranial nerves and improved visualization of not only the tumor but also the surrounding neurovasculature, which heralds the potential for improved surgical outcomes. All new techniques require a learning curve and this article describes the most important tenets that have proved useful to the authors regarding postoperative patient management as well as surgical practice.

A TEAM APPROACH BETWEEN OTOLARYNGOLOGY AND NEUROSURGERY

A cohesive collaboration between otolaryngology and neurosurgery is critical to the success of the development and performance of these surgical procedures. The most fundamental advances in open and endonasal cranial base surgery have been

[a] Department of Otolaryngology, Weill Medical College of Cornell University, New York-Presbyterian Hospital, 1305 York Avenue, Fifth Floor, New York, NY 10065, USA
[b] Department of Neurosurgery, Weill Medical College of Cornell University, New York-Presbyterian Hospital, 525 East 68th Street, PO Box 99, New York, NY 10065, USA
[c] Department of Neurology and Neuroscience, Weill Medical College of Cornell University, New York-Presbyterian Hospital, New York, 525 East 68th Street, PO Box 99, NY 10065, USA
* Corresponding author. Department of Otorhinolaryngology, Weill Medical College of Cornell University, 772 Park Avenue, Ground Floor, New York, NY 10021.
E-mail address: madeleine.schaberg@gmail.com

Otolaryngol Clin N Am 43 (2010) 945–954
doi:10.1016/j.otc.2010.04.022
0030-6665/10/$ – see front matter

realized as a result of this collaboration. The skull base is the frontier that bridges these two specialties and the combination of knowledge is essential for the advancement of endoscopic skull base surgery. Otolaryngologists have an intimate knowledge of nasal and paranasal sinus anatomy and its complex array of variations whereas neurosurgeons have an unparalleled knowledge of neurovascular anatomy. In tandem, these two specialties can work together, otolaryngologists navigating the pathway to tumors and neurosurgeons removing tumors intracranially. The closure of the resulting defect in the skull base is aided by the thought processes of two different surgical mentalities, both of which emphasize different aspects of the repair, one the watertight separation of sterile CSF from the bacteria-laden nasopharynx and the other the maintenance of mucosal integrity, ciliary transport, olfaction, and air flow.

METICULOUS REVIEW OF PREOPERATIVE CT AND MRI; THE USE OF IMAGE GUIDANCE INTRAOPERATIVELY

Systematic preoperative planning is essential in tackling lesions of the skull base. The first prerequisite for a successful approach is an understanding of the location of the lesion in 3-D.

CT provides critical information about the bony anatomic landmarks. CTs should be scrutinized for anatomic variations. The lamina papyracea should be examined for dehiscence. The degree of pneumatization of the sphenoid sinus should be evaluated to determine the amount of bone that must be removed to reach the pathology. The existence of any Onodi cells should be noted; these occur when the most posterior ethmoid cells are highly pneumatized, extending to the anterior wall of the sphenoid sinus and containing the optic nerve or carotid artery.[1] This is not a contraindication to surgery but must be appreciated prior to surgery to avoid neurovascular injury.

The intersinus septae of the sphenoid sinus must also be carefully examined. There is generally one septum separating the right and left sphenoid, but these can be multiple or asymmetric. The location of parasagittal septations with respect to the carotid artery and optic nerve are useful in identifying the location of these structures. The height and trajectory of the skull base should be noted; this is an often-discussed entity in safe sinus surgery and has value in skull base surgery as well. Keros has described 3 types of skull base conformations.[2] These categories relate to the risk of penetration of the skull base. In type 1, the olfactory sulcus is 1 to 3 mm deep, and the corresponding lateral lamella is short; this is the least hazardous configuration. In type 2, the olfactory sulcus is 3 to 7 mm deep, and in type 3 it is 7 to 16 mm deep. When the lateral lamella contributes significantly to the ethmoid roof, the risk of penetration of the skull base increases. By staying lateral to the insertion of the middle turbinate, a surgeon can avoid perforating the lamina cribosa inadvertently. The authors often use a CT angiogram to identify the precise course of the carotid artery with respect to the bony anatomy. The MRI, alternatively, is more sensitive to soft tissue and is invaluable in determining the location and extent of the pathology. The authors generally combine a CT angiogram and gadolinium-enhanced MRI for the purposes of image guidance to maximize the information available for surgical planning.

Image-guidance technology is a crucial adjunct when operating at the skull base. Contemporary image-guided surgery is not cumbersome and allows for rapid registration and calibration with accurate localization.[3] Image guidance is thought to be a valuable adjunct by many investigators.[4,5] The authors often obtain the CT angiography as an outpatient prior to surgery for coregistration with an MRI obtained the morning of surgery.

MUCOSA-SPARING SURGICAL TECHNIQUE WITH PRESERVATION OF THE MIDDLE TURBINATE

The authors advocate a minimally invasive approach with maximal preservation of normal intranasal structure and function. Preserving as much normal mucosa as possible and only removing that which is necessary promotes healthy postoperative ciliary movement and an earlier re-establishment of mucociliary flow. In most surgeries it is not necessary to remove the middle turbinate. These can easily be preserved with simple lateralization. A meticulous mucosa-sparing technique is critical in the postoperative course of these patients. With this approach there is decreased crusting, synechiae, and obstruction of natural ostia. If a nasoseptal flap is harvested, alternatively, the mucosa from the sphenoid must be completely removed to assure that a mucocele does not form behind the flap. Likewise, in certain circumstances, the superior, middle, or inferior turbinate must be removed to expose the skull base adequately, as in the transpterygoidal approach.

THE RELATIONSHIP OF THE SPHENOID SINUS SEPTATIONS WITH RESPECT TO THE CAROTID ARTERY AND CAROTID LOCALIZATION WITH A DOPPLER ULTRASOUND

As discussed previously, the exact insertion of the sphenoid sinus septae onto the posterior wall of the sphenoid sinus is an invaluable landmark for identifying the carotid artery intraoperatively. If the carotid artery is lateral to the insertion of the septum, surgeons can use as this a landmark intraoperatively and understand that as long as they are operating medial to the septum the carotid remains protected. The reverse is true if the carotid lies medial to the septum; if this is the case, surgeons must take special care to avoid injury because there is not an obvious septum protecting the carotid. It is also crucial to identify those septae that insert directly onto the carotid artery because removal of the septae in this case could lead to hemorrhage; thus, manipulation should be done with caution.

The use of intraoperative Doppler ultrasound is useful for carotid localization once the bone over the carotids has been removed and the anterior wall of the cavernous sinus is exposed. Although image guidance can also be used, the Doppler is superior because it measures blood flow in real time. This is useful if there is a question that the navigation may not be precise.

THE USE OF INTRATHECAL FLUOREOSCEIN FOR IDENTIFICATION OF INTRAOPERATIVE CSF LEAKS

Intrathecal fluorescein is a useful tool for the identification of intraoperative CSF leaks. Fluorescein is a green fluorescent dye that can be introduced intrathecally via lumbar puncture to alter the color of CSF. The dosage the authors recommend is 0.25 mL of injectable 10% solution mixed in 10 mL of CSF. Patients should first be premedicated with diphenhydramine (50 mg intravenously) and dexamethasone (10 mg intravenously) to reduce the risk of inflammatory or allergic reaction.

Clear CSF can often go unrecognized in a field of blood and secretions and this dye makes the identification and repair of subtle leaks possible, thus avoiding the risk of postoperative meningitis. The intrathecal application of fluorescein represents an off-label use of the product and requires informed consent discussion with the patient. There have been sporadic reports in the literature of adverse events associated with its use, including lower-extremity weakness and numbness, seizures, hemiparesis, cranial nerve palsies, and neuropathic pain.[6–9] The reported incidence is exceptionally low and most reports occurred after the use of higher and more concentrated doses than that used at the authors' institution without premedication. The efficacy and safety of intrathecal fluorescein has been demonstrated by the authors' group.[10,11]

MULTILAYERED WATERTIGHT SEAL FOR SKULLBASE CLOSURE

The endoscopic closure of small defects has a greater than 90% success rate during primary endoscopic surgery, rising to 97% at revision.[12,13]

Creating a watertight separation between the sinonasal and intracranial cavities is a challenge. Multilayered closure of the skull base defect remains the centerpiece of adequate reconstructive techniques, with or without the addition of a vascularized flap. The cornerstone of success in the closure of iatrogenic CSF leaks created in endoscopic skull base surgery is an impermeable seal. The consequences of an inadequate closure include the possibility for CSF leak, meningitis, pneumocephalus, and death.

The authors have previously described a technique for achieving a watertight skull base closure, called a gasket seal.[14] This involves an onlay fascia lata graft over the bony defect. A rigid buttress (vomer or Medpor implant) is then countersunk over the fascia lata graft, which countersinks the center of the fascia lata, allowing the circumference of the fascia to close the bone edges (**Fig. 1**). In addition, a nasoseptal flap can be placed over the gasket seal to achieve a vascularized flap closure at the skull base and a fat graft can be used intracranially to reduce pooling of CSF in the resection cavity. A final layer of tissue sealant, such as DuraSeal (Covidien, Hazelwood, Missouri), is then placed to keep the flap in place and maintain a watertight closure until the fibrous union of the graft materials occurs. Several other methods of closure, with varying success rates, have been described.[15–18] The gasket seal reduced the CSF leak from approximately 25%[17,19–21] to 0% in a preliminary small series of patients,[14] and, currently, in the authors' past 150 cases to 2.3% (Vijay K. Anand, MD and Theodore H. Schwartz, MD, unpublished data, 2009).

Many techniques exist for closing the skull base endonasally, all of which require a multilayer reconstruction, some sort of a buttress to keep the closure in place, and tissue sealants. CSF leak rates have continued to decrease over time to an acceptably low rate of less than 5% throughout centers with high volume.

CAREFUL CHOICE OF GRAFT MATERIAL AND USE OF THE VASCULARIZED NASOSEPTAL FLAP

An algorithmic approach can be applied to skull base repair depending on location of skull base defect, size of defect, pathology of lesion, and volume of leak.[21] A small

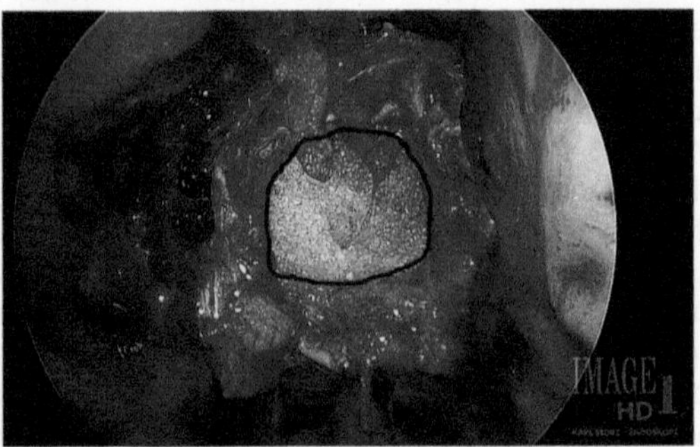

Fig. 1. Gasket seal closure. This is the Medpor implant (outlined in black), which is countersunk over the fascia lata in place over the defect in the skull base.

defect within the sella can be repaired with an allogenic fat graft, a rigid buttress to reconstruct the floor (vomer or Medpor implant), and tissue glue. A larger defect, however, with a high volume of CSF leak requires a more structurally sophisticated reconstruction.

The choice of material for closure is an important factor. The large variety in potential defect size and topography requires flexibility in the available materials. Autologous fat is the authors' primary tissue of choice for filling the tumor cavity in the case of a CSF leak. In the absence of a leak, the authors often simply use gelfoam. Fat can easily be harvested from the abdomen or thigh with little donor site morbidity. To reconstruct a large dural defect, the authors advocate the use of fascia lata. This is an autologous material that is easily harvested in large amounts. The alternative is acellular dermis or synthetic dura. The University of Miami group has published good results in a large series of patients with a variety of sizes of skull base defects in which acellular dermis (AlloDerm, LifeCell, Woodlands, TX, USA) was used as the primary graft material.[22] Both are pliable and easily tailored for ideal fit into the defect.

The next layer is a rigid buttress to keep the dural graft material in place. Refined vomer, synthetic Medpor implants, or absorbable or nonabsorbable miniplates can be used. The authors advocate the use of vomer or Medpor implants, because experience shows a tendency for miniplates to extrude; thus, the authors no longer use them in closure of the skull base (**Fig. 2**). The final tissue layer is the nasoseptal flap, which adds a blood supply to the closure and an additional vascular layer.

Free grafts, although exceptionally advantageous, are associated with an increased CSF leak rate for larger defects. A pedicled vascularized flap promotes rapid healing and the nasoseptal flap, described by Hadad and colleagues,[17] has become the workhorse of vascularized skull base repair. This flap is unique in that it has a large surface area and a robust pedicle and is adjacent to the operative field. The efficacy of the flap is demonstrated by the significant decrease in leak rate reported by Kassam and colleagues[20] in their recent series of 75 patients undergoing extended endonasal approaches, which decreased from 33% in their first 25 surgeries to 4% in their subsequent 50 surgeries. They attributed this to their technical improvement in flap harvesting over time. Additionally, Zanation and colleagues[23] recently published a series of 70 consecutive nasoseptal flaps for high-flow CSF leak closures, reporting a 94% successful closure rate. In the authors' most recent 150 cases, in which the nasoseptal flap was combined with a gasket seal, the leak rate was reduced to 2.3%, most likely attributable to technical advances and experience (Vijay K. Anand, MD and Theodore H. Schwartz, MD, unpublished data, 2009).

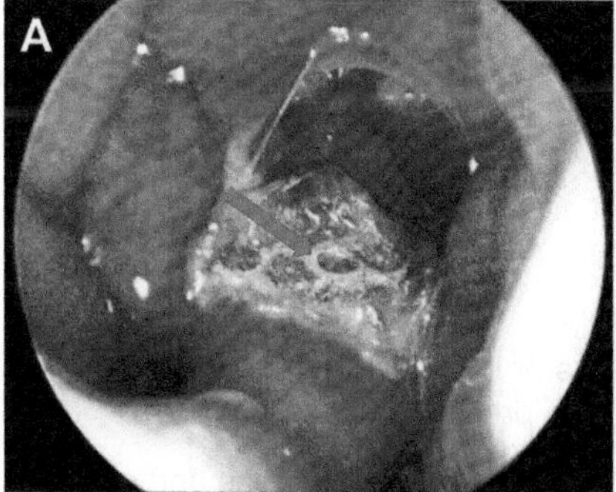

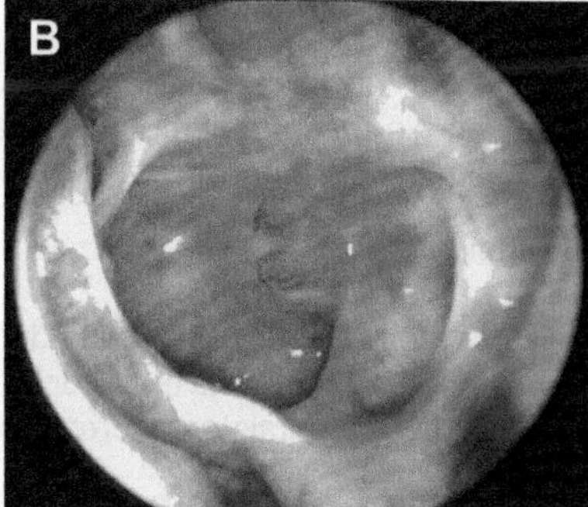

Fig. 2. (*A*) Exposed titanium plate with crusting extruded into floor of sphenoid sinus. (*B*) Partially exposed titanium plate in position over previous repair at anterior skull base.

The first crucial step is choosing the side on which to harvest the flap. It is generally easier to harvest the flap on the more concave side of the septum. It is also important to avoid large spurs, because mucosa tends to be thin here and can easily tear. The septum should be infiltrated with 1% lidocaine with epinephrine 1:100,000 but the sphenopalantine artery on the flap side should not be injected (this is to prevent vasospasm and ischemia of the flap). Removing the posterior tip of the inferior turbinate is also crucial in providing adequate room for the maneuvering of instruments when the posterior incisions are being made on the choanae. The sphenoid os should be identified and enlarged prior to the harvest of the flap, which serves as a landmark for the incisions. When making the septal incisions, the anterior incision should be made first, then the inferior incision. Lastly, the superior incision can be made. It is helpful to use the endoscopic microscissors for the superior incision. The superior incision should be the final one to avoid blood descending into the operative field when making the inferior incision. After the flap has been harvested and tucked into the posterior nasopharynx, it is necessary to remove the sphenoid rostrum. Although this is not in the surgical field, if this remains in place the nasoseptal flap, will not lie flat along the skull base. The authors generally drill down the floor of the sphenoid sinus to minimize the angulation of the flap as it passes over the inferior lip of the sinus onto the back wall. For large skull base defects, a Janus flap can be used by harvesting bilateral nasoseptal flaps.[24]

Finally, the authors advocate the use the use of a tissue sealant to secure the closure in lieu of placing a Foley balloon in the nasopharynx. A sealant, such as DuraSeal, serves the dual purpose of holding the flap in place and preventing minute amounts of CSF from leaking around the edges off the flap. The authors attach a 14-gauge angiocatheter to the tip of applicator and guide it into position with a ring-curette to facilitate application of the DuraSeal.

JUDICIOUS USE OF LUMBAR DRAIN WHEN NECESSARY TO DECREASE INTRACRANIAL PRESSURE

There are several factors that must be considered when deciding whether or not to place a lumbar drain preoperatively: pathology of the disease, amount of intracranial pressure, and size of skull base opening are critical elements.

The role of drains remains controversial and the low rates of CSF leak that can be achieved without the added complications of drains (immobility, spinal headache, and possible development of deep venous thrombosis) cautions that they should be used sparingly.[25]

For routine transsphenoidal surgery with small sellar openings for microadenomas, rathke cleft cysts, or small macroadenomas, the authors do not advocate the use of lumbar drains. Yet, there is a category of patients with a high risk of postoperative CSF leak, and in these patients placement of an intraoperative lumbar drain can be helpful. The most important factors include:

- Pathology
- Size of tumor
- Size of the projected skull base defect
- Presence of preoperative hydrocephalus or increased intracranial pressure
- Suspicion of a persistent increase in CSF pressure postoperatively.

The pathology of the disease is critical. Removal of meningiomas and craniopharyngiomas requires a wide opening of the arachnoid cistern and possibly entrance into the third ventricle with a subsequently greater chance of postoperative leak.

High preoperative intracranial pressure is often encountered in encephaloceles and these cases are also best managed with a postoperative lumbar drain. Additionally, if a large amount of dura is resected or if there is extensive opening of the cranial base, these patients benefit from lumbar drainage.

The authors' increased use of intraoperative lumbar drainage arose from experience in successfully managing patients' postoperative leaks with a lumbar drain. In addition, the drain is kept open during extubation to avoid the deleterious effect of the sudden increases in intracranial pressure that can occur on extubation, which might dislodge the closure.

CONSERVATIVE MANAGEMENT OF POSTOPERATIVE CSF LEAKS

Postoperative CSF leaks should be managed conservatively with lumbar drain placement, bed rest, head of bed elevation, and a bowel regimen.

In the authors' series of 127 patients reported in 2007, the CSF leak rate was 8.7%. Of the 11 patients with leaks, 10 were managed conservatively and had resolution of the leak, not requiring additional surgery.[21] Most recently, in the authors' series of 150 endoscopic skull base cases, the majority of postoperative CSF leaks were managed conservatively (Vijay K. Anand, MD and Theodore H. Schwartz, MD, unpublished data, 2009). This technique is recommended only if a multilayered closure has been performed. A low rate of lumbar drainage is recommended (5 mL/h) to avoid any risk of pneumocephalus and is indicated for 3 to 5 days. Serial CT scans should be used to monitor for the development of pneumocephalus.

It has been advocated by some investigators that CSF leaks should be immediately explored and repaired, and this is another option. Harvey and colleagues[26] demonstrate on 8.5% CSF leak rate in their large series of 106 patients all undergoing endoscopic skull base reconstruction. These were managed via endoscopic revision (3 patients), open craniotomy (2 patients), and ventriculoperitoneal shunt (2 patients). In the authors' experience, reoperation is not always necessary.

CONSCIENTIOUS POSTOPERATIVE CARE, WITH FREQUENT DÉBRIDEMENTS, AND NASAL TOILET UNTIL THE SKULL BASE IS COMPLETELY HEALED

Meticulous postoperative care is essential to healing after skull base reconstruction. The authors advocate that postoperative care begin 1 week after discharge from the hospital. At this early stage, the nasal cavity is lightly débrided. This entails

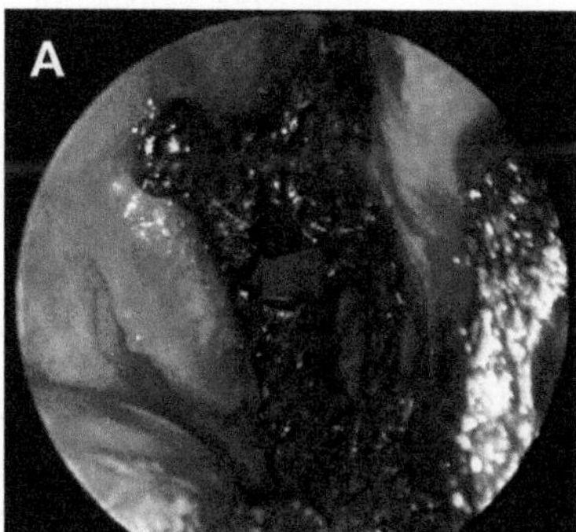

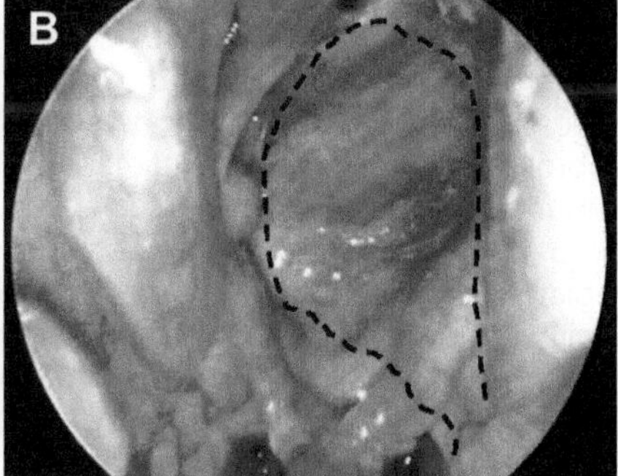

Fig. 3. (*A*) Amount of crusting exhibited at 2 weeks postoperatively in the nasal cavity after transsphenoidal tumor excision. (*B*) Healed skull base with left nasoseptal flap (*dashed line*) closure on the same patient at 6 weeks postoperatively.

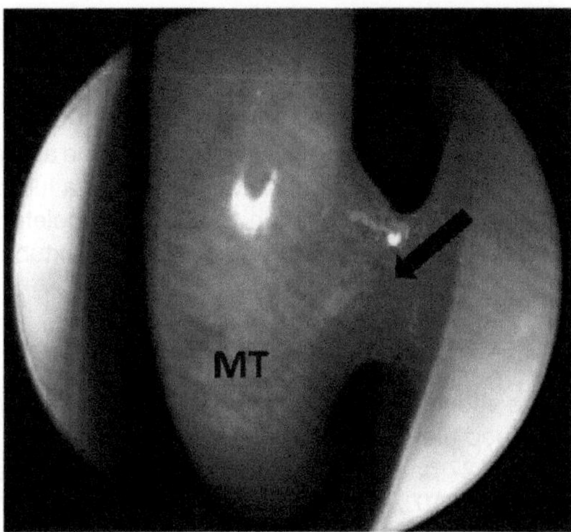

Fig. 4. Left nasal cavity endoscopy demonstrating synechiae (*arrow*) between middle turbinate (MT) and lateral nasal wall.

removing crusts, old blood, and breakdown products secondary to the use of hemostatic agents (**Fig. 3**). Gentle suctioning is performed without disruption of the skull base closure. Careful inspection of the operative bed is performed to ensure that the field has remained uninfected. In the first 2 weeks after surgery, the skull base should not be aggressively débrided because this may precipitate a CSF leak. At this time, patients are placed on gentamicin nasal spray (80 mg gentamicin in 1000 mL normal saline) for 1 month. This has been shown to decrease bacterial colony counts and improve mucociliary function.[27] Patients are subsequently seen 2 weeks later and at this time more aggressive débridement can be performed as needed. Close postoperative follow-up continues but is individualized based on the complexity of procedure and patients' individual wound healing ability. Most patients have complete healing of the skull base by 6 to 12 weeks postoperatively (see **Fig. 3**). Thorough postoperative care decreases the chance of infection, crusting, and the formation of synechiae (**Fig. 4**).

REFERENCES

1. Onodi A. The optic nerve and the accessory sinuses of the nose. London: Bailliere, Tindall and Cox; 1910. p. 1–26.
2. Keros P. Uber die praktische beteudung der Niveau-Unterschiede der lamina cribrosa des ethmoids. In: Naumann HH, editor. Head and neck surgery, Face and facial skull, vol. 1. Philadelphia: WB Saunders; 1980. p. 392.
3. Hardy SM, Melroy C, White DR, et al. A comparison of computer-aided surgery registration methods for endoscopic sinus surgery. Am J Rhinol 2006;20:48–52.
4. Smith T, Stewart M, Orlandi R, et al. Indications for image-guided surgery: the current evidence. Am J Rhinol 2007;21:80–3.
5. Citardi M, Batra P. Intraoperative surgical navigation for endoscopic sinus surgery: rationale and indications. Curr Opin Otolaryngol Head Neck Surg 2007;15:23–7.
6. Moseley JI, Carton CA, Stern WE. Spectrum of complications in the use of intrathecal fluorescein. J Neurosurg 1978;48:765–7.

7. Keerl R, Weber RK, Draf W, et al. Use of sodium fluorescein solution for detection of cerebrospinal fluid fistulas: an analysis of 420 administrations and reported complications in Europe and the United States. Laryngoscope 2004;114:266–72.
8. Mahaley MS Jr, Odom GL. Complication following intrathecal injection of flu- orescein. J Neurosurg 1966;25:298–9.
9. Locatelli D, Rampa F, Acchiardi I, et al. Endoscopic endonasal approaches for repair of cerebrospinal fluid leaks: nine-year experience. Neurosurgery 2006; 58:246–56.
10. Placantonakis DG, Tabaee A, Anand VK, et al. Safety of low-dose intrathecal fluorescein in endoscopic cranial base surgery. Neurosurgery 2007;61:161–5 [discussion: 165–6].
11. Tabaee A, Placantonakis DG, Schwartz TH, et al. Intrathecal fluorescein in endoscopic skull base surgery. Otolaryngol Head Neck Surg 2007;137:316–20.
12. Hegazy HM, Carrau RL, Snyderman CH, et al. Transnasal endoscopic repair of cerebrospinal fluid rhinorrhea: a meta-analysis. Laryngoscope 2000;110(7): 1166–72.
13. Nyquist GG, Anand VK, Mehra S, et al. Endoscopic endonasal repair of anterior skull base non-traumatic cerebrospinal fluid leaks, meningoceles, and encephaloceles. J Neurosurg 2009 Nov 20. [Epub ahead of print].
14. Leng LZ, Brown S, Anand VK, et al. "Gasket-seal" watertight closure in minimal-access endoscopic cranial base surgery. Neurosurgery 2008;62(5 Suppl 2): ONSE342–3 [discussion: ONSE343].
15. Cappabianca P, Cavallo LM, Esposito F, et al. Sellar repair in endoscopic endonasal transsphenoidal surgery: results of 170 cases. Neurosurgery 2002;51: 1365–72.
16. Leong JL, Citardi MJ, Batra PS. Reconstruction of skull base defects after minimally invasive endoscopic resection of anterior skull base neoplasms. Am J Rhinol 2006;20:476–82.
17. Hadad G, Bassagasteguy L, Carrau RL, et al. A novel reconstructive technique after endoscopic expanded endonasal approaches: vascular pedicle nasoseptal flap. Laryngoscope 2006;116:1882–6.
18. Kassam A, Carrau RL, Snyderman CH, et al. Evolution of reconstructive techniques following endo- scopic expanded endonasal approaches. Neurosurg Focus 2005;19:1–7.
19. Gardner PA, Kassam AB, Thomas A, et al. Endoscopic endonasal resection of anterior cranial base meningiomas. Neurosurgery 2008;63:36–52 [discussion: 52–4].
20. Kassam AB, Thomas A, Carrau RL, et al. Endoscopic reconstruction of the cranial base using a pedicled nasoseptal flap. Neurosurgery 2008;63:ONS44–52 [discussion: ONS52–3].
21. Tabaee A, Anand VK, Brown SM, et al. Algorithm for reconstruction after endoscopic pituitary and skull base surgery. Laryngoscope 2007;117:1133–7.
22. Germani RM, Vivero R, Herzallah IR, et al. Endoscopic reconstruction of large anterior skull base defects using acellular dermal allograft. Am J Rhinol 2007; 21(5):615–8.
23. Zanation AM, Carrau RL, Snyderman CH, et al. Nasoseptal flap reconstruction of high flow intraoperative cerebral spinal fluid leaks during endoscopic skull base surgery. Am J Rhinol Allergy 2009;23(5):518–21.
24. Nyquist GG, Anand VK, Singh A, et al. Otolaryngol Janus flap: bilateral nasoseptal flaps for anterior skull base reconstruction. Head Neck Surg 2010;142(3): 327–31.

25. Casiano RR, Jassir D. Endoscopic cerebral spinal fluid rhinorrhea repair: is a lumbar drain necessary? Otolaryngol Head Neck Surg 1999;121:745–50.
26. Harvey RJ, Smith JE, Wise SK, et al. Intracranial complications before and after endoscopic skull base reconstruction. Am J Rhinol 2008;22:516–21.
27. Kida Y. Gentamicin and CFTR. N Engl J Med 2003;349:2570.

Index

Note: Page numbers of article titles are in **boldface** type.

Otolaryngol Clin N Am 43 (2010) 955–963
doi:10.1016/S0030-6665(10)00133-7
0030-6665/10/$ – see front matter

D

E

F

M

N

O

Moving?

Make sure your subscription moves with you!

To notify us of your new address, find your **Clinics Account Number** (located on your mailing label above your name), and contact customer service at:

Email: journalscustomerservice-usa@elsevier.com

800-654-2452 **(subscribers in the U.S. & Canada)**
314-447-8871 **(subscribers outside of the U.S. & Canada)**

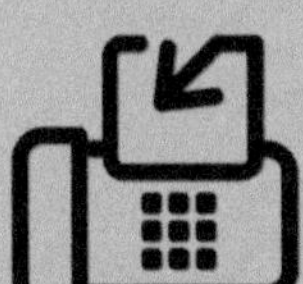

Fax number: 314-447-8029

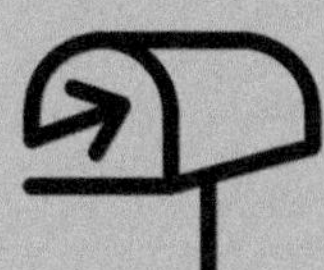

Elsevier Health Sciences Division
Subscription Customer Service
3251 Riverport Lane
Maryland Heights, MO 63043

*To ensure uninterrupted delivery of your subscription, please notify us at least 4 weeks in advance of move.

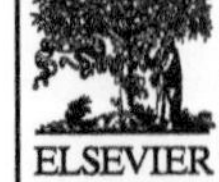